PORTABLE
ECG
Interpretation

PORTABLE
ECG
Interpretation

. Wolters Kluwer | Lippincott Williams & Wilkins
Health

Philadelphia · Baltimore · New York · London
Buenos Aires · Hong Kong · Sydney · Tokyo

STAFF

Executive Publisher
Judith A. Schilling McCann, RN, MSN

Editorial Director
David Moreau

Clinical Director
Joan M. Robinson, RN, MSN

Art Director
Mary Ludwicki

Senior Managing Editor
Jaime Stockslager Buss, MSPH, ELS

Clinical Project Manager
Jennifer Meyering, RN, BSN, MS, CCRN

Editors
Janeen Levine, Julie Munden,
Liz Schaeffer, Gale Thompson

Copy Editors
Kimberly Bilotta (supervisor),
Jane Bradford, Scotti Cohn,
Tom DeZego, Jeannine Fielding,
Shana Harrington, Liz Mooney,
Dorothy P. Terry, Pamela Wingrod

Designer
Arlene Putterman

Digital Composition Services
Diane Paluba (manager),
Joyce Rossi Biletz, Donna S. Morris

Associate Manufacturing Manager
Beth J. Welsh

Editorial Assistants
Megan L. Aldinger, Karen J. Kirk,
Jeri O'Shea, Linda K. Ruhf

Design Assistant
Georg W. Purvis IV

Indexer
Barbara Hodgson

Library of Congress
Cataloging-in Publication Data

Portable ECG interpretation.
    p. ; cm.
    Includes bibliographic references and index.
    1. Electrocardiography. 2. Nursing. 3.
Heart—Diseases—Nursing.
    [DNLM: 1. Electrocardiography—methods.
WG 140 P839 2008]
    RC683.5.E5P6779 2008
    616.1'207547—dc22
ISBN-13: 978-1-58255-677-2 (alk. paper)
ISBN-10: 1-58255-677-6 (alk. paper)
                                    2007008657

Contents

PART III
12-lead ECGs 243

PART IV
Practice strips 291

Contributors and consultants

Shelba Durston, RN, MSN, CCRN
Nursing Instructor
San Joaquin Delta College
Stockton, Calif.
Staff Nurse, San Joaquin General Hospital
French Camp, Calif.

Merita Konstantacos, RN, MSN
Nursing Consultant
Clinton, Ohio

Pamela Moody, APRN-BC, MSN, PhD, NHA
Nurse Practitioner Consultant,
Alabama Department of Public Health
Tuscaloosa

Susan L. Patterson, RN, MS, CCM, ACLS
Faculty, School of Nursing
PRN Staff—Cardiology
Carolinas College Health Sciences, CHS
Charlotte, N.C.

Bruce Austin Scott, APRN,BC, MSN
Nursing Instructor
San Joaquin Delta College
Staff Nurse
St. Josephs Medical Center
Stockton, Calif.

Allison J. Terry, RN, MSN, PhD
Director of Center for Nursing Workforce Research
Alabama Board of Nursing
Montgomery

Patricia Van Tine, RN, MA
Nursing Faculty
Mt. San Jacinto College
Menifee, Calif.

Wynona Wiggins, RN, MSN, CCRN
Assistant Professor of Nursing
Arkansas State University
State University

Lisa Wolf, RN, MSN
Clinical Educator
Mount Carmel West Hospital
Columbus, Ohio

PART

I

ECG overview

Cardiac anatomy and physiology

1

Knowing how to interpret an electrocardiogram (ECG) allows you to provide better patient care. For example, when caring for a patient with an arrhythmia or myocardial infarction, correctly interpreting an ECG can help you assess the patient's condition and, when necessary, begin life-saving measures. Having a clear understanding of cardiac anatomy and physiology is the first step toward developing these essential skills.

Cardiac anatomy

The heart is a hollow, muscular organ that lies obliquely in the chest behind the sternum in the mediastinum (the cavity between the lungs and in front of the spine). The top of the heart, called the *base*, lies just below the second rib. The bottom of the heart, called the *apex*, tilts forward and down toward the left side of the body and rests on the diaphragm. (See *Where the heart lies*, page 4.)

The heart varies in size, depending on the person's body size, but is roughly 5″ (12 cm) long and 3½″ (9 cm) wide, or about the size of the person's fist. The heart's weight, typically 9 to 12 oz (255 to 340 g), varies depending on the person's size, age, sex, and athletic conditioning. An athlete's heart usually weighs more than average, whereas an elderly person's heart weighs less. (See *Changes in the heart*, page 5.)

Heart wall

The heart wall contains three layers. The *epicardium*, the outermost layer, consists of squamous epithelial cells overlying connective tissue. The *myocardium*, the middle and thickest layer, forms the largest portion of the heart's wall. This layer of muscle tissue

Where the heart lies

The heart lies within the mediastinum, a cavity that contains the tissues and organs separating the two pleural sacs. In most people, two-thirds of the heart extends to the left of the body's midline.

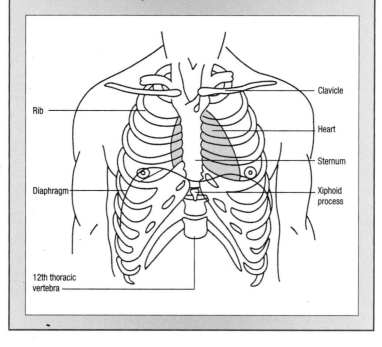

Rib

Clavicle

Heart

Sternum

Diaphragm

Xiphoid process

12th thoracic vertebra

contracts with each heartbeat. The *endocardium,* the heart wall's innermost layer, consists of a thin layer of endothelial tissue that lines the heart valves and chambers. (See *Layers of the heart wall,* page 6.)

Enveloping the heart is the *pericardium,* a fluid-filled sac that acts as a tough, protective covering. It consists of the fibrous pericardium and the serous pericardium. The fibrous pericardium is composed of tough, white, fibrous tissue, which fits loosely around the heart and protects it. The serous pericardium, the thin, smooth, inner portion, has two layers:

◆ the parietal layer, which lines the inside of the fibrous pericardium

◆ the visceral layer, which adheres to the surface of the heart.

The pericardial space separates the visceral and parietal

layers and contains 10 to 20 ml of thin, clear pericardial fluid that lubricates the two surfaces and cushions the heart. Excess pericardial fluid, a condition called *pericardial effusion*, can compromise the heart's ability to pump blood.

Heart chambers

The heart contains four chambers—two atria and two ventricles. (See *Inside a normal heart,* page 7.) The right atrium lies in front of and to the right of the smaller but thicker-walled left atrium. The right and left atria serve as volume reservoirs for blood being sent into the ventricles. An interatrial septum separates the two chambers and helps them contract, forcing blood into the ventricles.

The right and left ventricles serve as the pumping chambers of the heart. The right ventricle lies behind the sternum and forms the largest part of the heart's sternocostal surface and inferior border. The left ventricle forms the heart's apex, most of its left border, and most of its posterior and diaphragmatic surfaces. The interventricular septum separates the ventricles and helps them pump.

Because the atria act as reservoirs for the ventricles and pump the blood a shorter distance,

their walls are considerably thinner than the walls of the ventricles. Likewise, the left ventricle has a much thicker wall than the right ventricle because it works

---

Changes in the heart

The heart of the older adult

As a person ages, his heart usually becomes slightly smaller and loses its contractile strength and efficiency (although exceptions occur in people with hypertension or heart disease). By age 70, cardiac output at rest has diminished by about 30% to 35% in many people.

Irritable with age

As the myocardium of the aging heart becomes more irritable, extra systoles may occur, along with sinus arrhythmias and sinus bradycardias. In addition, increased fibrous tissue infiltrates the sinoatrial node and internodal atrial tracts, which may cause atrial fibrillation and flutter.

The heart of the child

The heart of an infant is positioned more horizontally in the chest cavity than an adult's is. As a result, the apex is positioned at the fourth left intercostal space. Until age 4, the apical impulse is left of the midclavicular line. By age 7, the heart is located in the same position as an adult's heart is.

Layers of the heart wall

This cross section of the heart wall shows its various layers.

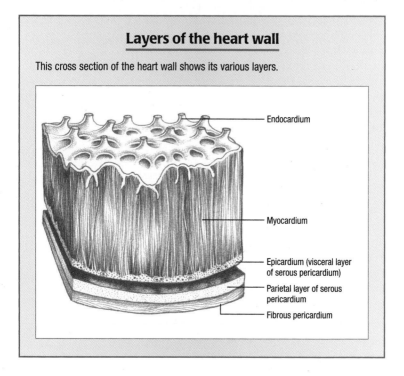

- Endocardium
- Myocardium
- Epicardium (visceral layer of serous pericardium)
- Parietal layer of serous pericardium
- Fibrous pericardium

harder, pumping blood against the higher pressures of the aorta.

Heart valves

The heart contains four valves—two atrioventricular (AV) valves (tricuspid and mitral) and two semilunar valves (aortic and pulmonic) (See *A view of the heart's valves,* page 8.) Each valve consists of cusps, or leaflets, that open and close in response to pressure changes within the chambers they connect. The primary function of the valves is to keep blood flowing through the

heart in a forward direction. When the valves close, they prevent backflow, or regurgitation, of blood from one chamber to another. Closure of the valves is associated with heart sounds.

Atrioventricular valves
The two AV valves are located between the atria and ventricles. The tricuspid valve, named for its three cusps, separates the right atrium from the right ventricle. The mitral valve, sometimes referred to as the bicuspid valve because of its two cusps, separates the left atrium from the

Inside a normal heart

This cross section shows the internal structure of a normal heart.

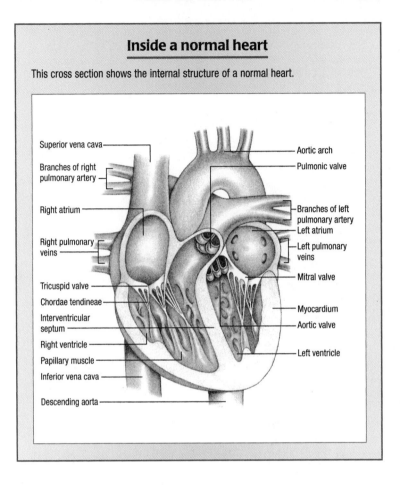

Superior vena cava

Branches of right pulmonary artery

Right atrium

Right pulmonary veins

Tricuspid valve

Chordae tendineae

Interventricular septum

Right ventricle

Papillary muscle

Inferior vena cava

Descending aorta

Aortic arch

Pulmonic valve

Branches of left pulmonary artery

Left atrium

Left pulmonary veins

Mitral valve

Myocardium

Aortic valve

Left ventricle

left ventricle. Closure of the AV valves is associated with S_1, or the first heart sound.

The cusps, or leaflets, of these valves are anchored to the papillary muscles of the ventricles by small tendinous cords called *chordae tendineae.* The papillary muscles and chordae tendineae work together to prevent the cusps from bulging backward into the atria during ventricular contraction. Disruption of either of these structures may prevent complete valve closure, allowing blood to flow backward into the atria. This backward blood flow may cause a heart murmur.

Semilunar valves
The semilunar valves receive their name from their three cusps

A view of the heart's valves

The illustration below shows the heart's four valves. The valves help prevent the backward flow of blood from one chamber to another.

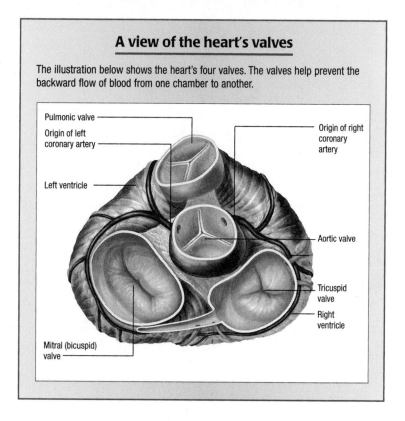

Pulmonic valve

Origin of left coronary artery

Left ventricle

Origin of right coronary artery

Aortic valve

Tricuspid valve

Right ventricle

Mitral (bicuspid) valve

---

that resemble half moons. The pulmonic valve, located where the pulmonary artery meets the right ventricle, permits blood to flow from the right ventricle to the pulmonary artery and prevents backflow into the right ventricle. The aortic valve, located where the left ventricle meets the aorta, allows blood to flow from the left ventricle to the aorta and prevents blood backflow into the left ventricle.

Increased pressure within the ventricles during ventricular sys-tole causes the pulmonic and aortic valves to open, allowing ejection of blood into the pulmonary and systemic circulation. Loss of pressure as the ventricular chambers empty causes the valves to close. Closure of the semilunar valves is associated with S_2, or the second heart sound. (See *Flow of blood through the heart.*)

Flow of blood through the heart

As shown in the illustrations below, blood follows a specific path as it flows through the heart. Keep in mind that right and left heart events occur simultaneously.

The right atrium receives deoxygenated blood returning from the body through the inferior and superior venae cavae and from the heart through the coronary sinus. The left atrium receives oxygenated blood flowing from the lungs through the pulmonary veins.

The increasing volume of blood in the right atrium raises the pressure in the chamber above the pressure in the right ventricle. This increased pressure causes the tricuspid valve to open and blood flows to the right ventricle. Simultaneously, as the volume of blood in the left atrium increases, the pressure in the left atrium exceeds the pressure in the left ventricle. The mitral valve opens and blood flows into the left ventricle.

The right ventricle pumps blood through the pulmonic valve into the pulmonary arteries and then into the lungs. There, oxygen is picked up and excess carbon dioxide is released. The blood returns, oxygenated, to the left atrium, completing pulmonic circulation.

The left ventricle pumps blood through the aortic valve into the aorta and then throughout the body. Deoxygenated blood returns to the right atrium, completing systemic circulation.

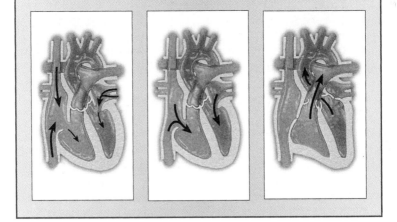

Coronary arteries

Like the brain and all other organs, the heart needs an adequate supply of oxygenated blood to survive. Two main coronary arteries—the right and the left—lie on the heart's surface, with smaller arterial branches penetrating into the cardiac muscle. The heart receives its blood supply almost entirely through these arteries. (See *Vessels that supply the heart.*)

Right coronary artery

The right coronary artery arises from the coronary ostia, small orifices located just above the aortic valve cusps. The right coronary artery fills the groove between the atria and ventricles, giving rise to the acute marginal artery and ending as the posterior descending artery. The right coronary artery supplies blood to the right atrium, the right ventricle, and the inferior wall of the left ventricle. This artery also supplies blood to the sinoatrial (SA) node in about 50% of the population and to the AV node in 90% of the population. The posterior descending artery supplies the posterior wall of the left ventricle in 80% to 90% of the population.

Left main coronary artery

The left main coronary artery also arises from the coronary ostia. Varying in length from a few millimeters to a few centimeters, it splits into two major branches: the left anterior descending (also known as the *interventricular*) and the left circumflex arteries. The left anterior descending artery runs down the anterior surface of the heart toward the apex. This artery and its branches—the diagonal arteries and the septal perforators—supply blood to the anterior wall of the left ventricle, the anterior interventricular septum, the bundle of His, the right bundle branch, and the anterior fasciculus of the left bundle branch.

The circumflex artery circles the left ventricle, ending on its posterior surface. The obtuse marginal artery arises from the circumflex artery. The circumflex artery provides oxygenated blood to the lateral wall of the left ventricle, the left atrium, the posterior wall of the left ventricle in 10% of the population, and the posterior fasciculus of the left bundle branch. In about 50% of the population, it supplies the SA node; in about 10% of the population, the AV node.

In most people, the right coronary artery supplies blood to the posterior wall via the posterior descending artery. This is described as right coronary dominance or as having a dominant right coronary artery. Likewise, when the left main coronary artery supplies blood to the posterior wall via the posterior descending artery, the terms left coronary dominance or dominant left coronary artery are used.

When two or more arteries supply the same region, they usually connect through anastomoses, junctions that provide al-

Vessels that supply the heart

The coronary circulation involves the arterial system of blood vessels that supply oxygenated blood to the heart and the venous system that removes oxygen-depleted blood from it.

ANTERIOR VIEW

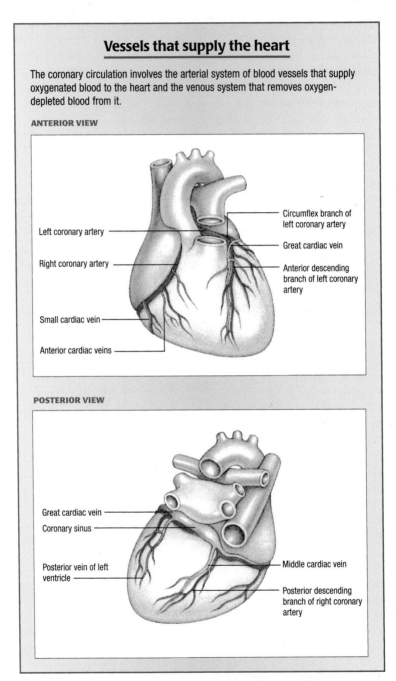

Left coronary artery

Right coronary artery

Small cardiac vein

Anterior cardiac veins

Circumflex branch of left coronary artery

Great cardiac vein

Anterior descending branch of left coronary artery

POSTERIOR VIEW

Great cardiac vein

Coronary sinus

Posterior vein of left ventricle

Middle cardiac vein

Posterior descending branch of right coronary artery

ternative routes of blood flow. This network of smaller arteries, called *collateral circulation,* provides blood to capillaries that directly feed the heart muscle. Collateral circulation commonly becomes so strong that even if major coronary arteries become narrowed with plaque, collateral circulation can continue to supply blood to the heart.

Coronary artery blood flow

In contrast to the other vascular beds in the body, the heart receives its blood supply primarily during ventricular relaxation or diastole, when the left ventricle is filling with blood. This occurs because the coronary ostia lie near the aortic valve and become partially occluded when the aortic valve opens during ventricular contraction or systole. When the aortic valve closes, the ostia are unobstructed and blood fills the coronary arteries. In addition, during contraction, the left ventricular muscle compresses the coronary vessels, impeding the flow of blood. Because the coronary arteries receive their blood supply during diastole, anything that shortens diastole, such as periods of increased heart rate or tachycardia, will also decrease coronary blood flow.

Cardiac veins

Just like the other parts of the body, the heart has its own veins, which remove oxygen-depleted blood from the myocardium. Approximately 75% of coronary venous blood leaves the left ventricle by way of the coronary sinus, an enlarged vessel that returns blood to the right atrium. Most of the venous blood from the right ventricle flows directly into the right atrium through the small anterior cardiac veins, not by way of the coronary sinus. A small amount of coronary blood flows back into the heart through the thebesian veins, minute veins that empty directly into all chambers of the heart.

Cardiac physiology

In this section, you'll find descriptions of the cardiac cycle; cardiac muscle innervation, depolarization and repolarization; and normal and abnormal impulse conduction.

The cardiac cycle

The cardiac cycle includes the cardiac events that occur from the beginning of one heartbeat to the beginning of the next. The cardiac cycle consists of ventricular diastole, or relaxation, and ventricular systole, or contraction. During *ventricular diastole,* blood flows from the atria through the open tricuspid and mitral valves into the relaxed ventricles. The aortic and pulmonic valves are closed during ventricular diastole. (See *Phases of the cardiac cycle,* page 14.)

During diastole, approximately 75% of the blood flows passively from the atria through the open tricuspid and mitral valves and into the ventricles even before the atria contract. Atrial contraction, or *atrial kick* as it's sometimes called, contributes another 25% to ventricular filling. Loss of effective atrial contraction occurs with some arrhythmias such as atrial fibrillation. This results in a subsequent reduction in cardiac output.

During *ventricular systole,* the mitral and tricuspid valves are closed as the relaxed atria fill with blood. As ventricular pressure rises, the aortic and pulmonic valves open. The ventricles contract, and blood is ejected into the pulmonic and systemic circulation.

Cardiac output

Cardiac output refers to the amount of blood pumped by the left ventricle in 1 minute. Cardiac output is determined by multiplying the heart rate by the stroke volume. Stroke volume is the amount of blood ejected with each ventricular contraction (usually about 70 ml).

Normal cardiac output is 4 to 8 L per minute, depending on body size. The heart pumps only as much blood as the body requires, based upon metabolic requirements. During exercise, for example, the heart increases cardiac output accordingly.

Three factors determine stroke volume: preload, afterload, and myocardial contractility. (See *Preload and afterload,* page 15.) *Preload* is the degree of stretch or tension on the muscle fibers when they begin to contract. It's usually considered to be the end-diastolic pressure when the ventricle has become filled.

Afterload is the load or amount of pressure the left ventricle must work against to eject blood during systole and corresponds to the systolic pressure. The greater this resistance, the greater the heart's workload. Afterload is also called the *systemic vascular resistance.*

Myocardial contractility is the ventricle's ability to contract, which is determined by the degree of muscle fiber stretch at the end of diastole. The more the muscle fibers stretch during ventricular filling, up to an optimal length, the more forceful the contraction.

Phases of the cardiac cycle

The cardiac cycle consists of the following phases.

1. Isovolumetric ventricular contraction—In response to ventricular depolarization, tension in the ventricles increases. The rise in pressure within the ventricles leads to closure of the mitral and tricuspid valves. The pulmonic and aortic valves stay closed during the entire phase.

2. Ventricular ejection—When ventricular pressure exceeds aortic and pulmonary artery pressures, the aortic and pulmonic valves open and the ventricles eject blood.

3. Isovolumetric relaxation—When ventricular pressure falls below the pressures in the aorta and pulmonary

artery, the aortic and pulmonic valves close. All valves are closed during this phase. Atrial diastole occurs as blood fills the atria.

4. Ventricular filling—Atrial pressure exceeds ventricular pressure, which causes the mitral and tricuspid valves to open. Blood then flows passively into the ventricles. About 75% of ventricular filling takes place during this phase.

5. Atrial systole—Known as the *atrial kick,* atrial systole (coinciding with late ventricular diastole) supplies the ventricles with the remaining 25% of the blood for each heartbeat.

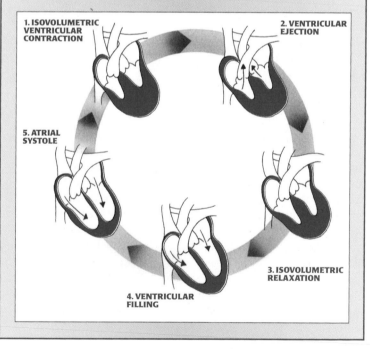

1. ISOVOLUMETRIC VENTRICULAR CONTRACTION

2. VENTRICULAR EJECTION

3. ISOVOLUMETRIC RELAXATION

4. VENTRICULAR FILLING

5. ATRIAL SYSTOLE

Preload and afterload

Preload refers to a passive stretching exerted by blood on the ventricular muscle fibers at the end of diastole. According to Starling's law, the more the cardiac muscles are stretched in diastole, the more forcefully they contract in systole.

Afterload refers to the pressure that the ventricles need to generate to overcome higher pressure in the aorta to eject blood into the systemic circulation. This systemic vascular resistance corresponds to the systemic systolic pressure.

PRELOAD

AFTERLOAD

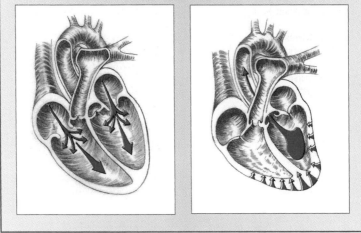

Autonomic innervation of the heart

The two branches of the autonomic nervous system—the sympathetic (or adrenergic) and the parasympathetic (or cholinergic)—abundantly supply the heart. Sympathetic fibers innervate all the areas of the heart, whereas parasympathetic fibers primarily innervate the SA and AV nodes.

Sympathetic nerve stimulation triggers the release of norepinephrine, which increases the heart rate by increasing SA node discharge, accelerates AV node conduction time, and increases the force of myocardial contraction and cardiac output. Parasympathetic (vagal) stimulation triggers the release of acetylcholine, which produces the opposite effects. The rate of SA node discharge is decreased, thus slowing heart rate and conduction through the AV node, and reducing cardiac output.

Transmission of electrical impulses

The generation and transmission of electrical impulses depend on four characteristics of cardiac cells: automaticity, excitability, conductivity, and contractility. Automaticity, excitability, and conductivity are electrical properties of a cell, whereas contractility is a mechanical response to electrical activity.

Automaticity refers to a cell's ability to spontaneously initiate an electrical impulse. A trait usually possessed by pacemaker cells, automaticity is the key factor in the development of cardiac rhythms. *Excitability* results from ion shifts across the cell membrane and refers to the cell's ability to respond to an electrical stimulus. *Conductivity* is the ability of a cell to transmit an electrical impulse from one cell to another. *Contractility* refers to the cell's ability to contract after receiving a stimulus by shortening and lengthening its muscle fibers.

Depolarization and repolarization

The transmission of electrical impulses results from the passage of ions (primarily sodium, potassium, and calcium) across cardiac cell membranes. Throughout the cardiac cycle, the permeability of the cell membrane changes, altering the passage of these ions into and out of the cell.

In a resting (or polarized) state, no electrical activity takes place and the cell has equal negative and positive charges inside and outside. Negatively charged ions then flow into the cell, creating an electrical difference across the membrane. This is known as *resting potential.* When the cell is stimulated by an electrical impulse, an action potential, or depolarization, occurs. At this point, sodium ions flow rapidly into the cell, causing the inside of the cell to become more positively charged than the outside. This change creates an impulse that causes myocardial contraction. After depolarization and contraction, the cell attempts to return to its resting state through the process of repolarization. (See *Understanding the depolarization-repolarization cycle,* pages 18 and 19, and *Action potential curves,* pages 20 and 21.)

Cardiac conduction system

After depolarization and repolarization, the resulting electrical impulse travels through the heart along a pathway called the *conduction system.* This system consists of the SA node, Bachmann's bundle, the AV node, the bundle of His, the bundle branches, and the Purkinje fibers. (See *Cardiac conduction system,* page 22.)

Sinoatrial node

The SA node—located in the right atrium near the superior vena cava—is the heart's main pacemaker. Under resting conditions, the SA node generates impulses from 60 to 100 beats/minute. The impulses usually don't travel backward because the cells can't respond to a stimulus immediately after depolarization.

From the SA node, the impulse travels through the right atrium by way of three internodal tracts: the anterior, the middle (or Wenckebach's), and the posterior (or Thorel's) internodal tracts. At the same time, the impulse travels to the left atrium by Bachmann's bundle (interatrial tracts of tissue extending from the SA node to the left atrium). Transmission through the right and left atria occurs so rapidly that the atria contract almost simultaneously.

Atrioventricular node

The AV node is located in the inferior right atrium near the ostium of the coronary sinus. Although the AV node doesn't possess pacemaker cells, the tissue surrounding it, referred to as junctional tissue, contains pacemaker cells that can fire at a rate of 40 to 60 beats/minute. As the AV node conducts the atrial impulse to the ventricles, it delays the impulse by 0.04 second. This delay allows the ventricles to complete their filling phase as the atria contract. It also allows the cardiac muscle to stretch to its fullest for peak cardiac output.

Bundle of His

Rapid conduction then resumes through the bundle of His into the ventricles. If the SA node fails to generate an impulse at a normal rate, or if the impulse fails to reach the AV junction, the bundle of His can fire at a rate between 40 and 60 beats/minute.

Right and left bundle branches

The bundle of His divides into the right and left bundle branches and extends down either side of the interventricular septum. The right bundle branch extends down the right side of the interventricular septum and through the right ventricle. The left bundle branch extends down the left side of the interventricular septum and through the left ventricle.

The left bundle branch then splits into two branches, or fasciculations. The left anterior fasciculus extends through the anterior portion of the left ventricle. The left posterior fasciculus ex-

(Text continues on page 20.)

Understanding the depolarization-repolarization cycle

The cycle of depolarization-repolarization consists of five phases. During phases 1 and 2 and the beginning of phase 3, no stimulus, no matter how strong, can excite the cell. During the last half of phase 3, the cell would be receptive to a very strong stimulus. By the end of phase 4, the cell is fully ready for another stimulus.

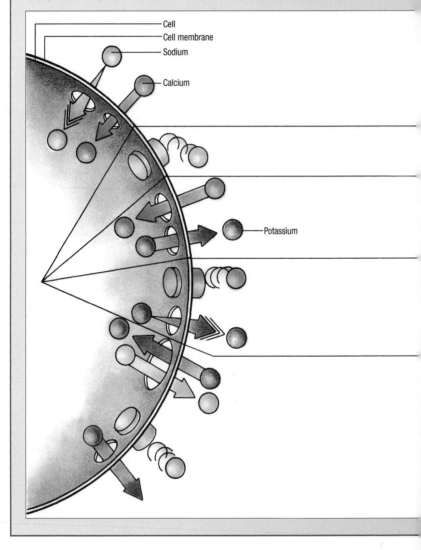

Cell
Cell membrane
Sodium
Calcium
Potassium

PHASE 0: RAPID DEPOLARIZATION
- ◆ Cardiac cell receives stimulus from a neighboring cell.
- ◆ Sodium moves rapidly into the cell.
- ◆ Calcium moves slowly into the cell.
- ◆ Myocardial contraction occurs.

PHASE 1: EARLY REPOLARIZATION
- ◆ Sodium channels close.
- ◆ Transmembrane potential falls slightly.

PHASE 2: PLATEAU PHASE
- ◆ Little change occurs in the cell's transmembrane potential.
- ◆ Calcium continues to flow in.
- ◆ Potassium flows out of the cell.

PHASE 3: RAPID REPOLARIZATION
- ◆ Calcium channels close.
- ◆ Potassium flows out rapidly.
- ◆ The cell returns to its original state.

PHASE 4: RESTING PHASE
- ◆ Active transport through the sodium-potassium pump begins restoring potassium to the inside of the cell and sodium to the outside.
- ◆ Cell membrane becomes impermeable to sodium.
- ◆ Potassium may move out of the cell.
- ◆ The cell is ready for another stimulus.

Action potential curves

An action potential curve shows the changes in a cell's electrical charge during the five phases of the depolarization-repolarization cycle. These graphs show electrical changes for nonpacemaker and pacemaker cells.

ACTION POTENTIAL CURVE: NONPACEMAKER CELL

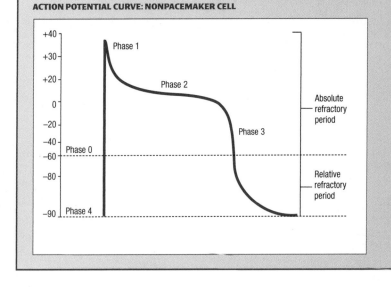

tends through the lateral and posterior portions of the left ventricle. Impulses travel much faster down the left bundle branch, which feeds the larger, thicker-walled left ventricle, than the right bundle branch, which feeds the smaller, thinner-walled right ventricle. The difference in the conduction speed allows both ventricles to contract simultaneously.

Purkinje fibers

After traveling through the left and right bundle branches, the impulses travel through the Purkinje fibers. Purkinje fibers—a diffuse muscle fiber network beneath the endocardium—transmit impulses quicker than any other part of the conduction system. This pacemaker site usually doesn't fire unless the SA and AV nodes fail to generate an impulse or if the normal impulse is blocked in both bundle branches. The automatic firing rate of the Purkinje fibers ranges from 20 to 40 beats/minute. The entire network of specialized nervous tissue that extends through the ventri-

As the graph below shows, the action potential curve for pacemaker cells, such as those in the sinoatrial node, differs from that of other myocardial cells. Pacemaker cells have a resting membrane potential of –60 mV (instead of –90 mV), and they begin to depolarize spontaneously. Called *diastolic depolarization,* this effect results primarily from calcium and sodium leakage into the cell.

ACTION POTENTIAL CURVE: PACEMAKER CELL

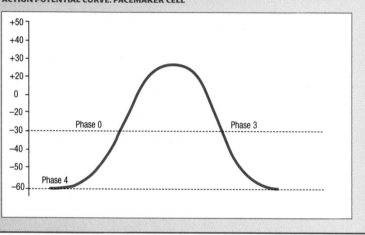

cles is known as the *His-Purkinje system.* (See *Pacemakers of the heart,* page 23.)

Abnormal impulse conduction

Causes of abnormal impulse conduction include altered automaticity, retrograde conduction of impulses, reentry abnormalities, and ectopy.

Altered automaticity

Automaticity, a special characteristic of pacemaker cells, allows them to generate electrical im-

pulses spontaneously. If a cell's automaticity is increased or decreased, an arrhythmia—or abnormality in the cardiac rhythm—can occur. Tachycardia and premature beats are commonly caused by an increase in the automaticity of pacemaker cells below the SA node. Likewise, a decrease in automaticity of cells in the SA node can cause the development of bradycardia or escape rhythms generated by lower pacemaker sites.

Cardiac conduction system

Specialized fibers send electrical impulses through the heart's cells, causing them to contract. This illustration shows the elements of the cardiac conduction system in the order that they contract (from 1 to 6). The firing of the sinoatrial (SA) node typically starts cardiac conduction.

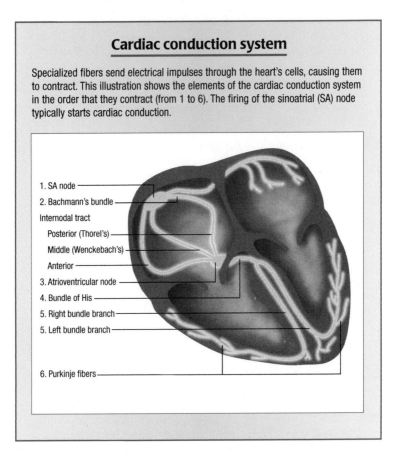

1. SA node
2. Bachmann's bundle
Internodal tract
 Posterior (Thorel's)
 Middle (Wenckebach's)
 Anterior
3. Atrioventricular node
4. Bundle of His
5. Right bundle branch
5. Left bundle branch

6. Purkinje fibers

Retrograde conduction

Impulses that begin below the AV node can be transmitted backward toward the atria. This backward, or retrograde, conduction usually takes longer than normal conduction and can cause the atria and ventricles to lose synchrony.

Reentry abnormalities

Reentry occurs when cardiac tissue is activated two or more times by the same impulse. This situation may happen when conduction speed is slowed or when the refractory periods for neighboring cells occur at different times. Impulses are delayed long enough that cells have time to repolarize. Therefore, the active

Pacemakers of the heart

Pacemaker cells in lower areas, such as the junctional tissue and the Purkinje fibers, normally remain dormant because they receive impulses from the sinoatrial (SA) node. They initiate an impulse only when they don't receive one from above, such as when the SA node is damaged from a myocardial infarction.

Firing rates

This illustration shows intrinsic firing rates of pacemaker cells located in three critical areas of the heart.

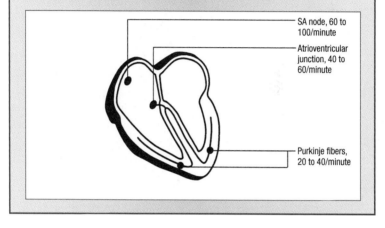

SA node, 60 to 100/minute

Atrioventricular junction, 40 to 60/minute

Purkinje fibers, 20 to 40/minute

impulse reenters the same area and produces another impulse.

Ectopy

Injured pacemaker (or nonpacemaker) cells may partially depolarize, rather than fully depolarize. Partial depolarization can lead to spontaneous or secondary depolarization, which involves repetitive ectopic firings called *triggered activity*.

The resultant depolarization is called afterdepolarization. Early afterdepolarization occurs before the cell is fully repolarized and can be caused by hypokalemia, slow pacing rates, or drug toxicity. If it occurs after the cell has been fully repolarized, it's called delayed afterdepolarization. These problems can be caused by digoxin toxicity, hypercalcemia, or increased catecholamine release. Atrial or ventricular tachycardias may result.

Cardiovascular assessment

2

Performed correctly, cardiovascular assessment can help to identify and evaluate changes in the patient's cardiac function. Complete cardiovascular assessment of a patient consists of obtaining an accurate, thorough history and performing a physical examination, including assessing the patient's heart and vascular system.

Obtaining a health history

To obtain a health history of a patient's cardiovascular system, begin by introducing yourself and explaining what will occur during the health history and physical examination. To take an effective history, you'll need to establish rapport with the patient. Ask open-ended questions and listen carefully to responses. Closely observe the patient's nonverbal behavior.

Chief complaint

You'll find that a patient with a cardiovascular problem typically cites specific complaints, such as:
◆ chest pain
◆ irregular heartbeat or palpitations
◆ shortness of breath on exertion, lying down, or at night
◆ cough
◆ cyanosis or pallor
◆ weakness
◆ fatigue
◆ unexplained weight change
◆ swelling of the extremities (see *Pregnancy and vein changes*)
◆ dizziness
◆ headache
◆ high or low blood pressure
◆ peripheral skin changes, such as decreased hair distribution, skin color changes, or a thin, shiny appearance to the skin
◆ pain in the extremities, such as leg pain or cramps.

Ask the patient how long he has had the problem, when it began, and how it affects his daily

◆

routine. Find out about any associated signs and symptoms. Ask about the location, radiation, intensity, and duration of any pain and any precipitating, exacerbating, or relieving factors. Ask him to rate the pain on a scale of 1 to 10, in which 1 means negligible pain and 10 means the worst pain imaginable. (See *Understanding chest pain,* pages 26 and 27.)

Let the patient describe his problem in his own words. Avoid leading questions. Use familiar expressions rather than medical terms whenever possible. If the patient isn't in distress, ask questions that require more than a yes-or-no response. Try to obtain as accurate a description as possible of any chest pain.

Because elderly patients have a higher risk of developing life-threatening conditions—such as a myocardial infarction (MI), angina, and aortic dissection— carefully evaluate chest pain in these patients. (See *Key questions for assessing cardiac function,* page 28.)

Abnormal findings

Orthopnea or dyspnea that occurs when the patient is lying down and improves when he sits up suggests left ventricular heart failure or mitral stenosis. It can also accompany obstructive lung disease. Fatigue in elderly pa-

---

Pregnancy and vein changes

Severe edema commonly occurs during the third trimester of pregnancy and in pregnant women who stand for long periods. You may observe 4+ pitting edema in the legs of a patient in her third trimester.

Varicose veins are another common finding during the third trimester.

---

tients may mask a more serious underlying condition.

Health history

Ask the patient about any history of cardiac-related disorders, such as hypertension, rheumatic fever, scarlet fever, diabetes mellitus, hyperlipidemia, congenital heart defects, and syncope. Other questions to ask include:
◆ Have you ever had severe fatigue not caused by exertion?
◆ Are you taking any prescription, over-the-counter, or illicit drugs?
◆ Are you allergic to any drugs, foods, or other products? If yes, describe the reaction you experienced.

In addition, ask the female patient:

(Text continues on page 28.)

Understanding chest pain

This chart outlines the different types of chest pain, including their location, exacerbating factors, and causes as well as measures used to alleviate them. Use this chart to accurately assess chest pain in a patient.

DESCRIPTION	LOCATION
Aching, squeezing, pressure, heaviness, burning pain; usually subsides within 10 minutes	Substernal; may radiate to jaw, neck, arms, and back
Tightness or pressure; burning, aching pain; possibly accompanied by shortness of breath, diaphoresis, weakness, anxiety, or nausea; sudden onset; lasts ½ to 2 hours	Typically across chest but may radiate to jaw, neck, arms, or back
Sharp and continuous; may be accompanied by friction rub; sudden onset	Substernal; may radiate to neck or left arm
Excruciating, tearing pain; may be accompanied by blood pressure difference between right and left arm; sudden onset	Retrosternal, upper abdominal, or epigastric; may radiate to back, neck, or shoulders
Sudden, stabbing pain; may be accompanied by cyanosis, dyspnea, or cough with hemoptysis	Over lung area
Sudden and severe pain; sometimes accompanied by dyspnea, increased pulse rate, decreased breath sounds, or deviated trachea	Lateral thorax
Dull, pressurelike, squeezing pain	Substernal, epigastric areas
Sharp, severe pain	Lower chest or upper abdomen
Burning feeling after eating sometimes accompanied by hematemesis or tarry stools; sudden onset that generally subsides within 15 to 20 minutes	Epigastric
Gripping, sharp pain; possibly nausea and vomiting	Right epigastric or abdominal areas; possible radiation to shoulders
Continuous or intermittent sharp pain; possibly tender to touch; gradual or sudden onset	Anywhere in chest
Dull or stabbing pain usually accompanied by hyperventilation or breathlessness; sudden onset; lasting less than a minute or as long as several days	Anywhere in chest

EXACERBATING FACTORS	CAUSES	ALLEVIATING MEASURES
Eating, physical effort, smoking, cold weather, stress, anger, hunger, lying down	Angina pectoris	Rest, nitroglycerin (Nitro-Dur) (*Note:* Unstable angina appears even at rest.)
Exertion, anxiety	Acute myocardial infarction	Opioid analgesics such as morphine (Duramorph), nitroglycerin
Deep breathing, supine position	Pericarditis	Sitting up, leaning forward, anti-inflammatory drugs
Not applicable	Dissecting aortic aneurysm	Analgesics, surgery
Inspiration	Pulmonary embolus	Analgesics
Normal respiration	Pneumothorax	Analgesics, chest tube insertion
Food, cold liquids, exercise	Esophageal spasm	Nitroglycerin, calcium channel blockers
Eating a heavy meal, bending, lying down	Hiatal hernia	Antacids, walking, semi-Fowler's position
Lack of food or highly acidic foods	Peptic ulcer	Food, antacids
Eating fatty foods, lying down	Cholecystitis	Rest and analgesics, surgery
Movement, palpation	Chest-wall syndrome	Time, analgesics, heat applications
Increased respiratory rate, stress or anxiety	Acute anxiety	Slowing of respiratory rate, stress relief

Key questions for assessing cardiac function

These questions and statements will help you to assess the patient more accurately:

◆ Are you still in pain? Where's it located? Point to where you feel it.

◆ Describe what the pain feels like. (If the patient needs prompting, ask if he feels a burning, tightness, or squeezing sensation in his chest.)

◆ Does the pain radiate to any other part of your body? Your arm? Neck? Back? Jaw?

◆ When did the pain begin? What relieves it? What makes it feel worse?

◆ Tell me about any other feelings you're experiencing. (If the patient needs prompting, suggest nausea, dizziness, fatigue, or sweating.)

◆ Tell me about any feelings of shortness of breath. Does a particular body position seem to bring this on? Which one? How long does any shortness of breath last? What relieves it?

◆ Has sudden breathing trouble ever awakened you from sleep? Tell me more about this.

◆ How many pillows do you sleep on at night?

◆ Do you ever wake up coughing? How often? Have you ever coughed up blood?

◆ Does your heart ever pound or skip a beat? If so, when does this happen?

◆ Do you ever feel dizzy or faint? What seems to bring this on?

◆ Tell me about any swelling in your ankles, feet, or hands. For example, do your rings or shoes feel tight? At what time of day?

◆ Does anything relieve the swelling?

◆ Have you noticed changes in color or sensation in your legs? If so, what are those changes?

◆ If you have sores or ulcers, how quickly do they heal?

◆ Do you stand or sit in one place for long periods at work?

◆ Do you urinate more frequently at night?

◆ Tell me how you feel while you're doing your daily activities. Have you had to limit your activities or rest more often while doing them?

◆ Have you begun menopause?

◆ Do you use hormonal contraceptives or estrogen?

◆ Have you experienced any medical problems during pregnancy? Have you ever had gestational hypertension?

Family history

Information about the patient's blood relatives may suggest a specific cardiac problem. Ask him if anyone in his family has ever had hypertension, MI, cardiomyopathy, diabetes mellitus, coronary artery disease (CAD), vascular disease, hyperlipidemia, or sudden death.

As you analyze a patient's problems, remember that age, gender, and race are essential considerations in identifying the risk of cardiovascular disorders. For example, CAD most commonly affects white men between ages 40 and 60. Hypertension occurs most commonly in blacks.

Women are also vulnerable to heart disease, especially postmenopausal women and those with diabetes mellitus. Many elderly people have increased systolic blood pressure because of an increase in the rigidity of their blood vessel walls with age. Overall, elderly people have a higher incidence of cardiovascular disease than do younger people.

Psychosocial history

Obtain information about your patient's occupation, educational background, living arrangements, daily activities, and family relationships.

Also, obtain information about:
◆ stress levels and how he deals with them
◆ current health habits, such as smoking, alcohol intake, caffeine intake, exercise, and dietary intake of fat and sodium
◆ environmental or occupational considerations

◆ activities of daily living.

During the history-taking session, note the appropriateness of the patient's responses, his speech clarity, and his mood so that you can better identify changes later.

Performing a cardiovascular assessment

Cardiovascular disease affects people of all ages and can take many forms. A consistent, methodical approach to your assessment will help you identify abnormalities. The key to accurate assessment is regular practice, which helps improve technique and efficiency.

When assessing the cardiovascular system, you must first assess the factors that reflect cardiovascular function. These include general appearance, body weight, vital signs, and related body structures.

Preparing for the assessment

Wash your hands and gather the necessary equipment. Choose a private room. Adjust the thermostat if necessary; cool temperatures may alter the patient's skin temperature and color, heart rate, and blood pressure. Make sure the room is quiet. If possible, close the door and windows and turn off radios and noisy equipment.

Combine parts of the assessment, as needed, to conserve time and the patient's energy. If the patient experiences cardiovascular difficulties, alter the order of your assessment as needed.

◆ **ALERT** If the patient develops chest pain and dyspnea, quickly check his vital signs and then auscultate the heart.

Assessing vital signs

Assessing vital signs includes measuring temperature, blood pressure, pulse rate, and respiratory rate.

Measuring temperature
Temperature is measured and documented in degrees Fahrenheit (° F) or degrees Celsius (° C). Choose the method of obtaining the patient's temperature (oral, tympanic, rectal, or axillary) based on the patient's age and condition. Normal body temperature ranges from 96.8° F to 99.5° F (36° C to 37.5° C).

Abnormal findings
An elevated temperature may indicate:
◆ cardiovascular inflammation or infection

◆ heightened cardiac workload (which may appear as tachycardia)
◆ MI or acute pericarditis (mild to moderate fever usually occurs 2 to 5 days after an MI when the healing infarct passes through the inflammatory stage)
◆ infections, such as infective endocarditis, which cause fever spikes (high fever).

In patients with lower than normal body temperatures, findings include poor perfusion and certain metabolic disorders.

Measuring blood pressure
First palpate and then auscultate the blood pressure in an arm or a leg. Wait 3 to 5 minutes between measurements. Normal blood pressure readings are less than 120/80 mm Hg in a resting adult and 78/46 to 114/78 mm Hg in a young child.

Emotional stress caused by physical examination may elevate blood pressure. If the patient's blood pressure is high, allow him to relax for several minutes and then measure again to rule out stress.

When assessing a patient's blood pressure for the first time, take measurements in both arms. If blood pressure is elevated in both arms, measure the pressure in the thigh. To do so, wrap a large cuff around the patient's upper leg at least 1″ (2.5 cm) above the knee. Place the stethoscope over the popliteal artery, located on the posterior surface slightly above the knee joint. Listen for sounds when the bladder of the cuff is deflated.

Abnormal findings
A difference of 10 mm Hg or more between the patient's arms may indicate thoracic outlet syndrome or other forms of arterial obstruction. High blood pressure in the patient's arms with normal or low pressure in the legs suggests aortic coarctation.

Determining pulse pressure
To calculate the patient's pulse pressure, subtract the diastolic pressure from the systolic pressure. This reflects arterial pressure during the resting phase of the cardiac cycle and normally ranges from 30 to 50 mm Hg.

Abnormal findings
Rising pulse pressure is seen with:
◆ increased stroke volume, which occurs with exercise, anxiety, and bradycardia
◆ declined peripheral vascular resistance or aortic distention, which occurs with anemia, hyperthyroidism, fever, hypertension, aortic coarctation, and aging.
    Diminishing pulse pressure occurs with:

◆ mitral or aortic stenosis, which occurs with mechanical obstruction
◆ constricted peripheral vessels, which occurs with shock
◆ declined stroke volume, which occurs with heart failure, hypovolemia, cardiac tamponade, or tachycardia.

Checking radial pulse
If you suspect cardiac disease, palpate for 1 full minute to detect arrhythmias. Normally, an adult's pulse ranges from 60 to 100 beats/minute. Its rhythm should feel regular, except for a subtle slowing on expiration, caused by changes in intrathoracic pressure and vagal response. Note whether the pulse feels weak, normal, or bounding.

Abnormal findings
A weak pulse may indicate increased peripheral vascular resistance or decreased stroke volume. A bounding pulse can indicate increased stroke volume, as with aortic insufficiency, or stiffness of arterial walls.

Evaluating respirations
Observe for eupnea—a regular, unlabored, and bilaterally equal breathing pattern.

Abnormal findings

In patients with irregular breathing, altered patterns may indicate:

◆ low cardiac output with tachypnea

◆ dyspnea, a possible indicator of heart failure (not evident at rest; however, pausing occurs after only a few words to take breaths)

◆ Cheyne-Stokes respirations, which may accompany severe heart failure (seen especially with coma)

◆ shallow breathing, which may occur with acute pericarditis as an attempt to reduce the pain associated with deep respirations.

Assessing appearance

Begin by observing the patient's general appearance, particularly noting weight and muscle composition. Is he well-developed, well-nourished, alert, and energetic? Document any departures from normal. Does the patient appear older than his chronological age or seem unusually tired or slow-moving? Does the patient appear comfortable or does he seem to be anxious or in distress?

Measuring height and body weight

Accurately measure and record the patient's height and weight. These measurements will help determine risk factors, calculate hemodynamic indexes (such as cardiac index), guide treatment plans, determine medication dosages, assist with nutritional counseling, and detect fluid overload.

◆ **ALERT** Fluctuations in weight may prove significant, especially when they're extreme (for example, a patient with developing heart failure who gains several pounds overnight).

Next, assess for cachexia—weakness and muscle wasting. Observe the amount of muscle bulk in the upper arms, thighs, and chest wall. For a more precise measurement, calculate the percentage of body fat. For men, this measurement should be 12%; for women, it should be 18%.

Abnormal findings

Loss of the body's energy stores slows healing and impairs immune function. A patient with chronic cardiac disease may develop cachexia, losing body fat and muscle mass. However, be aware that edema may mask these effects.

Assessing the skin

Inspect the skin color and note any cyanosis. Because normal skin color can vary widely among patients, ask him if his current skin tone is normal. Examine the underside of the tongue, buccal mucosa, and conjunctiva for signs of central cyanosis. Inspect the lips, tip of the nose, earlobes, and nail beds for signs of peripheral cyanosis.

In a dark-skinned patient, inspect the oral mucous membranes, such as the lips and gingivae, which normally appear pink and moist but would appear ashen if cyanotic. Because the color range for normal mucous membranes is narrower than that for the skin, it provides a more accurate assessment. When evaluating the patient's skin color, also observe for flushing, pallor, and rubor.

Next, assess the patient's perfusion by evaluating the arterial flow adequacy. With the patient lying down, elevate one leg 12″ (30.5 cm) above heart level for 60 seconds. Next, tell him to sit up and dangle both legs. Compare the color of both legs. The leg that was elevated should show mild pallor compared with the other leg. Color should return to the pale leg in about 10 seconds, and the veins should refill in about 15 seconds.

Touch the patient's skin. It should feel warm and dry. Then evaluate skin turgor by grasping and raising the skin between two fingers and then letting it go.

Normally, the skin immediately returns to its original position.

Observe the skin for signs of edema. Inspect the patient's arms and legs for symmetrical swelling. Because edema usually affects lower or dependent areas of the body first, be especially alert when assessing the arms, hands, legs, feet, and ankles of an ambulatory patient or the buttocks and sacrum of a bedridden patient. Determine the type of edema (pitting or nonpitting), its location, its extent, and its symmetry (unilateral or symmetrical). If the patient has pitting edema, assess the degree of pitting.

Finally, note the location, size, number, and appearance of any lesions.

Abnormal findings

Two types of cyanosis that may occur include:

◆ central cyanosis, suggesting reduced oxygen intake or transport from the lungs to the bloodstream, which may occur with heart failure

◆ peripheral cyanosis, suggesting constriction of peripheral arterioles, a natural response to cold or anxiety, hypovolemia, cardiogenic shock, or a vasoconstrictive disease.

Flushing can result from medications, excess heat, anxiety, or fear. Pallor can result from anemia or increased peripheral vascular resistance caused by atherosclerosis. Dependent rubor may be a sign of chronic arterial insufficiency. Suspect arterial insufficiency if the patient's foot shows marked pallor, delayed color return that ends with a mottled appearance, delayed venous filling, or marked redness.

Cool and clammy skin results from vasoconstriction, which occurs when cardiac output is low such as during shock. Warm, moist skin results from vasodilation, which occurs when cardiac output is high—for example during exercise.

Taut and shiny skin that can't be grasped may result from ascites or the marked edema that accompanies heart failure. Skin that doesn't immediately return to the original position exhibits tenting, a sign of decreased skin turgor, which may result from dehydration, especially if the patient takes diuretics. Tenting may also result from age, malnutrition, or an adverse reaction to corticosteroid treatment.

Edema can result from heart failure or venous insufficiency caused by varicosities or thrombophlebitis. Chronic right-sided heart failure may even cause ascites, which leads to generalized edema and abdominal distention. Venous compression may result in localized edema along the path of the compressed vessel.

Dry, open lesions on the patient's lower extremities accompanied by pallor, cool skin, and lack of hair growth signify arterial insufficiency, possibly caused by arterial peripheral vascular disease. Wet, open lesions with red or purplish edges that appear on the patient's legs may result from the venous stasis associated with venous peripheral vascular disease.

Assessing the arms and legs

Inspect the hair on the patient's arms and legs. Hair should be distributed symmetrically and should grow thicker on the anterior surface of the arms and legs. Also note whether the length of the arms and legs is proportionate to the length of the trunk.

Abnormal findings

Hair that isn't thicker on the anterior of the surface of the patient's arms and legs may indicate diminished arterial blood flow to these extremities. A patient with long, thin arms and legs may have Marfan syndrome, a congenital disorder that causes cardiovascular problems, such as aortic dissection, aortic valve incompetence, and cardiomyopathy.

Assessing the fingernails

Fingernails normally appear pinkish with no markings. To estimate the rate of peripheral blood flow, assess the capillary refill in the patient's fingernails (or toenails) by applying pressure to the nail for 5 seconds, then assessing the time it takes for color to return. In a patient with a good arterial supply, color should return in less than 3 seconds.

Assess the angle between the nail and the cuticle. Also evaluate the size of the patient's fingertips and palpate the nail bases. Nail bases should feel firm.

Evaluate the shape of the patient's nails. They should appear smooth and rounded. Finally, check for splinter hemorrhages— small, thin, red or brown lines that run from the base to the tip of the nail.

Abnormal findings

A bluish color in the nail beds indicates peripheral cyanosis. Delayed capillary refill suggests reduced circulation, a sign of low cardiac output that could lead to arterial insufficiency. An angle between the nail and the cuticle of 180 degrees or greater indicates finger clubbing, a sign of chronic tissue hypoxia. Enlarged fingertips and spongy nail bases also indicate early clubbing. A concave depression in the middle of a thin nail indicates koilonychia (spoon nail), a sign of iron deficiency anemia or Raynaud's disease, whereas thick, ridged nails can result from arterial insufficiency. Splinter hemorrhages may develop in patients with bacterial endocarditis.

Assessing the eyes

Inspect the eyelids, sclerae, and cornea for discolorations or lesions. Next, use an ophthalmoscope to examine the retinal structures, including the retinal vessels and background. The retina is normally light yellow to orange, and the background should be free from hemorrhages and exudates.

Abnormal findings

Xanthelasma—small, slightly raised, yellowish plaques on the eyelids, usually around the inner canthus—result from lipid deposits. They may signal severe hyperlipidemia, a risk factor of cardiovascular disease. Yellowish sclerae may be the first sign of jaundice, which occasionally results from liver congestion caused by right-sided heart failure. Arcus senilis—a thin grayish ring around the edge of the cornea—is a normal occurrence in older patients but can indicate hyperlipidemia in patients younger than age 65.

Identifying cardiovascular landmarks

These views show where to find critical landmarks used in cardiovascular assessment.

ANTERIOR THORAX

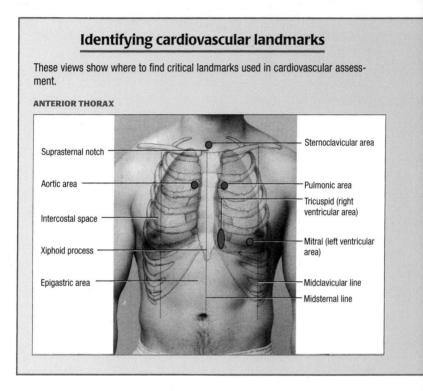

Suprasternal notch

Aortic area

Intercostal space

Xiphoid process

Epigastric area

Sternoclavicular area

Pulmonic area

Tricuspid (right ventricular area)

Mitral (left ventricular area)

Midclavicular line

Midsternal line

Changes in retinal structures, such as narrowing or blocking of a vein where an arteriole crosses over, indicate hypertension. Soft exudates may suggest hypertension or subacute bacterial endocarditis.

Assessing head movement

Assess the patient's head at rest and be alert for abnormal positioning or movements. Also check range of motion and rotation of the neck.

Abnormal findings

A slight, rhythmic bobbing of the patient's head in time with his heartbeat (Musset's sign) may signal aortic insufficiency or aneurysm.

Assessing the heart

Ask the patient to remove all clothing except his underwear and to put on an examination gown. Have the patient lie on his back, with the head of the examination table at a 30- to 45-degree angle. Stand on the patient's

LATERAL THORAX

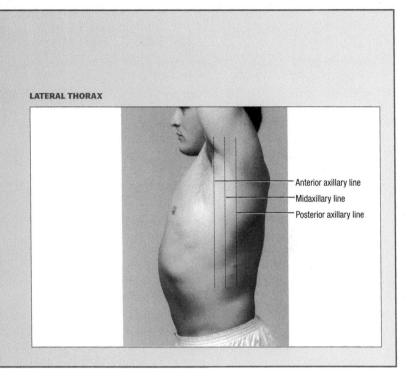

Anterior axillary line
Midaxillary line
Posterior axillary line

right side if you're right-handed or his left side if you're left-handed so you can auscultate more easily. If a female patient feels embarrassed about exposing her chest, explain each assessment step beforehand, use drapes appropriately, and expose only the area being assessed.

As with assessment of other body systems, you'll inspect, palpate, percuss, and auscultate in your assessment of the heart.

Inspection

Expose the anterior chest and observe its general appearance. Note landmarks you can use to describe your findings as well as structures underlying the chest wall. (See *Identifying cardiovascular landmarks*.) Note any deviations from typical chest shape. Normally, the lateral diameter is twice the anteroposterior diameter.

Next, look for pulsations, symmetry of movement, retractions, or heaves. A heave is a strong outward thrust of the chest wall and occurs during systole.

Position a light source, such as a flashlight or gooseneck lamp, so that it casts a shadow on the patient's chest. Note the location of the apical impulse. This is also usually the point of maximal impulse and should be located in the fifth intercostal space medial to the left midclavicular line. Because it corresponds to the apex of the heart, the apical impulse indicates how well the left ventricle is working.

The impulse can be seen in about 50% of adults. You'll notice the apical impulse more easily in children and in patients with thin chest walls. In thin adults and in children, you may see a slight sternal movement and pulsations over the pulmonary arteries or the aorta; you may also see pulsations in the epigastric area. To find the apical impulse in a woman with large breasts, displace the breasts during the examination.

Abnormal findings

On inspection you may discover irregularities in the patient's thorax and spine, some of which can impair cardiac output by preventing chest expansion and inhibiting heart muscle movement. These irregularities include:

◆ barrel chest (rounded thoracic cage caused by chronic obstructive pulmonary disease)
◆ pectus excavatum (depressed sternum)
◆ scoliosis (lateral curvature of the spine)
◆ pectus carinatum (protruding sternum)
◆ kyphosis (convex curvature of the thoracic spine)
◆ retractions (visible indentations of the soft tissue covering the chest wall) or the use of accessory muscles to breathe, which typically result from a respiratory disorder, but may also indicate congenital heart defect or heart failure
◆ visible pulsation to the right of the sternum, a possible indication of aortic aneurysm
◆ pulsation in the sternoclavicular or epigastric area, a possible indication of aortic aneurysm
◆ sustained, forceful apical impulse, a possible indication of left ventricular hypertrophy, which increases blood pressure and may cause cardiomyopathy and mitral insufficiency
◆ laterally displaced apical impulse, a possible sign of left ventricular hypertrophy.

Palpation

Maintain a gentle touch when you palpate so you won't obscure pulsations or similar findings. Follow a systematic palpation sequence covering the sternoclavicular, aortic, pulmonary right ventricular, left ventricular (apical), and epigastric areas. Use the pads of your fingers to effectively assess large pulse sites. Finger pads prove especially sensitive to vibrations. Start at the sternoclavicular area and move methodically through the palpation sequence down to the epigastric area.

At the sternoclavicular area, you may feel pulsations of the aortic arch, especially in a thin or average-build patient. In a thin patient, you may palpate a pulsation in the abdominal aorta over the epigastric area.

Using the ball of your hand, then your fingertips, palpate over the precordium to find the apical impulse. Note heaves or thrills, fine vibrations that feel like the purring of a cat. (See *Assessing the apical impulse*.) The apical impulse may be difficult to palpate in obese and pregnant patients and in patients with thick chest walls. If it's difficult to palpate with the patient lying on his back, have him lie on his left side or sit upright. It may also be helpful to have the patient exhale completely and hold his breath for a few seconds.

Abnormal findings

Palpation of the patient's chest may reveal:

> ## Assessing the apical impulse
>
> The apical impulse is associated with the first heart sound and carotid pulsation. To ensure that you're feeling the apical impulse and not a muscle spasm or some other pulsation, use one hand to palpate the patient's carotid artery and the other to palpate the apical impulse. Then compare the timing and regularity of the impulses. The apical impulse should roughly coincide with the carotid pulsation.
>
> Note the amplitude, size, intensity, location, and duration of the apical impulse. You should feel a gentle pulsation in an area about ½" to ¾" (1.5 to 2 cm) in diameter.

◆ apical impulse that exerts unusual force and lasts longer than one-third of the cardiac cycle—a possible indication of increased cardiac output
◆ displaced or diffuse impulse—a possible indication of left ventricular hypertrophy
◆ pulsation in the aortic, pulmonic, or right ventricular area—a sign of chamber enlargement or valvular disease
◆ pulsation in the sternoclavicular or epigastric area—a sign of aortic aneurysm
◆ palpable thrill (fine vibration)—an indication of blood

flow turbulence, usually related to valvular dysfunction (determine how far the thrill radiates and make a mental note to listen for a murmur at this site during auscultation)

◆ heave (a strong outward thrust during systole) along the left sternal border—an indication of right ventricular hypertrophy

◆ heave over the left ventricular area—a sign of a ventricular aneurysm (a thin patient may experience a heave with exercise, fever, or anxiety because of increased cardiac output and more forceful contraction)

◆ displaced point of maximal impulse—a possible indication of left ventricular hypertrophy caused by volume overload from mitral or aortic stenosis, septal defect, acute MI, or other disorder.

Percussion

Although percussion isn't as useful as other methods of assessment, this technique may help you locate cardiac borders. Begin percussing at the anterior axillary line, and percuss toward the sternum along the fifth intercostal space. The sound changes from resonance to dullness over the left border of the heart, normally at the midclavicular line.

In patients who are obese, percussion may be difficult because of the fat overlying the chest or in female patients because of breast tissue. In these cases, a chest X-ray can be used to provide information about the heart border.

Abnormal findings

If the cardiac border extends to the left of the midclavicular line, the patient's heart—and especially the left ventricle—may be enlarged. The right border of the heart is usually aligned with the sternum and can't be percussed.

Auscultation

Begin by warming the stethoscope in your hands, and then identify the sites where you'll auscultate: over the four cardiac valves and at Erb's point, the third intercostal space at the left sternal border. Use the bell to hear low-pitched sounds and the diaphragm to hear high-pitched sounds. (See *Auscultation sites*.)

Auscultate for heart sounds with the patient in three positions: lying on his back with the head of the bed raised 30 to 45 degrees, sitting up, and lying on his left side. You can start at the base and work downward or at the apex and work upward. Whichever approach you use, be consistent. (See *Auscultation tips*, page 42.)

Use the diaphragm to listen as you go in one direction; use the bell as you come back in the oth-

Auscultation sites

When auscultating for heart sounds, place the stethoscope over four different sites. Follow the same auscultation sequence during every cardiovascular assessment:

◆ Place the stethoscope in the second intercostal space along the right sternal border, as shown. In the aortic area, blood moves from the left ventricle during systole, crossing the aortic valve and flowing through the aortic arch.

◆ Move to the pulmonic area, located in the second intercostal space at the left sternal border. In the pulmonic area, blood ejected from the right ventricle during systole crosses the pulmonic valve and flows through the main pulmonary artery.

◆ In the third auscultation site, assess the tricuspid area, which lies in the fifth intercostal space along the left sternal border. In the tricuspid area, sounds reflect blood movement from the right atrium across the tricuspid valve, filling the right ventricle during diastole.

◆ Finally, listen in the mitral area, located in the fifth intercostal space near the midclavicular line. (If the patient's heart is enlarged, the mitral area may be closer to the anterior axillary line.) In the mitral (apical) area, sounds represent blood flow across the mitral valve and left ventricular filling during diastole.

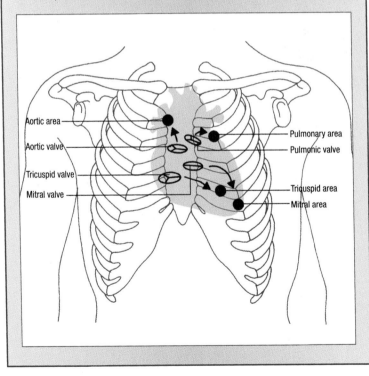

Auscultation tips

Follow these tips when you auscultate a patient's heart:
◆ Concentrate as you listen for each sound.
◆ Avoid auscultating through clothing or wound dressings because they can block sound.
◆ Avoid picking up extraneous sounds by keeping the stethoscope tubing off the patient's body and other surfaces.
◆ Until you become proficient at auscultation and can examine a patient quickly, explain to him that even though you may listen to his chest for a long period, it doesn't mean anything is wrong.
◆ Ask the patient to breathe normally and to hold his breath periodically to enhance sounds that may be difficult to hear.

systole. This sound corresponds to closure of the pulmonic and aortic valves and is generally described as sounding like "dub." It's a shorter, higher-pitched, louder sound than S_1. When the pulmonic valve closes later than the aortic valve during inspiration, you'll hear a split S_2.

From the base of the heart, move to the pulmonic area and then down to the tricuspid area. Then move to the mitral area, where S_1 is the loudest. S_1 is best heard at the apex of the heart. This sound corresponds to closure of the mitral and tricuspid valves and is generally described as sounding like "lub." It's low-pitched and dull. S_1 occurs at the beginning of ventricular systole. It may be split if the mitral valve closes just before the tricuspid.

er direction. Be sure to listen over the entire precordium, not just over the valves.

Note the heart rate and rhythm. Always identify the first heart sound (S_1) and the second heart sound (S_2). Then listen for adventitious sounds, such as third (S_3) and fourth heart sounds (S_4), murmurs, and rubs. (See *Cycle of heart sounds*, pages 44 and 45.)

Start auscultating at the aortic area where S_2 is loudest. S_2 is best heard at the base of the heart at the end of ventricular

Abnormal findings
Auscultation may detect S_1 and S_2 that are accentuated, diminished, or inaudible. These abnormalities may result from pressure changes, valvular dysfunctions, and conduction defects. A prolonged, persistent, or reversed split sound may result from a mechanical or electrical problem. Auscultation may also reveal an S_3, an S_4, or both. Other abnormal sounds include a click, an opening snap, and a summation gallop.

Recognizing abnormal heart sounds

With lots of practice, you'll be able to recognize these abnormal heart sounds upon auscultation.

Third heart sound

Also known as a *ventricular gallop,* S_3 is a low-pitched noise with a rhythm resembling a horse galloping and a cadence like the word "Ken-tuc-ky" ("lub-dub-by"). S_3 usually occurs during early diastole to mid-diastole, at the end of the passive-filling phase of either ventricle. The sound is best heart by placing the bell of the stethoscope at the apex of the heart while the patient is in a supine or left-lateral decubitus position. Listen for this sound immediately after S_2.

An S_3 may signify that the ventricle isn't compliant enough to accept the filling volume without additional force. If the right ventricle is noncompliant, the sound will occur in the tricuspid area; if the left ventricle is noncompliant, in the mitral area. A heave may be palpable when the sound occurs.

An S_3 may occur normally in a child or young adult. It may also occur during the last trimester of pregnancy. In a patient older than age 30, it usually indicates a disorder, such as right-sided heart failure, left-sided heart failure, pulmonary congestion, in-tracardiac shunting of blood, MI, anemia, or thyrotoxicosis.

Fourth heart sound

The fourth heart sound is an abnormal heart sound that occurs late in diastole, just before the pulse upstroke. It immediately precedes the S_1 of the next cycle and is associated with acceleration and deceleration of blood entering a chamber that resists additional filling. Known as the *atrial* or *presystolic gallop,* it occurs during atrial contraction.

S_4 shares the same cadence as the word "Ten-nes-see" ("le-lub-dub"). Heard best with the bell of the stethoscope and with the patient in a supine position, S_4 may occur in the tricuspid or mitral area, depending on which ventricle is dysfunctional.

Although rare, S_4 may occur normally in a young patient with a thin chest wall. More commonly, it indicates cardiovascular disease, such as acute MI, hypertension, CAD, cardiomyopathy, angina, anemia, elevated left ventricular pressure, or aortic stenosis. If the sound persists, it may indicate impaired ventricular compliance or volume overload. S_4 commonly appears in elderly patients with age-related systolic hypertension and aortic stenosis.

(Text continues on page 46.)

Cycle of heart sounds

Heart sounds are generated by events in the cardiac cycle. When valves close or blood fills the ventricles, vibrations of the heart muscle can be heard through the chest wall.

Varying sound patterns

The phonogram at right shows how heart sounds vary in duration and intensity. For instance, S_2 (which occurs when the semilunar valves snap shut) is a shorter-lasting sound than S_1 because the semilunar valves take less time to close than the atrioventricular valves, which cause S_1.

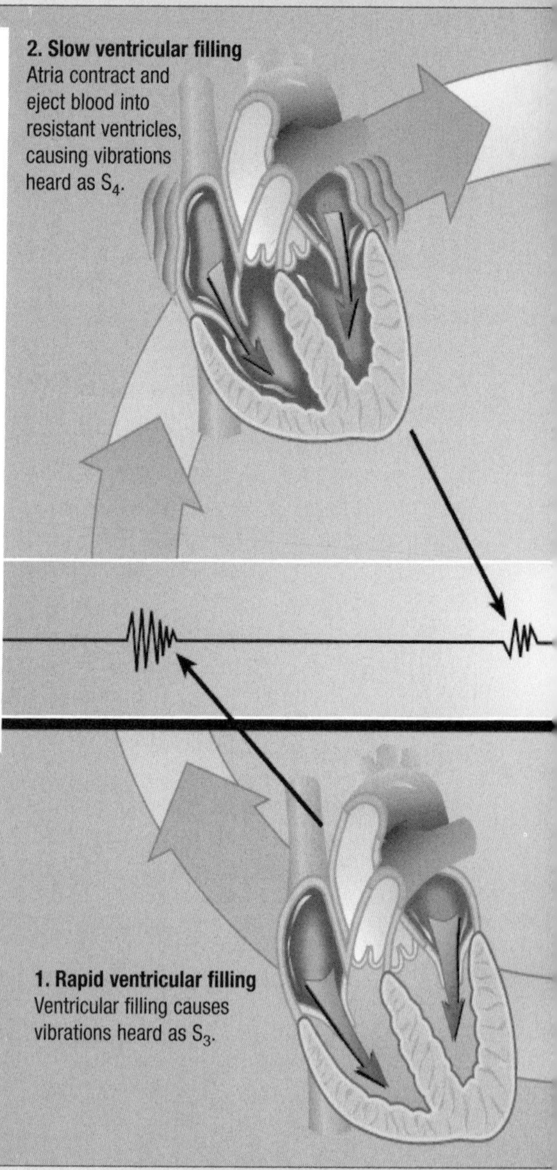

2. Slow ventricular filling
Atria contract and eject blood into resistant ventricles, causing vibrations heard as S_4.

1. Rapid ventricular filling
Ventricular filling causes vibrations heard as S_3.

Diastole

Systole

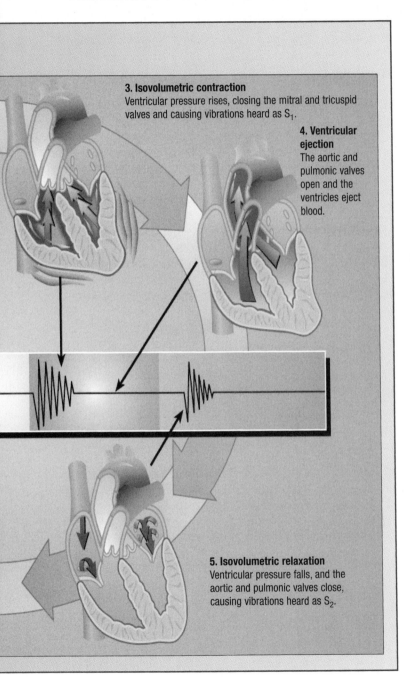

3. Isovolumetric contraction
Ventricular pressure rises, closing the mitral and tricuspid valves and causing vibrations heard as S_1.

4. Ventricular ejection
The aortic and pulmonic valves open and the ventricles eject blood.

5. Isovolumetric relaxation
Ventricular pressure falls, and the aortic and pulmonic valves close, causing vibrations heard as S_2.

Summation gallop

Occasionally, a patient may have both S_3 and S_4. Auscultation may reveal two separate abnormal heart sounds and two normal sounds. Usually, the patient has tachycardia and diastole is shortened. S_3 and S_4 occur so close together that they appear to be one sound—a summation gallop.

Clicks

Clicks are high-pitched abnormal heart sounds that result from tensing of the chordae tendineae structures and mitral valve cusps. Initially, the mitral valve closes securely, but a large cusp prolapses into the left atrium. The click usually precedes a late systolic murmur caused by regurgitation of a little blood from the left ventricle into the left atrium. Clicks occur in 5% to 10% of young adults and affect more women than men.

To detect the high-pitched click of mitral valve prolapse, place the stethoscope diaphragm at the apex and listen during midsystole to late systole. To enhance the sound, change the patient's position to sitting or standing, and listen along the lower left sternal border.

Snaps

Upon placing the stethoscope diaphragm dial at the apex along the lower left sternal border, you may detect an opening snap immediately after S_2. The snap resembles the normal S_1 and S_2 in quality; its high pitch helps differentiate it from an S_3. Because the opening snap may accompany mitral or tricuspid stenosis, it usually precedes a middiastolic to late diastolic murmur—a classic sign of stenosis. It results from the stenotic valve attempting to open.

Rubs

To detect a pericardial friction rub, use the diaphragm of the stethoscope to auscultate in the third left intercostal space along the lower left sternal border. Listen for a harsh, scratchy, scraping, or squeaking sound that occurs throughout systole, diastole, or both. To enhance the sound, have the patient sit upright and lean forward or exhale. A rub usually indicates pericarditis.

Murmurs

Longer than a heart sound, a murmur occurs as a vibrating, blowing, or rumbling noise. Just as turbulent water in a stream babbles as it passes through a narrow point, turbulent blood flow produces a murmur. (See *Understanding murmurs*.)

An innocent or functional murmur may appear in a patient without heart disease. Best heard in the pulmonic area, it occurs

Understanding murmurs

Normally, heart valves close tightly and then open completely to let blood flow through. However, various conditions may alter blood flow through the valves, causing murmurs and, in many cases, increasing the heart's workload.

The first two illustrations show a normal valve open and closed. The other illustrations portray three common reasons for the development of murmurs.

NORMAL VALVE OPEN

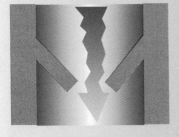

NORMAL VALVE CLOSED

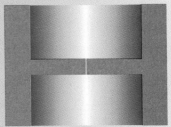

HIGH BLOOD FLOW

High blood flow through a normal valve may cause a murmur. Examples include an aortic systolic murmur, which can be caused by anemia and a subsequent compensatory increase in cardiac output.

DECREASED BLOOD FLOW

Low blood flow through a stenotic valve can cause a murmur. The valves can't open or close properly because they're thickened, fibrotic, or calcified. Common examples include aortic and mitral stenosis.

BACKFLOW OF BLOOD

A backflow of blood through an insufficient or incompetent valve can cause a murmur. Because the valve can't close properly, blood can leak back or regurgitate into the heart chamber from which it came. Common examples include aortic and mitral insufficiency.

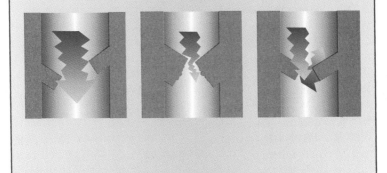

Positioning the patient for auscultation

If heart sounds are faint or if you hear abnormal sounds, try listening to them with the patient lying on his left side (left lateral recumbent position) or seated and leaning forward.

Left lateral recumbent
The left lateral recumbent position is best suited for hearing low-pitched sounds, such as mitral valve murmurs and extra heart sounds. To hear these sounds, place the bell of the stethoscope over the apical area, as shown.

Leaning forward
To auscultate for high-pitched heart sounds related to semilunar valve problems, such as aortic and pulmonic valve murmurs, lean the patient forward. Place the diaphragm of the stethoscope over the aortic and pulmonic areas in the right and left second intercostal spaces, as shown.

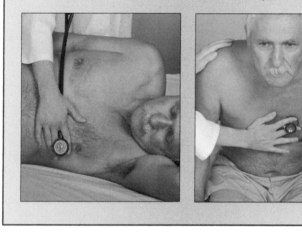

early in systole and seldom exceeds grade 2 in intensity. When the patient changes from a supine to a sitting position, the murmur may disappear. If fever, exercise, anemia, anxiety, pregnancy, or other factors increase cardiac output, the murmur may increase in intensity.

Innocent murmurs affect up to 25% of all children but usually disappear by adolescence. Similarly, elderly patients who experience changes in the aortic valve structures and the aorta also experience a nonpathologic murmur—a short systolic murmur, best heard at the left sternal border.

Pathologic murmurs may occur during systole or diastole and may affect any heart valve. These murmurs may result from valvular stenosis (inability of the heart valves to open properly), valvular insufficiency (inability of the heart valves to close properly, allowing regurgitation of blood), or a septal defect (a defect in the septal wall separating two heart chambers). The best way to hear murmurs is with the patient sitting up and leaning forward. You can also have him lie on his left side. (See *Positioning the patient for auscultation*.)

If you detect a murmur, identify where it's loudest, pinpoint the time it occurs during the cardiac cycle, and describe its pitch, pattern, quality, and intensity. (See *Tips for describing murmurs*.)

Location and timing
Murmurs may occur in any cardiac auscultatory site and may radiate from one site to another. (See *Identifying heart murmurs*, pages 50 and 51.) To identify the radiation area, auscultate from the site where the murmur seems loudest to the farthest site it's still heard. Note the anatomic landmark of this farthest site.

Determine if the murmur occurs during systole (between S_1 and S_2) or diastole (between S_2 and the next S_1). Pinpoint when in the cardiac cycle the murmur

occurs—for example, during mid-diastole or late systole. A murmur that's heard throughout systole is called *holosystolic* or *pansystolic*, whereas a murmur heard throughout diastole is called a *pandiastolic murmur*. Occasionally, murmurs occur during both portions of the cycle (continuous murmur).

Pitch
Depending on rate and pressure of blood flow, pitch may be high, medium, or low. You can best hear a low-pitched murmur with the bell of the stethoscope, a high-pitched murmur with the diaphragm, and a medium-pitched murmur with both.

Tips for describing murmurs

Describing murmurs can be tricky. After you've auscultated a murmur, list the terms you would use to describe it. Then check the patient's chart to see how others have described it or ask an experienced colleague to listen and describe the murmur. Compare the descriptions and then auscultate for the murmur again, if necessary, to confirm the description.

Identifying heart murmurs

Heart murmurs can occur as a result of various conditions and have wide-ranging characteristics. Here's a list of some conditions and their associated murmurs.

Aortic stenosis

In a patient with aortic stenosis, the aortic valve has calcified and restricts blood flow, causing a midsystolic, low-pitched, harsh murmur that radiates from the valve to the carotid artery. The murmur shifts from crescendo to decrescendo and back.

The crescendo-decrescendo murmur of aortic stenosis results from the turbulent, highly pressured flow of blood across stiffened leaflets and through a narrowed opening.

Pulmonic stenosis

During auscultation, listen for a murmur near the pulmonic valve. In a patient with this type of murmur it might indicate pulmonic stenosis, a condition in which the pulmonic valve has calcified and interferes with the flow of blood out of the right ventricle. The murmur is medium-pitched, systolic, and harsh and shifts from crescendo to decrescendo and back. The murmur is caused by turbulent blood flow across a stiffened, narrowed valve.

Aortic insufficiency

In a patient with aortic insufficiency, the blood flows backward through the aortic valve and causes a high-pitched, blowing, decrescendo, diastolic murmur. The murmur radiates from the aortic valve area to the left sternal border.

Pulmonic insufficiency

In a patient with pulmonic insufficiency, the blood flows backward through the pulmonic valve, causing a blowing, diastolic, decrescendo murmur at Erb's point (at the left sternal border of the third intercostal space). If the patient has a higher-than-normal pulmonary pressure, the murmur is high-pitched. If not, it will be low-pitched.

Mitral stenosis

In a patient with mitral stenosis, the mitral valve has calcified and is blocking blood flow out of the left atrium. Listen for a low-pitched, rumbling, crescendo-decrescendo murmur in the mitral valve area. This murmur results from turbulent blood flow across the stiffened, narrowed valve.

Pattern

Crescendo occurs when the velocity of blood flow increases and the murmur becomes louder. Decrescendo occurs when velocity decreases and the murmur becomes quieter. A crescendo-decrescendo pattern describes a murmur with increasing loudness followed by increasing softness.

Quality

The volume of blood flow, the force of the contraction, and the degree of valve compromise all contribute to murmur quality.

Mitral insufficiency

In a patient with mitral insufficiency, blood regurgitates into the left atrium. The regurgitation produces a high-pitched, blowing murmur throughout systole (pansystolic or holosystolic). The murmur may radiate from the mitral area to the left axillary line. You can hear it best at the apex.

Tricuspid stenosis

In a patient with tricuspid stenosis, the tricuspid valve has calcified and is blocking blood flow through the valve from the right atrium. Listen for a low, rumbling, crescendo-decrescendo murmur in the tricuspid area. The murmur results from turbulent blood flow across the stiffened, narrowed valvular leaflets.

Tricuspid insufficiency

In a patient with tricuspid insufficiency, blood regurgitates into the right atrium. This backflow of blood through the valve causes a high-pitched, blowing murmur throughout systole in the tricuspid area. The murmur becomes louder when the patient inhales.

Grading murmurs

Use the system outlined here to describe a murmur's intensity. When recording your findings, use Roman numerals as part of a fraction, always with VI as the denominator. For instance, a grade III murmur would be recorded as "grade III/VI."

◆ Grade I is barely audible.
◆ Grade II is audible but quiet and soft.
◆ Grade III is moderately loud, without a thrust or thrill.
◆ Grade IV is loud, with a thrill.
◆ Grade V is very loud, with a thrust or a thrill.
◆ Grade VI is loud enough to be heard before the stethoscope comes into contact with the chest.

Terms used to describe quality include musical, blowing, harsh, rasping, rumbling, or machine-like.

Intensity

Murmurs range in intensity from barely audible to loud enough to be heard without a stethoscope. Use a standard, six-level grading scale to describe the murmur's intensity. (See *Grading murmurs*.)

Assessing the vascular system

Assessment of the vascular system is an important part of a full cardiovascular assessment.

Inspection

Start your assessment of the vascular system the same way you start an assessment of the cardiac system—by making general observations. Are the patient's

Jugular vein distention

Inspecting the jugular veins helps provide information about the blood volume and the pressure in the right side of the heart. Normally, the highest pulsation occurs no more than 1½″ (3.8 cm) above the sternal notch. Pulsations above that point indicate an elevation in central venous pressure and jugular vein distention.

If the patient has jugular vein distention, characterize it as mild, moderate, or severe. Determine the level of distention in fingerbreadths above the clavicle or in relation to the jaw or clavicle. Also, note the amount of distention in relation to head elevation.

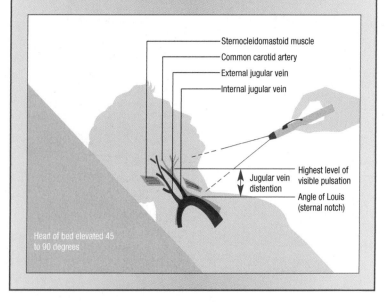

Sternocleidomastoid muscle
Common carotid artery
External jugular vein
Internal jugular vein

Jugular vein distention

Highest level of visible pulsation
Angle of Louis (sternal notch)

Head of bed elevated 45 to 90 degrees

arms equal in size? Are the legs symmetrical? Examination of the patient's arms and legs can reveal arterial or venous disorders. Examine the patient's arms when you take his vital signs. Check the legs later during the physical examination, when the patient is lying on his back. Remember to evaluate leg veins when the patient is standing.

Inspect the patient's skin color. Note how body hair is distributed. Note lesions, scars, clubbing, and edema of the extremities. If the patient is bedridden, be sure to check the sacrum for swelling. Examine the fingernails and toenails for abnormalities.

Next, observe the vessels in the patient's neck. The carotid artery should show a brisk, local-

Findings in arterial and venous insufficiency

Assessment findings differ in patients with arterial insufficiency and those with chronic venous insufficiency.

Arterial insufficiency

In a patient with arterial insufficiency, pulses may be decreased or absent. His skin is cool, pale, and shiny, and he may have pain in his legs and feet. Ulcerations typically occur in the area around the toes, and the foot usually turns deep red when dependent. Nails may be thick and ridged.

Chronic venous insufficiency

In a patient with chronic venous insufficiency, check for ulcerations around the ankle. Pulses are present but may be difficult to find because of edema. The foot may become cyanotic when dependent.

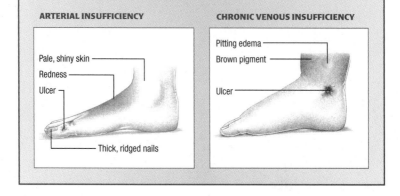

ARTERIAL INSUFFICIENCY

Pale, shiny skin
Redness
Ulcer
Thick, ridged nails

CHRONIC VENOUS INSUFFICIENCY

Pitting edema
Brown pigment
Ulcer

---

ized pulsation. The carotid pulsation doesn't decrease when the patient is upright, when he inhales, or when you palpate the carotid. Note whether carotid pulsations are weak or bounding.

Inspect the jugular veins. The internal jugular vein has a softer, undulating pulsation. Unlike the pulsation of the carotid artery, pulsation of the internal jugular vein changes in response to position, breathing, and palpation.

To check the jugular venous pulse, have the patient lie on his back. Elevate the head of the bed 30 to 45 degrees, and turn the patient's head slightly away from you. (See *Jugular vein distention*.)

Abnormal findings

Upon inspection of the patient's vascular system you may uncover irregularities, including:

Assessing arterial pulses

To assess arterial pulses, apply pressure with your index and middle fingers. The following illustrations show where to position your fingers when palpating for various pulses.

Carotid pulse

Lightly place your fingers just medial to the trachea and below the jaw angle. Never palpate both carotid arteries at the same time.

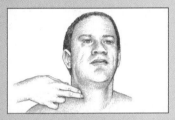

Brachial pulse

Position your fingers medial to the biceps tendon.

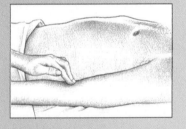

Radial pulse

Apply gentle pressure to the medial and ventral side of the wrist, just below the base of the thumb.

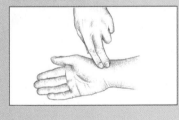

Femoral pulse

Press relatively hard at a point inferior to the inguinal ligament. For an obese patient, palpate in the crease of the groin, halfway between the pubic bone and the hip bone.

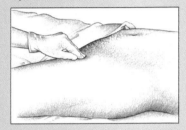

Popliteal pulse

Press firmly in the popliteal fossa at the back of the knee.

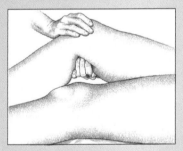

Posterior tibial pulse

Apply pressure behind and slightly below the malleolus of the ankle.

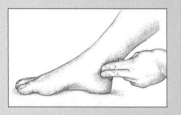

Dorsalis pedis pulse

Place your fingers on the medial dorsum of the foot while the patient points his toes down. *(Note:* The pulse is difficult to detect here and may be nonpalpable in healthy patients.)

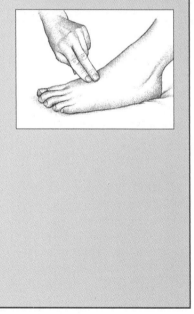

◆ cyanosis, pallor, or cool or cold skin, indicating poor cardiac output and tissue perfusion
◆ warm skin caused by fever or increased cardiac output
◆ absence of body hair on the patient's arms or legs, indicating diminished arterial blood flow to those areas (see *Findings in arterial and venous insufficiency*, page 53.)
◆ swelling or edema, indicating heart failure or venous insufficiency, or varicosities or thrombophlebitis
◆ ascites and generalized edema, indicating chronic right-sided heart failure
◆ localized swelling, indicating compressed veins
◆ swelling in the lower legs, indicating right-sided heart failure.

Palpation

The first step in palpating the vascular system is to assess skin temperature, texture, and turgor. Then check capillary refill time by assessing the nail beds of the fingers and toes. Refill time should be no more than 3 seconds, or long enough to say "capillary refill."

Palpate the patient's arms and legs for temperature and edema. Edema is graded on a four-point scale. If your finger leaves a slight imprint, the edema is recorded as +1. If your finger leaves a deep imprint that only

Pulse waveforms

To identify abnormal arterial pulses, check the waveforms below and see which one matches the patient's peripheral pulse.

Weak pulse

A weak pulse has a decreased amplitude with a slower upstroke and downstroke. Possible causes of a weak pulse include increased peripheral vascular resistance, such as happens in cold weather or severe heart failure, and decreased stroke volume, as with hypovolemia or aortic stenosis.

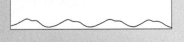

Bounding pulse

A bounding pulse has a sharp upstroke and downstroke with a pointed peak. The amplitude is elevated. Possible causes of a bounding pulse include increased stroke volume, as with aortic insufficiency, or stiffness of arterial walls, as with aging.

Pulsus alternans

Pulsus alternans has a regular, alternating pattern of a weak and a strong pulse. This pulse is associated with left-sided heart failure.

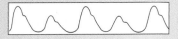

Pulsus bigeminus

Pulsus bigeminus is similar to alternating pulse but occurs at irregular intervals. This pulse is caused by premature atrial or ventricular beats.

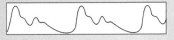

---

slowly returns to normal, the edema is recorded as +4.

Using the pads of your index and middle fingers, palpate for arterial pulses. (See *Assessing arterial pulses,* pages 54 and 55.) Start at the top of the patient's body at the temporal artery, and work your way down. Check the carotid, brachial, radial, femoral, popliteal, posterior tibial, and dorsalis pedis pulses. Palpate for the pulses on each side of the body, comparing pulse volume and symmetry. If you haven't put on gloves for the examination, do so when you palpate the femoral arteries.

◆ **ALERT** Don't palpate both carotid arteries at the same time or press too firmly. If you do, the patient may faint or become bradycardic.

All pulses should be regular in rhythm and equal in strength. Pulses are graded on the follow-

Pulsus paradoxus

Pulsus paradoxus has increases and decreases in amplitude associated with the respiratory cycle. Marked decreases occur when the patient inhales. Pulsus paradoxus is associated with pericardial tamponade, advanced heart failure, and constrictive pericarditis.

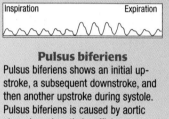

Inspiration — Expiration

Pulsus biferiens

Pulsus biferiens shows an initial upstroke, a subsequent downstroke, and then another upstroke during systole. Pulsus biferiens is caused by aortic stenosis and aortic insufficiency.

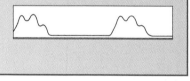

ing scale: 4 + is bounding, 3 + is increased, 2 + is normal, 1 + is weak, and 0 is absent.

Abnormal findings

A weak arterial pulse may indicate decreased cardiac output or increased peripheral vascular resistance, both pointing to arterial atherosclerotic disease.

Elderly patients commonly have weak pedal pulses. Strong or bounding pulsations usually occur in patients with conditions that cause increased cardiac output, such as hypertension, hypoxia, anemia, exercise, or anxiety. (See *Pulse waveforms.*)

Auscultation

After you palpate, use the bell of the stethoscope to begin auscultating the vascular system. Following the palpation sequence, listen over each artery. You shouldn't hear sounds over the carotid arteries.

Next, assess the upper abdomen for abnormal pulsations. Finally, auscultate the femoral and popliteal pulses, checking for a bruit or other abnormal sounds.

Abnormal findings

If you hear a bruit during arterial auscultation, the patient may have occlusive arterial disease or an arteriovenous fistula. Various high cardiac output conditions— such as anemia, hyperthyroidism, and pheochromocytoma— may also cause bruits. Abnormal pulsations over the upper abdomen could indicate an abdominal aortic aneurysm. (See *The cardiovascular system: Interpreting your findings,* pages 58 to 60.)

The cardiovascular system: Interpreting your findings

This chart shows some common groups of findings for signs and symptoms of cardiovascular system disorders, along with their probable causes.

SIGN OR SYMPTOM AND FINDINGS	PROBABLE CAUSE

Chest pain

◆ A feeling of tightness or pressure in the chest described as pain or a sensation of indigestion or expansion ◆ Pain may radiate to the neck, jaw, and arms; classically to the inner aspect of the left arm ◆ Pain begins gradually, reaches a maximum, then slowly subsides ◆ Pain is provoked by exertion, emotional stress, or a heavy meal ◆ Pain typically lasts 2 to 10 minutes (usually no more than 20 minutes) ◆ Dyspnea ◆ Nausea and vomiting ◆ Tachycardia ◆ Dizziness ◆ Diaphoresis	Angina
◆ Crushing substernal pain, unrelieved by rest or nitroglycerin ◆ Pain that may radiate to the left arm, jaw, neck, or shoulder blades ◆ Pain that lasts from 15 minutes to hours ◆ Pallor ◆ Clammy skin ◆ Dyspnea ◆ Diaphoresis ◆ Feeling of impending doom	Myocardial infarction
◆ Sharp, severe pain aggravated by inspiration, coughing, or pressure ◆ Shallow, splinted breaths ◆ Dyspnea ◆ Cough ◆ Local tenderness and edema	Rib fracture

The cardiovascular system:
Interpreting your findings (continued)

SIGN OR SYMPTOM AND FINDINGS	PROBABLE CAUSE
Fatigue	
◆ Fatigue following mild activity ◆ Pallor ◆ Tachycardia ◆ Dyspnea	Anemia
◆ Persistent fatigue unrelated to exertion ◆ Headache ◆ Anorexia ◆ Constipation ◆ Sexual dysfunction ◆ Loss of concentration ◆ Irritability	Depression
◆ Progressive fatigue ◆ Cardiac murmur ◆ Exertional dyspnea ◆ Cough ◆ Hemoptysis	Valvular heart disease
Palpitations	
◆ Paroxysmal palpitations ◆ Diaphoresis ◆ Facial flushing ◆ Trembling ◆ Impending sense of doom ◆ Hyperventilation ◆ Dizziness	Acute anxiety attack
◆ Paroxysmal or sustained palpitations ◆ Dizziness ◆ Weakness ◆ Fatigue ◆ Irregular, rapid, or slow pulse rate ◆ Decreased blood pressure ◆ Confusion ◆ Diaphoresis	Arrhythmias
◆ Sustained palpitations ◆ Fatigue ◆ Irritability ◆ Hunger ◆ Cold sweats ◆ Tremors ◆ Anxiety	Hypoglycemia

(continued)

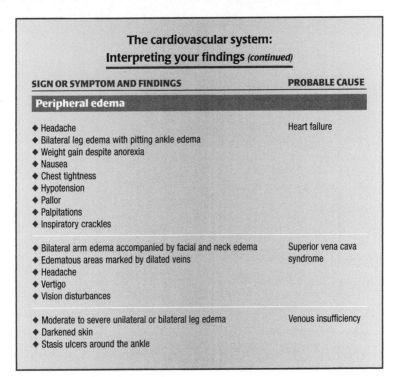

The cardiovascular system:
Interpreting your findings *(continued)*

SIGN OR SYMPTOM AND FINDINGS	PROBABLE CAUSE
Peripheral edema	
◆ Headache ◆ Bilateral leg edema with pitting ankle edema ◆ Weight gain despite anorexia ◆ Nausea ◆ Chest tightness ◆ Hypotension ◆ Pallor ◆ Palpitations ◆ Inspiratory crackles	Heart failure
◆ Bilateral arm edema accompanied by facial and neck edema ◆ Edematous areas marked by dilated veins ◆ Headache ◆ Vertigo ◆ Vision disturbances	Superior vena cava syndrome
◆ Moderate to severe unilateral or bilateral leg edema ◆ Darkened skin ◆ Stasis ulcers around the ankle	Venous insufficiency

ECG basics

3

One of the most valuable diagnostic tools available, an electrocardiogram (ECG) records the heart's electrical activity as waveforms. By interpreting these waveforms accurately, you can identify rhythm disturbances, conduction abnormalities, and electrolyte imbalances. An ECG aids in diagnosing and monitoring such conditions as myocardial infarction (MI) and pericarditis.

To interpret an ECG correctly, you must first recognize its key components. Next, you need to analyze the key components separately. Then you can put your findings together to reach a conclusion about the heart's electrical activity. This chapter explains that analytic process, beginning with some fundamental information about electrocardiography.

The heart's electrical activity produces currents that radiate through the surrounding tissue to the skin. When electrodes are at-

tached to the skin, they sense the electrical currents and transmit them to the electrocardiograph. This electrical activity is transformed into waveforms that represent the heart's depolarization-repolarization cycle.

Myocardial depolarization occurs when a wave of stimulation passes through the heart and causes the heart muscle to contract. Repolarization is the relaxation phase. An ECG shows the precise sequence of electrical events occurring in the cardiac cells throughout that process and identifies rhythm disturbances and conduction abnormalities.

Leads and planes

Because the electrical currents from the heart radiate to the skin in many directions, electrodes are placed at different locations to get a total picture of the heart's electrical activity. The ECG can

Current direction and waveform deflection

This illustration shows possible directions of electrical current and the corresponding waveform deflections. The direction of the electrical current determines the upward or downward deflection of an electrocardiogram waveform.

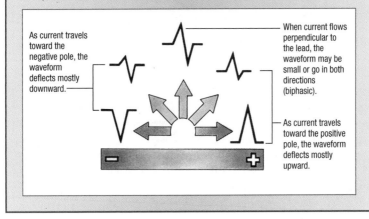

As current travels toward the negative pole, the waveform deflects mostly downward.

When current flows perpendicular to the lead, the waveform may be small or go in both directions (biphasic).

As current travels toward the positive pole, the waveform deflects mostly upward.

then record information from different perspectives, which are called *leads* and *planes.*

Leads

A lead provides a view of the heart's electrical activity between two points, or poles. Each lead consists of one positive and one negative pole. Between the two poles lies an imaginary line representing the lead's *axis,* a term that refers to the direction of the current moving through the heart. Because each lead measures the heart's electrical potential from different directions, each lead generates its own char-

acteristic tracing. (See *Current direction and waveform deflection.*)

The direction in which the electric current flows determines how the waveforms appear on the ECG tracing. When the current flows along the axis toward the positive pole of the electrode, the waveform deflects upward and is called a *positive deflection.* When the current flows away from the positive pole, the waveform deflects downward, below the baseline, and is called a *negative deflection.* When the current flows perpendicular to the axis, the wave may go in both directions or be unusually small. When electrical activity is absent or too small to measure, the waveform is a straight line, also called an *isoelectric deflection.*

Planes

A plane is a cross section of the heart that provides a different view of the heart's electrical activity. In the frontal plane—a vertical cut through the middle of the heart from top to bottom—electrical activity is viewed from an anterior to posterior approach. The six limb leads are viewed from the frontal plane.

In the horizontal plane—a transverse cut through the middle of the heart dividing it into upper and lower portions—electrical activity can be viewed from a superior or an inferior approach. The six precordial leads are viewed from the horizontal plane.

Types of ECG recordings

The two main types of ECG recordings are the 12-lead ECG and the rhythm strip. Both types give valuable information about the heart's electrical activity.

12-lead ECG

A 12-lead ECG records information from 12 different views of

the heart and provides a complete picture of electrical activity. These 12 views are obtained by placing electrodes on the patient's limbs and chest. The limb leads and the chest, or *precordial*, leads reflect information from the different planes of the heart.

Different leads provide different information. The six limb leads—I, II, III, augmented vector right (aV_R), augmented vector left (aV_L), and augmented vector foot (aV_F)—provide information about the heart's frontal plane. Leads I, II, and III require a negative and positive electrode for monitoring, which makes these leads bipolar. The augmented leads—aV_R, aV_L, and aV_F— are *unipolar,* meaning they need only a positive electrode.

The six precordial, or V, leads—V_1, V_2, V_3, V_4, V_5, and V_6—provide information about the heart's horizontal plane. Like the augmented leads, the precordial leads are unipolar, requiring only a positive electrode. The negative pole of these leads, which is in the center of the heart, is calculated by the ECG.

Rhythm strip

A rhythm strip provides continuous information about the heart's electrical activity from one or more leads simultaneously. Commonly monitored leads include lead II, V_1, and V_6. A rhythm strip is used to monitor cardiac status. Chest electrodes pick up the heart's electrical activity for display on the monitor. The monitor also displays heart rate and other measurements and can print out strips of cardiac rhythms.

ECG monitoring systems

The type of ECG monitoring system used—hardwire monitoring or telemetry—depends on the patient's clinical status. With hardwire monitoring, the electrodes are connected directly to the cardiac monitor. Most hardwire monitors are mounted permanently on a shelf or wall near the patient's bed. Some monitors are mounted on an I.V. pole for portability, and some may include a defibrillator.

The monitor provides a continuous cardiac rhythm display and transmits the ECG tracing to a console at the nurses' station. Both the monitor and the console have alarms and can print rhythm strips to show ectopic beats, for example, or other arrhythmias. Hardwire monitors also have the ability to track pulse oximetry, blood pressure, hemodynamic measurements, and other parameters through various attachments to the patient.

Hardwire monitoring is generally used in critical care units and emergency departments because it permits continuous observation of one or more patients from more than one area in the unit. However, this type of monitoring has disadvantages, including limited mobility because the patient is tethered to a monitor.

With telemetry monitoring, the patient carries a small, battery-powered transmitter that sends electrical signals to another location, where the signals are displayed on a monitor screen. This type of ECG monitoring frees the patient from cumbersome wires and cables and protects him from the electrical leakage and accidental shock occasionally associated with hardwire monitoring.

Telemetry monitoring still requires skin electrodes to be placed on the patient's chest. Each electrode is connected by a thin wire to a small transmitter box that's carried in a pocket or pouch. Telemetry monitoring is especially useful for detecting arrhythmias that occur at rest or during sleep, exercise, or stressful situations. Most systems, however, can monitor only heart rate and rhythm.

Electrode placement

Electrode placement is different for each lead, and different leads provide different views of the heart. A lead may be chosen to highlight a particular part of the ECG complex or the electrical events of a specific area of the heart.

Although leads II, V_1, and V_6 are among the most commonly used leads for continuous monitoring, lead placement is varied according to the patient's clinical status. If your monitoring system has the capability, you may also monitor the patient in more than one lead. (See *Dual lead monitoring.*)

Dual lead monitoring

Monitoring in two leads provides a more complete picture than monitoring in only one lead. With simultaneous dual monitoring, you'll generally review the first lead—usually designated as the primary lead—for arrhythmias.

A two-lead view helps detect ectopic beats or aberrant rhythms. Leads II and V_1 are the leads most commonly monitored simultaneously.

LEAD II

LEAD V₁

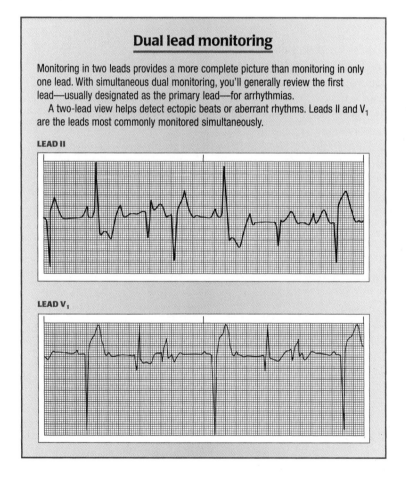

Standard limb leads

All standard limb leads or bipolar limb leads have a third electrode, known as the *ground*, which is placed on the chest to prevent electrical interference from appearing on the ECG recording.

Lead I provides a view of the heart that shows current moving from right to left. Because current flows from negative to positive, the positive electrode for this lead is placed on the left arm or on the left side of the chest; the negative electrode is placed on the right arm. Lead I produces a positive deflection on ECG tracings and is helpful in monitoring atrial rhythms.

Lead II produces a positive deflection. The positive electrode is placed on the patient's left leg and the negative electrode on the right arm. For continuous monitoring, place the electrodes on the torso for convenience, with the positive electrode below the lowest palpable rib at the left midclavicular line and the negative electrode below the right clavicle. The current travels down and to the left in this lead. Lead II tends to produce a positive, high-voltage deflection, resulting in tall P, R, and T waves. This lead is commonly used for routine monitoring and is useful for detecting sinus node and atrial arrhythmias and monitoring the inferior wall of the left ventricle.

Lead III usually produces a positive deflection. The positive electrode is placed on the left leg and the negative electrode on the left arm. Along with lead II, this lead is useful for detecting changes associated with an inferior wall of the left ventricle.

The axes of the three bipolar limb leads—I, II, and III—form a triangle around the heart and provide a frontal plane view of the heart. (See *Einthoven's triangle.*)

Augmented unipolar leads

Leads aV_R, aV_L, and aV_F are called *augmented leads* because the small waveforms that normally would appear from these unipolar leads are enhanced by the ECG. (See *Augmented leads,* page 68.)

In lead aV_R, the positive electrode is placed on the right arm and produces a negative deflection because the heart's electrical activity moves away from the lead. In lead aV_L, the positive electrode is on the left arm and usually produces a positive deflection on the ECG. In lead aV_F, the positive electrode is on the left leg (despite the name aV_F) and produces a positive deflection. These three limb leads also

May we have your comments?

Please fill out and mail this postpaid card. Thanks!

Product title _____

Your comments _____

_____

Would you like to be placed on our mailing list? ☐ Yes ☐ No

☐ You have permission to use my name and comments in advertising.

Name _____

(please print)

Address _____ Apt. _____

City _____ State _____ Zip _____

E-mail address _____

☐ You have my permission to alert me by E-mail to special savings and product updates from Lippincott Williams & Wilkins.

N-CC2Q06

Einthoven's triangle

The axes of the three bipolar limb leads (I, II, and III) form a triangle, known as *Einthoven's triangle.* Because the electrodes for these leads are about equidistant from the heart, the triangle is equilateral.

The axis of lead I extends from shoulder to shoulder, with the right arm lead being the negative electrode and the left arm lead being the positive electrode. The axis of lead II runs from the negative right arm lead electrode to the positive left leg lead electrode. The axis of lead III extends from the negative left arm lead electrode to the positive left leg lead electrode.

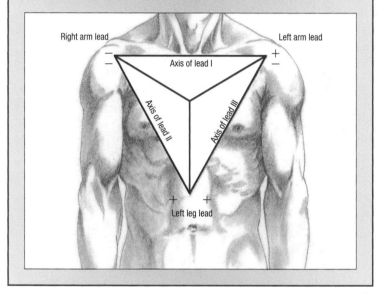

provide a view of the heart's frontal plane.

Precordial unipolar leads

The six unipolar precordial leads are placed in sequence across the chest and provide a view of the heart's horizontal plane. (See *Precordial views,* page 69.)

The precordial lead V_1 electrode is placed on the right side of the sternum at the fourth intercostal rib space. This lead shows the P wave, QRS complex, and ST segment particularly well. It helps to distinguish between right and left ventricular ectopic beats that result from myocardial irritation or other cardiac stimulation outside the normal con-

Augmented leads

Leads aV$_R$, aV$_L$, and aV$_F$ are called augmented leads. They measure electrical activity between one limb and a single electrode. Lead aV$_R$ provides no specific view of the heart because the heart's electrical activity moves away from the lead. Lead aV$_L$ shows electrical activity coming from the heart's lateral wall. Lead aV$_F$ shows electrical activity coming from the heart's inferior wall.

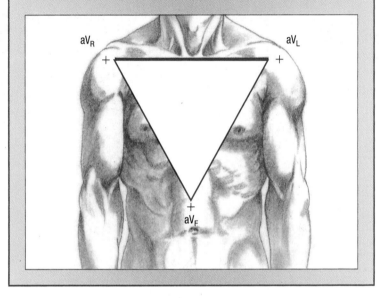

duction system. Lead V$_1$ is also useful in monitoring ventricular arrhythmias, ST-segment changes, and bundle-branch blocks.

Lead V$_2$ is placed to the left of the sternum at the fourth intercostal space.

Lead V$_3$ goes between V$_2$ and V$_4$ at the fifth intercostal space. Leads V$_1$, V$_2$, and V$_3$ are biphasic, with positive and negative deflections. Leads V$_2$ and V$_3$ can

be used to detect ST-segment elevation.

Lead V$_4$ is placed at the fifth intercostal space at the midclavicular line and produces a positive deflection.

Lead V$_5$ is placed between lead V$_4$ and V$_6$ anterior to the axillary line. Lead V$_5$ produces a positive deflection on the ECG and, along with V$_4$, can show changes in the ST segment or T wave.

Precordial views

These illustrations show the different views of the heart obtained from each precordial (chest) lead.

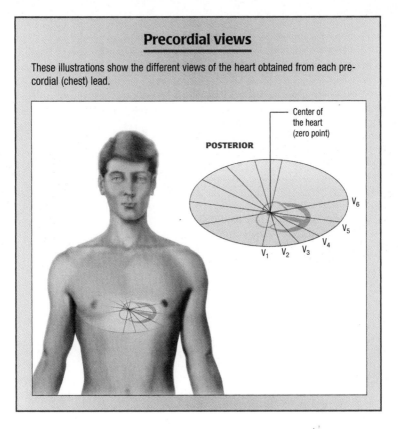

Lead V_6, the last of the precordial leads, is placed level with lead V_4 at the midaxillary line. Lead V_6 produces a positive deflection on the ECG.

Modified chest leads

MCL stands for modified chest lead. Modification of the chest lead involves placing the negative electrode on the left side of the chest rather than having the center of the heart function as the negative lead. MCL_1 is created by placing the negative electrode on the left upper chest, the positive electrode on the right side of the chest, and the ground electrode usually on the right upper chest. The MCL_1 lead most closely approximates the ECG pattern produced by the chest lead V_1.

When the positive electrode is on the right side of the heart and the electrical current travels toward the left ventricle, the waveform has a negative deflection. As a result, ectopic or abnormal beats deflect in a positive direction.

Choose MCL_1 to assess QRS-complex arrhythmias. You can use this lead to monitor premature ventricular beats and to distinguish different types of tachycardia, such as ventricular and supraventricular tachycardia. MCL_1 can also be used to assess bundle-branch defects and P-wave changes and to confirm pacemaker wire placement.

MCL_6 is an alternative to MCL_1 and most closely approximates the ECG pattern produced by the chest lead V_6. Like MCL_1, it monitors ventricular conduction changes. The positive lead in MCL_6 is placed at the midaxillary line of the left fifth intercostal space, the negative electrode below the left shoulder, and the ground below the right shoulder.

Leadwire systems

A three- or five-electrode system may be used for cardiac monitoring. (See *Leadwire systems.*) Both systems use a ground electrode to prevent accidental electrical shock to the patient.

A three-electrode system has one positive electrode, one negative electrode, and a ground. The popular five-electrode system is an extension of the four-electrode system and uses an additional exploratory chest lead to allow you to monitor any six modified chest leads as well as the standard limb leads. (See *Using a five-leadwire system,* page 73.) This system uses standardized chest placement. Wires that attach to the electrodes are usually color-coded to help you to place them correctly on the patient's chest.

Remember the needs of the patient when applying chest electrodes. For example, if defibrillation is anticipated, avoid placing the electrodes to the right of the sternum and under the left breast, where the paddles would be placed.

Application of electrodes

Before attaching electrodes to your patient, make sure he knows you're monitoring his heart rate and rhythm, not controlling them. Tell him not to become upset if he hears an alarm during the procedure; it probably just means a leadwire has come loose.

Explain the electrode placement procedure to the patient, provide privacy, and wash your hands. Expose the patient's chest and select electrode sites for the chosen lead. Choose sites over

Leadwire systems

These illustrations show the correct electrode positions for some of the leads you'll use most often—the five-leadwire, three-leadwire, and telemetry systems. The abbreviations used are RA for the right arm, LA for the left arm, RL for the right leg, LL for the left leg, C for the chest, and G for the ground.

Electrode positions

In the three- and five-leadwire systems, electrode positions for one lead may be identical to those for another lead. When that happens, change the lead selector switch to the setting that corresponds to the lead you want. In some cases, you'll need to reposition the electrodes.

Telemetry

In a telemetry monitoring system, you can create the same leads as the other systems with just two electrodes and a ground wire.

FIVE-LEADWIRE SYSTEM **THREE-LEADWIRE SYSTEM** **TELEMETRY SYSTEM**

LEAD I

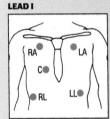 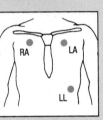 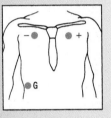

LEAD II

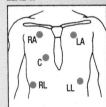 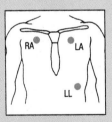 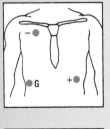

LEAD III

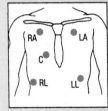 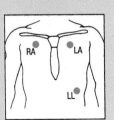 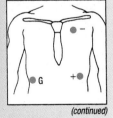

(continued)

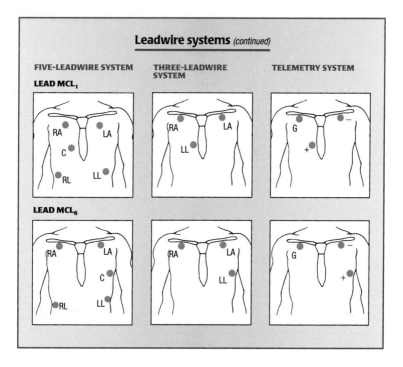

Leadwire systems *(continued)*

FIVE-LEADWIRE SYSTEM

LEAD MCL₁

THREE-LEADWIRE SYSTEM

TELEMETRY SYSTEM

LEAD MCL₆

soft tissues or close to bone, not over bony prominences, thick muscles, or skin folds. Those areas can produce ECG artifacts— waveforms not produced by the heart's electrical activity.

Skin preparation

Wash the chest with soap and water and dry it thoroughly. Hair may interfere with electrical contact; therefore, it may be necessary to clip areas with dense hair.

To prepare the patient's skin, use a special rough patch on the back of the electrode, a dry washcloth, or a gauze pad to briskly rub each site until the skin reddens. Make sure you don't damage or break the skin. Brisk scrubbing helps to remove dead skin cells and improves electrical contact.

If the patient has oily skin, clean each site with an alcohol pad and let it air-dry. This ensures proper adhesion and prevents alcohol from becoming trapped beneath the electrode, which can irritate the skin and cause skin breakdown.

Application of electrode pads

To apply the electrodes, remove the backing and make sure each pregelled electrode is still moist.

Using a five-leadwire system

This illustration shows the correct placement of the leadwires for a five-leadwire system. The chest electrode shown is located in the lead V_1 position, but you can place it in any of the chest-lead positions. The electrodes are color-coded as follows.

◆ White—right arm (RA)
◆ Black—left arm (LA)
◆ Green—right leg (RL)
◆ Red—left leg (LL)
◆ Brown—chest (C)

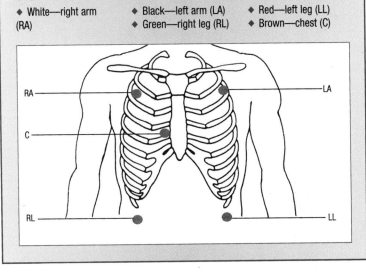

If an electrode has become dry, discard it and select another. A dry electrode decreases electrical contact and interferes with waveforms.

Apply one electrode to each prepared site using this method:
◆ Press one side of the electrode against the patient's skin, pull gently, and then press the opposite side of the electrode against the skin.
◆ Using two fingers, press the adhesive edge around the outside of the electrode to the patient's chest. This fixes the gel and stabilizes the electrode.
◆ Repeat this procedure for each electrode.
◆ Every 24 hours, remove the electrodes, assess the patient's skin, and replace the old electrodes with new ones.

Attaching leadwires

You'll also need to attach leadwires, or cable connections, to the monitor. Then, attach leadwires to the electrodes. Leadwires may clip on or, more commonly, snap on. If you're using the snap-on type, attach the electrode to the leadwire immediately before applying it to the patient's chest. This will help to prevent patient discomfort and disturbances of the contact between the electrode and the skin. When you use a clip-on leadwire, apply it after the electrode has been secured to the patient's skin. That way, applying the clip won't interfere with the electrode's contact with the skin.

Observing cardiac rhythm

After the electrodes are in proper position, the monitor is on, and the necessary cables are attached, observe the screen. You should see the patient's ECG waveform. Although some monitoring systems allow you to make adjustments by touching the screen, most require you to manipulate knobs and buttons. If the waveform appears too large or too small, change the size by adjusting the gain control. If the waveform appears too high or too low on the screen, adjust the position dial.

Verify that the monitor detects each heartbeat by comparing the patient's apical rate with the rate displayed on the monitor. Set the upper and lower limits of the heart rate according to your facil-

ity's policy and the patient's condition. Heart rate alarms are generally set 10 to 20 beats per minute higher or lower than the patient's heart rate.

Monitors with arrhythmia detection generate a rhythm strip automatically whenever the alarm goes off. You can obtain other views of your patient's cardiac rhythm by selecting different leads with the lead selector button or switch.

To get a printout of the patient's cardiac rhythm, press the record control on the monitor. The ECG strip will be printed at the central console. Some systems print the rhythm from a recorder box on the monitor itself.

Most monitors can input the patient's information as a permanent record; however, if the monitor you're using can't do this, label the rhythm strip with the patient's name, room number, date, time, and rhythm interpretation. Add appropriate clinical information to the ECG strip, such as any medication administered, presence of chest pain, or patient activity at the time of the recording. Be sure to place the rhythm strip in the appropriate section of the patient's medical record.

Waveforms produced by the heart's electrical current are

ECG grid

This electrocardiogram (ECG) grid shows the horizontal axis and vertical axis and their respective measurement values.

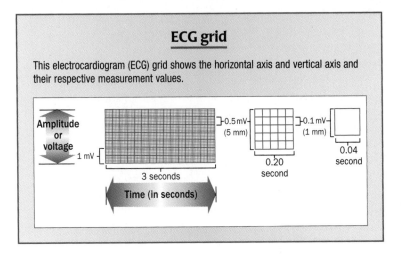

recorded on graphed ECG paper by a heated stylus. ECG paper consists of horizontal and vertical lines forming a grid. A piece of ECG paper is called an *ECG strip* or *tracing*. (See *ECG grid.*)

The horizontal axis of the ECG strip represents time. Each small block equals 0.04 second, and five small blocks form a large block, which equals 0.2 second. This time increment is determined by multiplying 0.04 second (for one small block) by 5, the number of small blocks that compose a large block. Five large blocks equal 1 second (5 × 0.2). When measuring or calculating a patient's heart rate, a 6-second strip consisting of 30 large blocks is usually used.

The ECG strip's vertical axis measures amplitude in millimeters (mm) or electrical voltage in

millivolts (mV). Each small block represents 1 mm or 0.1 mV; each large block, 5 mm or 0.5 mV. To determine the amplitude of a wave, segment, or interval, count the number of small blocks from the baseline to the highest or lowest point of the wave, segment, or interval.

Troubleshooting monitor problems

For optimal cardiac monitoring, you need to recognize problems that can interfere with obtaining a reliable ECG recording. (See *Common monitor problems,* pages 76 and 77.) Causes of interference include artifact from patient movement and poorly placed or poorly functioning equipment.

(Text continues on page 78.)

Common monitor problems

These illustrations present the most commonly encountered monitor problems, including how to identify them, their possible causes, and interventions.

WAVEFORM	POSSIBLE CAUSE	INTERVENTIONS

Artifact (waveform interference)

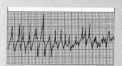

	◆ Patient experiencing seizures, chills, or anxiety	◆ If the patient is having a seizure, notify the practitioner and intervene as ordered. ◆ Keep the patient warm and encourage him to relax.
	◆ Dirty or corroded connections	◆ Replace dirty or corroded wires.
	◆ Improper electrode application	◆ Check the electrodes and reapply them if needed. Clean the patient's skin well because skin oils and dead skin cells inhibit conduction.
	◆ Dry electrode gel	◆ Check the electrode gel. If the gel is dry, apply new electrodes.
	◆ Short circuit in leadwires or cable	◆ Replace broken equipment.
	◆ Electrical interference from other equipment in the room	◆ Make sure that all electrical equipment is attached to a common ground. Check all three-pronged plugs to ensure that none of the prongs are loose. Notify biomedical department.
	◆ Static electricity interference from inadequate room humidity	◆ Regulate room humidity to 40% if possible.

False high-rate alarm

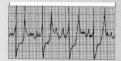

	◆ Gain setting too high, particularly with MCL_1 setting	◆ Assess the patient for signs and symptoms of hyperkalemia. ◆ Reset gain.
	◆ HIGH alarm set too low, or LOW alarm set too high	◆ Set alarm limits according to the patient's heart rate.

Common monitor problems (continued)

WAVEFORM	POSSIBLE CAUSE	INTERVENTIONS

Weak signals

	◆ Improper electrode application	◆ Reapply the electrodes.
	◆ QRS complex too small to register	◆ Reset gain so that the height of the complex is greater than 1 mV.
		◆ Try monitoring the patient on another lead.
	◆ Wire or cable failure	◆ Replace faulty wires or cables.

Wandering baseline

	◆ Patient restless	◆ Encourage the patient to relax.
	◆ Chest wall movement during respiration	◆ Make sure that tension on the cable isn't pulling the electrode away from the patient's body.
	◆ Improper electrode application; electrode positioned over bone	◆ Reposition improperly placed electrodes.

Fuzzy baseline (electrical interference)

	◆ Electrical interference from other equipment in the room	◆ Ensure that all electrical equipment is attached to a common ground.
		◆ Check all three-pronged plugs to make sure none of the prongs are loose.
	◆ Improper grounding of the patient's bed	◆ Ensure that the bed ground is attached to the room's common ground.
	◆ Electrode malfunction	◆ Replace the electrodes.

Baseline (no waveform)

	◆ Improper electrode placement (perpendicular to axis of heart)	◆ Reposition improperly placed electrodes.
	◆ Electrode disconnected	◆ Check if electrodes are disconnected.
	◆ Dry electrode gel	◆ Check electrode gel. If the gel is dry, apply new electrodes.
	◆ Wire or cable failure	◆ Replace faulty wires or cables.

Artifact, also called *waveform interference,* may be seen with excessive movement (*somatic tremor*). The baseline of the ECG appears wavy, bumpy, or tremulous. Dry electrodes may also cause this problem due to poor contact.

Electrical interference or AC interference, also called *60-cycle interference,* is caused by electrical power leakage. It may also occur due to interference from other room equipment or improperly grounded equipment. As a result, the lost current pulses at a rate of 60 cycles per second. This interference appears on the ECG as a baseline that is thick and unreadable.

A wandering baseline undulates, meaning that all waveforms are present but the baseline isn't stationary. Movement of the chest wall during respiration, poor electrode placement, or poor electrode contact usually causes this problem.

Faulty equipment, such as broken leadwires and cables, can also cause monitoring problems. Excessively worn equipment can cause improper grounding, putting the patient at risk for accidental shock.

Be aware that some types of artifact resemble arrhythmias and the monitor will interpret them as such. For example, the monitor may sense a small movement, such as the patient brushing his teeth, as a potentially lethal ventricular tachycardia. So, remember to treat the patient, not the monitor. The more familiar you become with your unit's monitoring system—and with your patient—the more quickly you can recognize and interpret problems and act appropriately.

Rhythm strip interpretation

4

An electrocardiogram (ECG) complex represents the electrical events occurring in one cardiac cycle. A complex consists of five waveforms labeled with the letters P, Q, R, S, and T. The middle three letters—Q, R, and S—are referred to as a unit, the QRS complex. ECG tracings represent the conduction of electrical impulses from the atria to the ventricles. (See *ECG waveform components*.)

P wave

The P wave is the first component of a normal ECG waveform. It represents atrial depolarization

---

ECG waveform components

This illustration shows the components of a normal electrocardiogram (ECG) waveform.

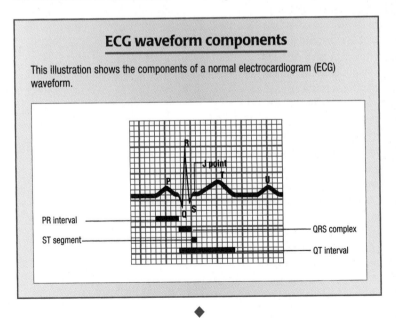

or conduction of an electrical impulse through the atria. When evaluating a P wave, look closely at its characteristics, especially its location, configuration, and deflection. A normal P wave has these characteristics:

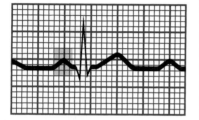

◆ *Location:* precedes the QRS complex
◆ *Amplitude:* 2 to 3 mm high
◆ *Duration:* 0.06 to 0.12 second
◆ *Configuration:* usually rounded and upright
◆ *Deflection:* positive or upright in leads I, II, aV_F, and V_2 to V_6; usually positive but may vary in leads III and aV_L; negative or inverted in lead aV_R; biphasic or variable in lead V_1.

If the deflection and configuration of a P wave are normal—for example, if the P wave is upright in lead II and is rounded and smooth—and if the P wave precedes each QRS complex, you can assume that this electrical impulse originated in the sinoatrial (SA) node. The atria start to contract partway through the P wave, but you won't see this on the ECG. Remember that the ECG records electrical activity only, not mechanical activity or contraction.

Peaked, notched, or enlarged P waves may represent atrial hypertrophy or enlargement associated with chronic obstructive pulmonary disease, pulmonary emboli, valvular disease, or heart failure. Inverted P waves may signify retrograde or reverse conduction from the atrioventricular junction toward the atria. Whenever an upright sinus P wave becomes inverted, consider retrograde or reverse conduction as possible conditions.

Varying P waves indicate that the impulse may be coming from different sites, as with a wandering pacemaker rhythm, irritable atrial tissue, or damage near the SA node. Absent P waves may signify conduction by a route other than the SA node, as with a junctional or atrial fibrillation rhythm. When a P wave doesn't precede the QRS complex, complete heart block may be present. Absence of a P wave doesn't mean that there isn't atrial depolarization. The P wave may be buried or hidden in the T wave or the QRS complex.

PR interval

The PR interval tracks the atrial impulse from the atria through the atrioventricular (AV) node, bundle of His, and right and left bundle branches. When evaluating a PR interval, look especially at its duration. Changes in the PR interval indicate an altered impulse formation or a conduction delay, as seen in AV block. A normal PR interval has these characteristics (amplitude, configuration, and deflection aren't measured):

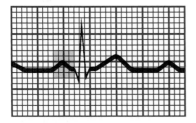

◆ *Location:* from the beginning of the P wave to the beginning of the QRS complex

◆ *Duration:* 0.12 to 0.20 second.

Short PR intervals (less than 0.12 second) indicate that the impulse originated somewhere other than the SA node. This variation is associated with junctional arrhythmias and preexcitation syndromes. Prolonged PR intervals (greater than 0.20 second) may represent a conduction de-lay through the atria or AV junction due to digoxin toxicity, common cardiac medications (such as beta and calcium channel blockers), or heart block—slowing related to ischemia or conduction tissue disease.

QRS complex

The QRS complex follows the P wave and represents depolarization of the ventricles, or impulse conduction. Immediately after the ventricles depolarize, as represented by the QRS complex, they contract. That contraction ejects blood from the ventricles and pumps it through the arteries, creating a pulse.

Whenever you're monitoring cardiac rhythm, remember that the waveform you see represents the heart's electrical activity only. It doesn't guarantee a mechanical contraction of the heart and a subsequent pulse. The contraction could be weak, as occurs with premature ventricular contractions, or absent, as occurs with pulseless electrical activity. So, before you treat the strip, check the patient.

Pay special attention to the duration and configuration when evaluating a QRS complex. A

QRS waveform variety

These illustrations show the various configurations of QRS complexes. When documenting the QRS complex, use uppercase letters to indicate a wave with a normal or high amplitude (greater than 5 mm) and lowercase letters to indicate one with a low amplitude (less than 5 mm).

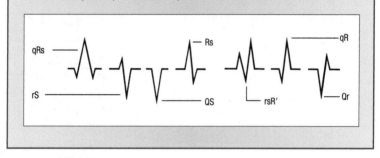

normal complex has these characteristics:

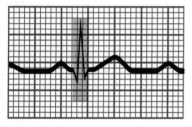

◆ *Location:* follows the PR interval

◆ *Amplitude:* 5 to 30 mm high, but differs for each lead used

◆ *Duration:* 0.06 to 0.10 second, or one-half of the PR interval. Duration is measured from the beginning of the Q wave to the end of the S wave or from the beginning of the R wave if the Q wave is absent.

◆ *Configuration:* consists of the Q wave (the first negative deflection, or deflection below the baseline, after the P wave), the R wave (the first positive deflection after the Q wave), and the S wave (the first negative deflection after the R wave). You may not always see all three waves. The ventricles depolarize quickly, minimizing contact time between the stylus and the ECG paper, so the QRS complex typically appears thinner than other ECG components. The QRS complex may also look different in each lead. (See *QRS waveform variety.*)

◆ *Deflection:* positive (with most of the complex above the baseline) in leads I, II, III, aV_L, aV_F, and V_4 to V_6; negative in leads

aV_R and V_1 to V_2; and biphasic in lead V_3.

Remember that the QRS complex represents intraventricular conduction time. That's why identifying and correctly interpreting this complex is so crucial. If no P wave appears with the QRS complex, then the impulse may have originated in the ventricles, indicating a ventricular arrhythmia.

Deep, wide Q waves may represent myocardial infarction. In this case, the Q wave amplitude (depth) is greater than or equal to 25% of the height of the succeeding R wave, or the duration of the Q wave is 0.04 second or more. A notched R wave may signify a bundle-branch block. A widened QRS complex (greater than 0.12 second) may signify a ventricular conduction delay. A missing QRS complex may indicate atrioventricular block or ventricular standstill.

ST segment

The ST segment represents the end of ventricular conduction or depolarization and the beginning of ventricular recovery or repolarization. The point that marks the end of the QRS complex and the beginning of the ST segment is known as the *J point*.

Pay special attention to the deflection of an ST segment. A normal ST segment has these characteristics (amplitude, duration, and configuration aren't observed):

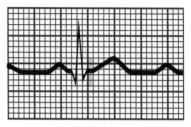

◆ *Location:* extends from the S wave to the beginning of the T wave
◆ *Deflection:* usually isoelectric (neither positive nor negative); may vary from –0.5 to +1 mm in some precordial leads.

A change in the ST segment may indicate myocardial injury or ischemia. An ST segment may become either elevated or depressed. (See *Changes in the ST segment,* page 84.)

T wave

The peak of the T wave represents the relative refractory period of repolarization or ventricular recovery. When evaluating a T wave, look at the amplitude, configuration, and deflection.

Normal T waves have these characteristics (duration isn't measured):

Changes in the ST segment

Closely monitoring the ST segment on a patient's electrocardiogram can help you detect ischemia or injury before infarction develops.

ST-SEGMENT DEPRESSION
An ST segment is considered depressed when it's 0.5 mm or more below the baseline. A depressed ST segment may indicate myocardial ischemia or digoxin toxicity.

ST-SEGMENT ELEVATION
An ST segment is considered elevated when it's 1 mm or more above the baseline. An elevated ST segment may indicate myocardial injury.

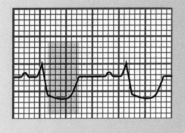

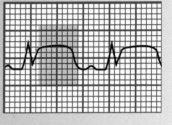

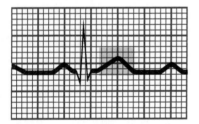

◆ *Location:* follows the ST segment
◆ *Amplitude:* 0.5 mm in leads I, II, and III and up to 10 mm in the precordial leads
◆ *Configuration:* typically rounded and smooth
◆ *Deflection:* usually positive or upright in leads I, II, and V_2 to V_6; inverted in lead aV_R; variable leads III and V_1.

The T wave's peak represents the relative refractory period of ventricular repolarization, a period during which cells are especially vulnerable to extra stimuli. Bumps in a T wave may indicate that a P wave is hidden in it. If a P wave is hidden, atrial depolarization has occurred, the impulse having originated at a site above the ventricles.

Tall, peaked, or "tented" T waves may indicate myocardial injury or electrolyte imbalances such as hyperkalemia. Hypokalemia can cause flattened T waves. Inverted T waves in leads I, II, aV_L, aV_F, or V_2 through V_6 may represent myocardial ischemia. Heavily notched or pointed T waves in an adult may indicate pericarditis.

QT interval

The QT interval measures the time needed for ventricular depolarization and repolarization. The length of the QT interval varies according to heart rate. The faster the heart rate, the shorter the QT interval. When checking the QT interval, look closely at the duration.

A normal QT interval has these characteristics (amplitude, configuration, and deflection aren't observed):

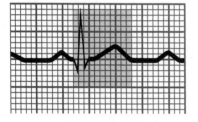

◆ *Location:* extends from the beginning of the QRS complex to the end of the T wave
◆ *Duration:* varies according to age, sex, and heart rate; usually lasts from 0.36 to 0.44 second; shouldn't be greater than one-half the distance between the two consecutive R waves (called *the R-R interval*) when the rhythm is regular.

The QT interval measures the time needed for ventricular depolarization and repolarization. Prolonged QT intervals indicate that ventricular repolarization time is slowed, meaning that the relative refractory or vulnerable period of the cardiac cycle is longer.

This variation is also associated with certain medications such as class I antiarrhythmics. Prolonged QT syndrome is a congenital conduction-system defect present in certain families. Short QT intervals may result from digoxin toxicity or electrolyte imbalances such as hypercalcemia.

U wave

The U wave represents repolarization of the His-Purkinje system or ventricular conduction fibers. It isn't present on every rhythm strip. The configuration is the most important characteristic of the U wave

When present, a normal U wave has these characteristics (amplitude and duration aren't measured):

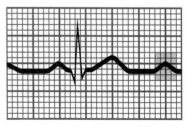

◆ *Location:* follows the T wave
◆ *Configuration:* typically upright and rounded
◆ *Deflection:* upright.

Recognizing normal sinus rhythm

Normal sinus rhythm, shown below, represents normal impulse conduction through the heart.

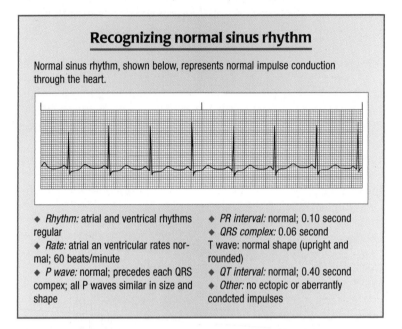

◆ *Rhythm:* atrial and ventrical rhythms regular
◆ *Rate:* atrial an ventricular rates normal; 60 beats/minute
◆ *P wave:* normal; precedes each QRS compex; all P waves similar in size and shape

◆ *PR interval:* normal; 0.10 second
◆ *QRS complex:* 0.06 second
T wave: normal shape (upright and rounded)
◆ *QT interval:* normal; 0.40 second
◆ *Other:* no ectopic or aberrantly condcted impulses

The U wave may not appear on an ECG. A prominent U wave may be due to hypercalcemia, hypokalemia, or digoxin toxicity.

Normal sinus rhythm

Before you can recognize an arrhythmia, you first need to be able to recognize a normal cardiac rhythm. The term *arrhythmia* literally means an absence of rhythm. The more-accurate term *dysrhythmia* means an abnormality in rhythm. These terms, however, are frequently used interchangeably.

Normal sinus rhythm (NSR) occurs when an impulse starts in the SA node and progresses to the ventricles through a normal conduction pathway—from the SA node to the atria and AV node, through the bundle of His, to the bundle branches, and on to the Purkinje fibers. There are no premature or aberrant contractions. NSR is the standard against which all other rhythms are compared. (See *Recognizing normal sinus rhythm.*)

Practice the 8-step method to analyze an ECG strip showing NSR. The ECG characteristics of NSR include:
◆ *Rhythm:* atrial and ventricular rhythms are regular

ECG changes in the older adult

Always keep the patient's age in mind when interpreting the electrocardiogram (ECG). Changes that might be seen in the ECG of an older adult include increased PR, QRS, and QT intervals, decreased amplitude of the QRS complex, and a shift of the QRS axis to the left.

◆ *Rate:* atrial and ventricular rates are 60 to 100 beats/minute, the SA node's normal firing rate
◆ *P wave:* normally shaped (round and smooth) and upright in lead II; all P waves similar in size and shape; a P wave for every QRS complex
◆ *PR interval:* within normal limits (0.12 to 0.20 second)
◆ *QRS complex:* within normal limits (0.06 to 0.10 second)
◆ *T wave:* normally shaped; upright and rounded in lead II
◆ *QT interval:* within normal limits (0.36 to 0.44 second)
◆ *Other:* no ectopic or aberrant beats. (See *ECG changes in the older adult.*)

The 8-step method

Analyzing a rhythm strip is a skill developed through practice. You can use one of several methods, as long as you're consistent. Rhythm strip analysis requires a sequential and systematic approach such as the eight steps outlined here.

Step 1: Determine rhythm

To determine the heart's atrial and ventricular rhythms, use either the paper-and-pencil method or the caliper method. (See *Methods of measuring rhythm,* page 88.)

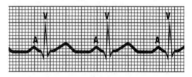

For atrial rhythm, measure the P-P intervals; that is, the intervals between consecutive P waves. These intervals should occur regularly, with only small variations associated with respirations. Then compare the P-P intervals in several cycles. Consistently similar P-P intervals indicate regular atrial rhythm; dissimilar P-P intervals indicate irregular atrial rhythm.

To determine the ventricular rhythm, measure the intervals between two consecutive R waves in the QRS complexes. If an R wave isn't present, use either the Q wave or the S wave of consecutive QRS complexes. The

Methods of measuring rhythm

You can use either of these methods to determine atrial or ventricular rhythm.

Paper-and-pencil method

Place the ECG strip on a flat surface. Then position the straight edge of a piece of paper along the strip's baseline. Move the paper up slightly so the straight edge is near the peak of the R wave.

With a pencil, mark the paper at the R waves of two consecutive QRS complexes, as shown. This is the R-R interval. Next, move the paper across the strip lining up the two marks with succeeding R-R intervals. If the distance for each R-R interval is the same, the ventricular rhythm is regular. If the distance varies, the rhythm is irregular.

Use the same method to measure the distance between the P waves (the P-P interval) and determine whether the atrial rhythm is regular or irregular.

Caliper method

With the ECG on a flat surface, place one point of the calipers on the peak of the first R wave of two consecutive QRS complexes. Then adjust the caliper legs so the other point is on the peak of the next R wave, as shown. This distance is the R-R interval.

Now pivot the first point of the calipers toward the third R wave and note whether it falls on the peak of that wave. Check succeeding R-R intervals in the same way. If they're all the same, the ventricular rhythm is regular. If they vary, the rhythm is irregular.

Using the same method, measure the P-P intervals to determine whether the atrial rhythm is regular or irregular.

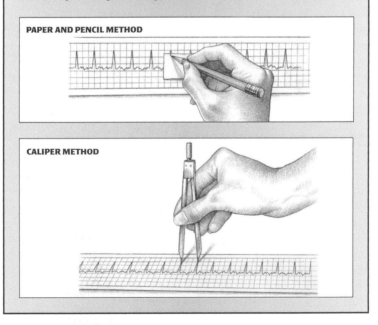

PAPER AND PENCIL METHOD

CALIPER METHOD

R-R intervals should occur regularly. Then compare R-R intervals in several cycles. As with atrial rhythms, consistently similar intervals mean a regular rhythm; dissimilar intervals point to an irregular rhythm.

After completing your measurements, ask yourself:
◆ Is the rhythm regular or irregular? Consider a rhythm with only slight variations, up to 0.04 second, to be regular.
◆ If the rhythm is irregular, is it slightly irregular or markedly so? Does the irregularity occur in a pattern (a regularly irregular pattern)?

Step 2: Calculate rate

You can use one of three methods to determine atrial and ventricular heart rates from an ECG waveform. Although these methods can provide accurate information, you shouldn't rely solely on them when assessing your patient. Keep in mind that the ECG waveform represents electrical, not mechanical, activity. Therefore, although an ECG can show you that ventricular depolarization has occurred, it doesn't mean that ventricular contraction has occurred. To do this, you must assess the patient's pulse. So remember, always check a pulse to correlate it with the heart rate on the ECG.

Times-ten method
The simplest, quickest, and most common way to calculate rate is the times-ten method, especially if the rhythm is irregular. ECG paper is marked in increments of 3 seconds, or 15 large boxes. To calculate the atrial rate, obtain a

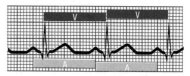

6-second strip, count the number of P waves on it, and multiply by 10. Ten 6-second strips equal 1 minute. Calculate ventricular rate the same way, using the R waves.

1,500 method
If the heart rhythm is regular, use the 1,500 method, so named because 1,500 small squares equals 1 minute. Count the number of small squares between identical points on two consecutive P waves, and then divide 1,500 by that number to get the atrial rate. To obtain the ventricular rate, use the same method with two consecutive R waves.

Sequence method
The third method of estimating heart rate is the sequence method, which requires memorizing a sequence of numbers. For atrial rate, find a P wave that peaks on a heavy black line and

assign the following numbers to the next six heavy black lines: 300, 150, 100, 75, 60, and 50. Then find the next P wave peak and estimate the atrial rate, based on the number assigned to the nearest heavy black line. Estimate the ventricular rate the same way, using the R wave.

Step 3: Evaluate P wave

When examining a rhythm strip for P waves, ask yourself:

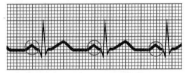

◆ Are P waves present?
◆ Do the P waves have a normal configuration?
◆ Do all the P waves have a similar size and shape?
◆ Is there one P wave for every QRS complex?

Step 4: Determine PR interval duration

To measure the PR interval, count the small squares between the start of the P wave and the start of the QRS complex; then multiply the number of squares by 0.04 second. After performing this calculation, ask yourself:

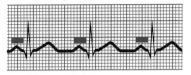

◆ Does the duration of the PR interval fall within normal limits, 0.12 to 0.20 second (or 3 to 5 small squares)?
◆ Is the PR interval constant?

Step 5: Determine QRS complex duration

When determining QRS complex duration, make sure that you measure straight across from the end of the PR interval to the end of the S wave, not just to the peak. Remember, the QRS complex has no horizontal components. To calculate duration, count the number of small squares between the beginning and end of the QRS complex and multiply this number by 0.04 second. Then ask yourself:

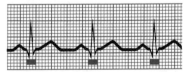

◆ Does the duration of the QRS complex fall within normal limits, 0.06 to 0.10 second?
◆ Are all QRS complexes the same size and shape? (If not, measure each one and describe them individually.)

◆ Does a QRS complex appear after every P wave?

Step 6: Evaluate T wave

Examine the ECG strip. Then ask yourself:

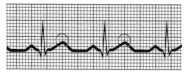

◆ Are T waves present?
◆ Do all of the T waves have a normal shape?
◆ Could a P wave be hidden in a T wave?
◆ Do all T waves have a normal amplitude?
◆ Do the T waves have the same deflection as the QRS complexes?

Step 7: Determine QT interval duration

Count the number of small squares between the beginning of the QRS complex and the end of the T wave, where the T wave returns to the baseline. Multiply this number by 0.04 second. Ask yourself:

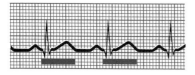

◆ Does the duration of the QT interval fall within normal limits, 0.36 to 0.44 second?

Step 8: Evaluate other components

Note the presence of ectopic or aberrantly conducted beats or other abnormalities. Also check the ST segment for abnormalities, and look for the presence of a U wave.

Now, interpret your findings by classifying the rhythm strip according to one or all of the following factors:

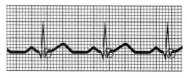

◆ *Site of origin of the rhythm:* for example, SA node, atria, AV node, or ventricles
◆ *Rate:* normal (60 to 100 beats/minute), bradycardia (less than 60 beats/minute), or tachycardia (greater than 100 beats/minute) (See *Pediatric rates and intervals,* page 92.)
◆ *Rhythm:* normal or abnormal; for example, flutter, fibrillation, heart block, escape rhythm, or other arrhythmias.

Pediatric rates and intervals

The hearts of infants and children beat faster than those of adults because children have smaller ventricular size and higher metabolic needs. The fast heart rate and small size produce short PR intervals and QRS duration.

AGE	HEART RATE (BEATS/MINUTE)	PR INTERVAL (SECOND)	QRS DURATION (SECOND)
1 to 3 weeks	100 to 180	0.07 to 0.14	0.03 to 0.07
1 to 6 months	100 to 185	0.07 to 0.16	0.03 to 0.07
7 to 11 months	100 to 170	0.08 to 0.16	0.03 to 0.08
1 to 3 years	90 to 150	0.09 to 0.16	0.03 to 0.08
4 to 5 years	70 to 140	0.09 to 0.16	0.03 to 0.08
6 to 7 years	65 to 130	0.09 to 0.16	0.03 to 0.08
8 to 11 years	60 to 110	0.09 to 0.16	0.03 to 0.09
12 to 16 years	60 to 100	0.09 to 0.18	0.03 to 0.09

PART

II

ECG arrhythmias and abnormalities

Sinus node arrhythmias

5

When the heart functions normally, the sinoatrial (SA) node (also called the *sinus node*), acts as the primary pacemaker. The sinus node assumes this role because its automatic firing rate exceeds that of the heart's other pacemakers. In an adult at rest, the sinus node has an inherent firing rate of 60 to 100 times per minute.

In approximately 50% of the population, the SA node's blood supply comes from the right coronary artery, and from the left circumflex artery in the other 50% of the population. The autonomic nervous system (ANS) richly innervates the sinus node through the vagal nerve, a parasympathetic nerve, and several sympathetic nerves. Stimulation of the vagus nerve decreases the node's firing rate, and stimulation of the sympathetic system increases it.

Changes in the automaticity of the sinus node, alterations in its blood supply, and ANS influences may all lead to sinus node arrhythmias. This chapter will help you to identify sinus node arrhythmias on an electrocardiogram (ECG). It will also help you to determine the causes, clinical significance, and signs and symptoms of each arrhythmia as well as the interventions associated with them.

The 8-step method to analyze the ECG strip will be used for each of the following arrhythmias.

Sinus arrhythmia

In sinus tachycardia and sinus bradycardia, the cardiac rate falls outside the normal limits. In sinus arrhythmia, the rate stays within normal limits but the rhythm is irregular and corresponds to the respiratory cycle. Sinus arrhythmia can occur normally in athletes, children, and

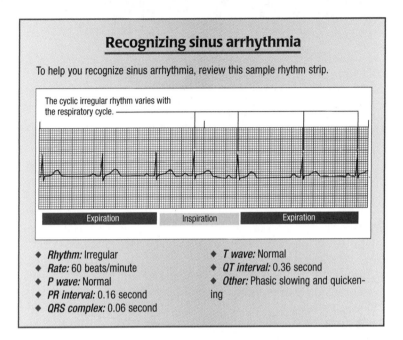

Recognizing sinus arrhythmia

To help you recognize sinus arrhythmia, review this sample rhythm strip.

The cyclic irregular rhythm varies with the respiratory cycle.

Expiration   Inspiration   Expiration

- ◆ **Rhythm:** Irregular
- ◆ **Rate:** 60 beats/minute
- ◆ **P wave:** Normal
- ◆ **PR interval:** 0.16 second
- ◆ **QRS complex:** 0.06 second
- ◆ **T wave:** Normal
- ◆ **QT interval:** 0.36 second
- ◆ **Other:** Phasic slowing and quickening

older adults, but it rarely occurs in infants.

Causes

Sinus arrhythmia, the heart's normal response to respirations, results from an inhibition of reflex vagal activity, or tone. During inspiration, an increase in the flow of blood back to the heart reduces vagal tone, which increases the heart rate. ECG complexes fall closer together, which shortens the P-P interval. During expiration, venous return decreases, which in turn increases vagal tone, slows the heart rate, and lengthens the P-P interval.

(See *Recognizing sinus arrhythmia.*)

Conditions unrelated to respiration may also produce sinus arrhythmia, including heart disease; inferior wall myocardial infarction (MI); the use of certain drugs, such as digoxin and morphine; and conditions involving increased intracranial pressure.

Clinical significance

Sinus arrhythmia usually isn't significant and produces no symptoms. A marked variation in P-P intervals in an older adult, however, may indicate sick sinus syndrome—a related, but potentially more serious, phenomenon.

ECG characteristics

◆ *Rhythm:* Atrial rhythm is irregular, corresponding to the respiratory cycle. The P-P interval is shorter during inspiration, longer during expiration. The difference between the longest and shortest P-P interval exceeds 0.12 second. Ventricular rhythm is also irregular, corresponding to the respiratory cycle. The R-R interval is shorter during inspiration, longer during expiration. The difference between the longest and shortest R-R interval exceeds 0.12 second.

◆ *Rate:* Atrial and ventricular rates are within normal limits (60 to 100 beats/minute) and vary with respiration. Typically, the heart rate increases during inspiration and decreases during expiration.

◆ *P wave:* Normal size and configuration; P wave precedes each QRS complex.

◆ *PR interval:* May vary slightly within normal limits.

◆ *QRS complex:* Normal duration and configuration.

◆ *T wave:* Normal size and configuration.

◆ *QT interval:* May vary slightly, but usually within normal limits.

◆ *Other:* None.

Signs and symptoms

The patient's peripheral pulse rate increases during inspiration and decreases during expiration. Sinus arrhythmia is easier to detect when the heart rate is slow; it may disappear when the heart rate increases, as with exercise.

If the arrhythmia is caused by an underlying condition, you may note signs and symptoms of that condition. Marked sinus arrhythmia may cause dizziness or syncope in some cases.

Interventions

Unless the patient is symptomatic, treatment usually isn't necessary. If sinus arrhythmia is unrelated to respirations, the underlying cause may require treatment.

When caring for a patient with sinus arrhythmia, observe the heart rhythm during respiration to determine whether the arrhythmia coincides with the respiratory cycle. Check the monitor carefully to avoid an inaccurate interpretation of the waveform.

If sinus arrhythmia is induced by medications, such as morphine and other sedatives, the practitioner may decide to continue to give the patient the medications because discontinuing them may be worse for the patient than the rhythm itself.

◆ **ALERT** If sinus arrhythmia develops suddenly in a patient taking digoxin, notify the practitioner immediately. The patient may be experiencing digoxin toxicity.

Sinus bradycardia

Sinus bradycardia is characterized by a sinus rate below 60 beats/minute and a regular rhythm. All impulses originate in the SA node. This arrhythmia's significance depends on the symptoms and the underlying cause. Unless the patient shows symptoms of decreased cardiac output, no treatment is necessary. (See *Recognizing sinus bradycardia* and *Bradycardia and tachycardia in children,* page 100.)

Causes

Sinus bradycardia usually occurs as the normal response to a reduced demand for blood flow. In this case, vagal stimulation increases and sympathetic stimulation decreases. As a result, *automaticity* (the tendency of cells to initiate their own impulses) in the SA node diminishes. It may occur normally during sleep or in a person with a well-conditioned heart—an athlete, for example.

Sinus bradycardia may be caused by:
◆ noncardiac disorders, such as hyperkalemia, increased intracranial pressure, hypothyroidism, hypothermia, and glaucoma
◆ conditions producing excess vagal stimulation or decreased sympathetic stimulation, such as sleep, deep relaxation, Valsalva's maneuver, carotid sinus massage, and vomiting
◆ cardiac diseases, such as SA node disease, cardiomyopathy, myocarditis, and myocardial ischemia, can also occur immediately following an inferior wall MI that involves the right coronary artery, which supplies blood to the SA node
◆ certain drugs, especially beta-adrenergic blockers, digoxin, calcium channel blockers, lithium, and antiarrhythmics, such as sotalol (Betapace), amiodarone (Cordarone), propafenone (Rhythmol), and quinidine.

Clinical significance

The clinical significance of sinus bradycardia depends on how low the rate is and whether the patient is symptomatic. For example, most adults can tolerate a sinus bradycardia of 45 to 59 beats/minute but are less tolerant of a rate below 45 beats/minute.

Usually, sinus bradycardia doesn't produce symptoms and is

Recognizing sinus bradycardia

To help you recognize sinus bradycardia, review this sample rhythm strip.

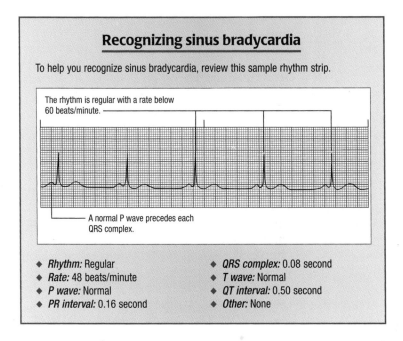

The rhythm is regular with a rate below 60 beats/minute.

A normal P wave precedes each QRS complex.

◆ *Rhythm:* Regular
◆ *Rate:* 48 beats/minute
◆ *P wave:* Normal
◆ *PR interval:* 0.16 second

◆ *QRS complex:* 0.08 second
◆ *T wave:* Normal
◆ *QT interval:* 0.50 second
◆ *Other:* None

insignificant. Many athletes develop sinus bradycardia because their well-conditioned hearts can maintain a normal stroke volume with less-than-normal effort. Sinus bradycardia also occurs normally during sleep as a result of circadian variations in heart rate.

When sinus bradycardia produces symptoms, however, prompt attention is critical. The heart of a patient with underlying cardiac disease may not be able to compensate for a drop in rate by increasing its stroke volume. The resulting drop in cardiac output produces such signs and symptoms as hypotension and dizziness. Bradycardia may

also predispose some patients to more serious arrhythmias, such as ventricular tachycardia and ventricular fibrillation.

In a patient with acute inferior wall MI, sinus bradycardia is considered a favorable prognostic sign, unless it's accompanied by hypotension. Because sinus bradycardia rarely affects children, it's considered a poor prognostic sign in ill children.

ECG characteristics

◆ *Rhythm:* Atrial and ventricular rhythms are regular.

Bradycardia and tachycardia in children

Evaluate bradycardia and tachycardia in children in context. Bradycardia (less than 90 beats/minute) may occur in the healthy infant during sleep, and tachycardia may occur when the child is crying or otherwise upset. Because the heart rate varies considerably from the neonate to the adolescent, neither bradycardia nor tachycardia can be assigned a single definition that can be used for all children.

◆ *Rate:* Atrial and ventricular rates are less than 60 beats/minute.
◆ *P wave*: Normal size and configuration; P wave precedes each QRS complex.
◆ *PR interval:* Within normal limits and constant.
◆ *QRS complex:* Normal duration and configuration.
◆ *T wave:* Normal size and configuration.
◆ *QT interval:* Within normal limits, but may be prolonged.
◆ *Other:* None.

Signs and symptoms

The patient will have a pulse rate of less than 60 beats/minute,

with a regular rhythm. As long as he's able to compensate for the decreased cardiac output, he's likely to remain asymptomatic. If compensatory mechanisms fail, however, signs and symptoms of declining cardiac output usually appear, including:
◆ hypotension
◆ cool, clammy skin
◆ altered mental status
◆ dizziness
◆ blurred vision
◆ crackles, dyspnea, and third heart sound (S_3), indicating heart failure
◆ chest pain
◆ syncope.

Palpitations and pulse irregularities may occur if the patient experiences ectopy such as premature atrial, junctional, or ventricular contractions. This is because the SA node's increased relative refractory period permits ectopic firing. Bradycardia-induced syncope (Stokes-Adams attack) may also occur.

Interventions

If the patient is asymptomatic and his vital signs are stable, treatment generally isn't necessary. Continue to observe his heart rhythm, monitoring the progression and duration of the bradycardia. Evaluate his tolerance of the rhythm at rest and with activity. Review the medications he's taking. Check with the practitioner about stopping medications that may be depressing the SA node, such as digoxin, beta-adrenergic blockers, or calcium channel blockers. Before giving these drugs, make sure the heart rate is within a safe range.

If the patient is symptomatic, treatment aims to identify and correct the underlying cause. Meanwhile, the heart rate must be maintained with a transcutaneous pacemaker. Use drugs, such as atropine, epinephrine, or dobutamine (Dobutrex) while awaiting a pacemaker or if pacing is ineffective.

Keep in mind that a patient with a transplanted heart won't respond to atropine and may require pacing for emergency treatment. Treatment of chronic, symptomatic sinus bradycardia requires insertion of a permanent pacemaker.

Sinus tachycardia

Sinus tachycardia is an acceleration of the firing of the SA node beyond its normal discharge rate. Sinus tachycardia in an adult is characterized by a sinus rate of more than 100 beats/minute. The rate rarely exceeds 180 beats/minute except during strenuous exercise; the maximum rate achievable with exercise decreas-

es with age. (See *Recognizing sinus tachycardia,* page 102.)

Causes

Sinus tachycardia may be a normal response to exercise, pain, stress, fever, or strong emotions, such as fear and anxiety. Other causes of sinus tachycardia include:
◆ certain cardiac conditions, such as heart failure, cardiogenic shock, and pericarditis
◆ other conditions, such as shock, anemia, respiratory distress, pulmonary embolism, sepsis, and hyperthyroidism in which the increased heart rate serves as a compensatory mechanism
◆ drugs, such as atropine, isoproterenol (Isuprel), aminophylline, dopamine (Inocor), dobutamine, epinephrine, alcohol, caffeine, nicotine, and amphetamines.

Clinical significance

The clinical significance of sinus tachycardia depends on the underlying cause. The arrhythmia may be the body's response to exercise or high emotional states and of no clinical significance. It may also occur with hypovolemia, hemorrhage, or pain. When the stimulus for the tachycardia

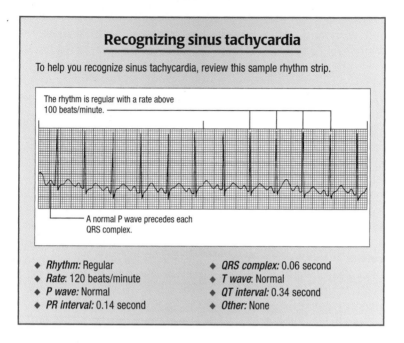

Recognizing sinus tachycardia

To help you recognize sinus tachycardia, review this sample rhythm strip.

The rhythm is regular with a rate above 100 beats/minute.

A normal P wave precedes each QRS complex.

- ◆ *Rhythm:* Regular
- ◆ *Rate:* 120 beats/minute
- ◆ *P wave:* Normal
- ◆ *PR interval:* 0.14 second

- ◆ *QRS complex:* 0.06 second
- ◆ *T wave:* Normal
- ◆ *QT interval:* 0.34 second
- ◆ *Other:* None

is removed, the arrhythmia generally resolves spontaneously.

Although sinus tachycardia commonly occurs without serious adverse effects, persistent sinus tachycardia can be serious, especially if it occurs in the setting of an acute MI. Tachycardia can lower cardiac output by reducing ventricular filling time and stroke volume. Normally, ventricular volume reaches 120 to 130 ml during diastole. In tachycardia, decreased ventricular volume leads to decreased cardiac output with subsequent hypotension and decreased peripheral perfusion.

Tachycardia worsens myocardial ischemia by increasing the heart's demand for oxygen and reducing the duration of diastole, the period of greatest coronary blood flow. Sinus tachycardia occurs in about 30% of patients after an acute MI and is considered a poor prognostic sign because it may be associated with massive heart damage.

An increase in heart rate can also be detrimental for patients with obstructive types of heart conditions, such as aortic stenosis and hypertrophic cardiomyopathy. Persistent tachycardia may also signal impending heart failure or cardiogenic shock. Sinus tachycardia can also cause angina in patients with coronary artery disease.

ECG characteristics

◆ *Rhythm:* Atrial and ventricular rhythms are regular.
◆ *Rate:* Atrial and ventricular rates are greater than 100 beats/minute, usually between 100 and 160 beats/minute.
◆ *P wave:* Normal size and configuration, but it may increase in amplitude. The P wave precedes each QRS complex, but as the heart rate increases, the P wave may be superimposed on the preceding T wave and difficult to identify.
◆ *PR interval:* Within normal limits and constant.
◆ *QRS complex:* Normal duration and configuration.
◆ *T wave:* Normal size and configuration.
◆ *QT interval:* Within normal limits, but commonly shortened.
◆ *Other:* None.

Signs and symptoms

The patient will have a peripheral pulse rate above 100 beats/minute, but with a regular rhythm. Usually, he'll be asymptomatic. However, if his cardiac output falls and compensatory mechanisms fail, he may experience hypotension, syncope, and blurred vision. He may report chest pain and palpitations, commonly described as a pounding chest or a sensation of skipped heartbeats. He may also report a sense of nervousness or anxiety. If heart failure develops, he may exhibit crackles, an extra heart sound (S_3), and jugular vein distention.

Interventions

When treating the asymptomatic patient, focus on determining the cause of the tachycardia. The focus of treatment in the symptomatic patient with sinus tachycardia is to maintain adequate cardiac output and tissue perfusion and to identify and correct the underlying cause. For example, if the tachycardia is caused by hemorrhage, treatment includes stopping the bleeding and replacing blood and fluid losses.

If tachycardia leads to cardiac ischemia, treatment may include medications to slow the heart rate. The most commonly used medications include beta-adrenergic blockers, such as metoprolol (Lopressor) and atenolol (Tenormin), and calcium channel blockers such as verapamil (Calan) and diltiazem (Cardizem).

Check the patient's medication history. Over-the-counter sympathomimetic agents, which mimic the effects of the sympathetic nervous system, may contribute to the sinus tachycardia. Sympathomimetic agents may be contained in nose drops and cold formulas.

Also question the patient about the use of caffeine, nicotine, and alcohol, each of which can trigger tachycardia. Advise him to avoid these substances. Ask about the use of illicit drugs, such as cocaine and amphetamines, which can also cause tachycardia.

Here are other steps you should take for the patient with sinus tachycardia:

◆ Because sinus tachycardia can lead to injury of the heart muscle, assess the patient for signs and symptoms of angina. Also assess for signs and symptoms of heart failure, including crackles, an S_3 heart sound, and jugular vein distention.

◆ Monitor intake and output, along with daily weight.

◆ Check the patient's level of consciousness to assess cerebral perfusion.

◆ Provide the patient with a calm environment. Help to reduce fear and anxiety, which can aggravate the arrhythmia.

◆ Teach about procedures and treatments. Include relaxation techniques in the information you provide.

◆ Be aware that a sudden onset of sinus tachycardia after an MI may signal extension of the infarction. Prompt recognition is vital so treatment can be started.

◆ Keep in mind that tachycardia is frequently the initial sign of pulmonary embolism. Maintain a high index of suspicion, especially if your patient has predisposing risk factors for thrombotic emboli.

Sinus arrest and sinoatrial exit block

Although sinus arrest and SA or sinus exit block are two separate arrhythmias with different etiologies, they're discussed together because distinguishing the two can be difficult. In addition, there's no difference in their clinical significance and treatment.

In sinus arrest, the normal sinus rhythm is interrupted by an occasional, prolonged failure of the SA node to initiate an impulse. Therefore, sinus arrest is caused by episodes of failure in the automaticity or impulse formation of the SA node. The atria aren't stimulated, and an entire PQRST complex is missing from the ECG strip. Except for this missing complex, or pause, the ECG usually remains normal. (See *Recognizing sinus arrest.*)

Recognizing sinus arrest

To help you recognize sinus arrest, review this sample rhythm strip.

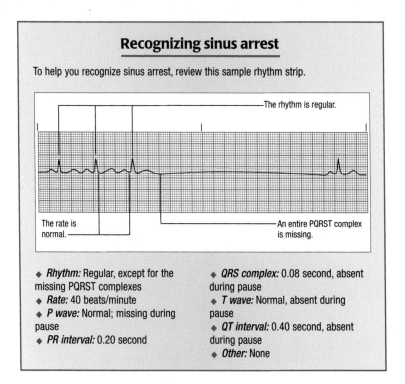

The rhythm is regular.

The rate is normal.

An entire PQRST complex is missing.

◆ *Rhythm:* Regular, except for the missing PQRST complexes
◆ *Rate:* 40 beats/minute
◆ *P wave:* Normal; missing during pause
◆ *PR interval:* 0.20 second

◆ *QRS complex:* 0.08 second, absent during pause
◆ *T wave:* Normal, absent during pause
◆ *QT interval:* 0.40 second, absent during pause
◆ *Other:* None

In sinus exit block, the SA node discharges at regular intervals, but some impulses are delayed or blocked from reaching the atria, resulting in long sinus pauses. Blocks result from failure to conduct impulses, whereas sinus arrest results from failure to form impulses in the SA node. Both arrhythmias cause atrial activity to stop. In sinus arrest, the pause commonly ends with a junctional escape beat. In sinus exit block, the pause occurs for an indefinite period and ends with a sinus rhythm. (See *Recognizing sinoatrial exit block,* page 106.)

Causes

Causes of sinus arrest and sinus exit block include:
◆ acute infection
◆ sick sinus syndrome
◆ sinus node diseases, such as fibrosis and idiopathic degeneration
◆ increased vagal tone, such as with Valsalva's maneuver, carotid sinus massage, and vomiting

Recognizing sinoatrial exit block

To help you recognize sinoatrial (SA) exit block, review this sample rhythm strip.

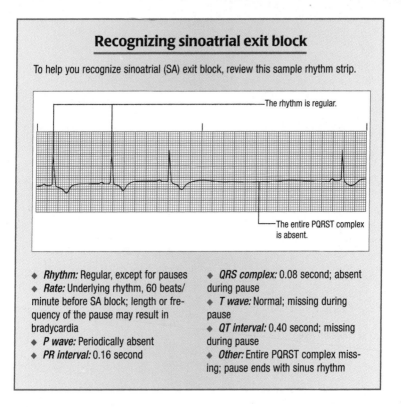

The rhythm is regular.

The entire PQRST complex is absent.

◆ *Rhythm:* Regular, except for pauses
◆ *Rate:* Underlying rhythm, 60 beats/minute before SA block; length or frequency of the pause may result in bradycardia
◆ *P wave:* Periodically absent
◆ *PR interval:* 0.16 second

◆ *QRS complex:* 0.08 second; absent during pause
◆ *T wave:* Normal; missing during pause
◆ *QT interval:* 0.40 second; missing during pause
◆ *Other:* Entire PQRST complex missing; pause ends with sinus rhythm

◆ digoxin, quinidine, procainamide (Procain), and salicylate toxicity
◆ excessive doses of beta-adrenergic blockers, such as metoprolol and propranolol (Inderal)
◆ cardiac disorders, such as coronary artery disease (CAD), acute myocarditis, cardiomyopathy, hypertensive heart disease, and acute inferior wall MI.

Clinical significance

The clinical significance of these two arrhythmias depends on the patient's symptoms. If the pauses are short and infrequent, the patient will most likely be asymptomatic and won't require treatment. He may have a normal sinus rhythm for days or weeks between episodes of sinus arrest or sinus exit block, and he may be totally unaware of the arrhythmia. Pauses of 2 to 3 seconds normally occur in healthy adults during sleep and occasionally in patients with increased vagal tone or hypersensitive carotid sinus disease.

If either of the arrhythmias is frequent or prolonged, however, the patient will most likely experience symptoms related to low cardiac output. The arrhythmias can produce syncope or near-syncopal episodes usually within 7 seconds of asystole.

During a prolonged pause, the patient may fall and injure himself. Other situations are potentially just as serious. For example, a symptom-producing arrhythmia that occurs while the patient is driving a car could result in a fatal accident. Extremely slow rates can also give rise to other arrhythmias.

ECG characteristics

Sinus arrest and SA exit block share these ECG characteristics:
◆ *Rhythm:* Atrial and ventricular rhythms are usually regular except when sinus arrest or SA exit block occurs.
◆ *Rate:* The underlying atrial and ventricular rates are usually within normal limits (60 to 100 beats/minute) before the arrest or SA exit block occurs. The length or frequency of the pause may result in bradycardia.
◆ *P wave:* Periodically absent, with entire PQRST complex missing. However, when present, the P wave is normal in size and configuration and precedes each QRS complex.
◆ *PR interval:* Within normal limits and constant when a P wave is present.
◆ *QRS complex:* Normal duration and configuration, but absent during a pause.
◆ *T wave:* Normal size and configuration, but absent during a pause.
◆ *QT interval:* Usually within normal limits, but absent during a pause.

To differentiate between these two rhythms, compare the length of the pause with the underlying P-P or R-R interval. If the underlying rhythm is regular, determine if the underlying rhythm resumes on time following the pause. With sinus exit block, because the regularity of the SA node discharge is blocked, not interrupted, the underlying rhythm will resume on time following the pause. In addition, the length of the pause will be a multiple of the underlying P-P or R-R interval.

In sinus arrest, the timing of the SA node discharge is interrupted by the failure of the SA node to initiate an impulse. The result is that the underlying rhythm doesn't resume on time after the pause and the length of the pause is not a multiple of the previous R-R intervals.

Signs and symptoms

You won't be able to detect a pulse or heart sounds when sinus arrest or sinus exit block occurs. Short pauses usually produce no symptoms. Recurrent or prolonged pauses may cause signs of decreased cardiac output, such as low blood pressure; altered mental status; cool, clammy skin; or syncope. The patient may also complain of dizziness or blurred vision.

Interventions

An asymptomatic patient needs no treatment. Symptomatic patients are treated according to the guidelines for patients with symptom-producing bradycardia. Treatment will also focus on the cause of the sinus arrest or sinus exit block. This may involve discontinuing medications that contribute to SA node discharge or conduction, such as digoxin, beta-adrenergic blockers, and calcium channel blockers.

Examine the circumstances under which the pauses occur. Both SA arrest and SA exit block may be insignificant if detected while the patient is sleeping. If the pauses are recurrent, assess the patient for evidence of decreased cardiac output, such as altered mental status, low blood pressure, and cool, clammy skin.

Ask him whether he's dizzy or light-headed or has blurred vision. Does he feel as if he has passed out? If so, he may be experiencing syncope from a prolonged sinus arrest or sinus exit block.

Document the patient's vital signs and how he feels during pauses as well as the activities he was involved in at the time. Activities that increase vagal stimulation, such as Valsalva's maneuver or vomiting, increase the likelihood of sinus pauses.

Assess for a progression of the arrhythmia. Notify the practitioner immediately if the patient becomes unstable. If appropriate, be alert for signs of digoxin, quinidine, or procainamide toxicity. Obtain a serum digoxin level and a serum electrolyte level.

Sick sinus syndrome

Also known as *sinoatrial syndrome, sinus nodal dysfunction,* and *Stokes-Adams syndrome,* sick sinus syndrome (SSS) refers to a wide spectrum of SA node arrhythmias. This syndrome is caused by disturbances in the way impulses are generated or in the ability to conduct impulses to the atria. These disturbances may be either intrinsic or mediated by the ANS.

Recognizing sick sinus syndrome

To help you identify sick sinus syndrome, review this sample rhythm strip.

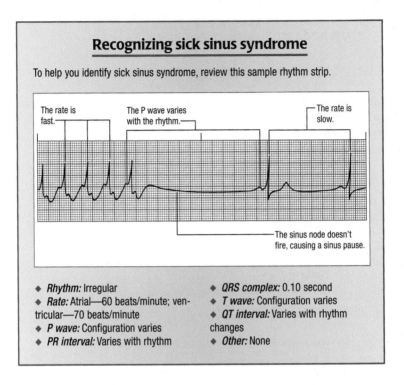

The rate is fast.

The P wave varies with the rhythm.

The rate is slow.

The sinus node doesn't fire, causing a sinus pause.

- ◆ *Rhythm:* Irregular
- ◆ *Rate:* Atrial—60 beats/minute; ventricular—70 beats/minute
- ◆ *P wave:* Configuration varies
- ◆ *PR interval:* Varies with rhythm

- ◆ *QRS complex:* 0.10 second
- ◆ *T wave:* Configuration varies
- ◆ *QT interval:* Varies with rhythm changes
- ◆ *Other:* None

SSS usually shows up as bradycardia, with episodes of sinus arrest and SA block interspersed with sudden, brief periods of rapid atrial fibrillation. Patients are also prone to paroxysms of other atrial tachyarrhythmias, such as atrial flutter and ectopic atrial tachycardia, a condition sometimes referred to as *bradycardia-tachycardia* (or *"brady-tachy") syndrome.*

Most patients with SSS are older than age 60, but anyone can develop the arrhythmia. It's rare in children except after open-heart surgery that results in SA

node damage. The arrhythmia affects men and women equally. The onset is progressive, insidious, and chronic. (See *Recognizing sick sinus syndrome.*)

Causes

SSS results either from a dysfunction of the sinus node's automaticity or from abnormal conduction or blockages of impulses coming out of the nodal region. These conditions, in turn, stem from a degeneration of the area's ANS and partial destruction of the sinus node, as may occur with an interrupted blood supply after an inferior wall MI.

In addition, certain conditions can affect the atrial wall surrounding the SA node and cause exit blocks. Conditions that cause inflammation or degeneration of atrial tissue can also lead to SSS. In many patients, though, the exact cause is never identified.

Causes of SSS include:
◆ conditions leading to fibrosis of the SA node, such as increased age, atherosclerotic heart disease, hypertension, and cardiomyopathy
◆ trauma to the SA node caused by open heart surgery (especially valvular surgery), pericarditis, or rheumatic heart disease
◆ autonomic disturbances affecting autonomic innervation, such as hypervagotonia or degeneration of the autonomic system
◆ cardioactive medications, such as digoxin, beta-adrenergic antagonists, and calcium channel blockers.

Clinical significance

The significance of SSS depends on the patient's age, the presence of other diseases, and the type and duration of the specific arrhythmias that occur. If atrial fibrillation is involved, the prognosis is worse, most likely because of the risk of thromboembolic complications.

If prolonged pauses are involved with SSS, syncope may occur. The length of a pause needed to cause syncope varies with the patient's age, posture at the time, and cerebrovascular status. Any pause that lasts 2 to 3 seconds or more should be considered significant.

A significant part of the diagnosis is whether the patient experiences symptoms while the disturbance occurs. Because the syndrome is progressive and chronic, a symptomatic patient will need lifelong treatment. In addition, thromboembolism may develop as a complication of SSS, possibly resulting in stroke or peripheral embolization.

ECG characteristics

SSS encompasses several potential rhythm disturbances that may be intermittent or chronic. SSS may include one, or a combination, of these rhythm disturbances:
◆ sinus bradycardia
◆ SA block
◆ sinus arrest
◆ sinus bradycardia alternating with sinus tachycardia
◆ episodes of atrial tachyarrhythmias, such as atrial fibrillation and atrial flutter
◆ failure of the sinus node to increase heart rate with exercise.

SSS displays these ECG characteristics:

◆ *Rhythm:* atrial and ventricular rhythms irregular because of sinus pauses and abrupt rate changes

◆ *Rate:* atrial and ventricular rates are fast or slow or alternate between fast and slow; and interrupted by a long sinus pause

◆ *P wave:* varies with the prevailing rhythm; may be normal size and configuration or may be absent; when present, a P wave usually precedes each QRS complex

◆ *PR interval:* usually within normal limits; varies with change in rhythm

◆ *QRS complex:* duration usually within normal limits; may vary with changes in rhythm; usually normal configuration

◆ *T wave:* usually normal size and configuration

◆ *QT interval:* usually within normal limits; varies with rhythm changes

◆ *Other:* usually more than one arrhythmia on a 6-second strip.

Signs and symptoms

The patient's pulse rate may be fast, slow, or normal, and the rhythm may be regular or irregular. You can usually detect an irregularity on the monitor or when palpating the pulse, which may feel inappropriately slow, then rapid.

If you monitor the patient's heart rate during exercise or exertion, you may observe an inappropriate response to exercise, such as a failure of the heart rate to increase. You may also detect episodes of brady-tachy syndrome, atrial flutter, atrial fibrillation, SA block, or sinus arrest on the monitor.

Other assessment findings depend on the patient's condition. For example, he may have crackles in the lungs, S_3, or a dilated and displaced left ventricular apical impulse if he has underlying cardiomyopathy. The patient may also show signs and symptoms of decreased cardiac output, such as fatigue, hypotension, blurred vision, and syncope, a common experience with this arrhythmia. Syncopal episodes, when related to SSS, are referred to as *Stokes-Adams attacks.*

◆ **ALERT** When caring for a patient with SSS, be alert for signs and symptoms of thromboembolism, especially if the patient has atrial fibrillation. Blood clots or thrombi forming in the heart can dislodge and travel through the bloodstream, resulting in decreased blood supply to the lungs, heart, brain, kidneys, intestines, or other organs.

Assess the patient for neurologic changes (such as confusion), vision disturbances, weakness, chest pain, dyspnea, tachypnea, tachycardia, and acute onset of pain. Early recognition allows for prompt treatment.

◆ **ALERT** Because the older adult with SSS may have mental status changes, be sure to perform a thorough assessment to rule out such disor-ders as stroke, delirium, or dementia.

Interventions

As with other sinus node arrhythmias, no treatment is generally necessary for SSS if the patient is asymptomatic. If the patient is symptomatic, however, treatment aims to alleviate signs and symptoms and correct the underlying cause of the arrhythmia.

Atropine or epinephrine may be given initially for symptom-producing bradycardia. A temporary pacemaker may be required until the underlying disorder resolves. Tachyarrhythmias may be treated with antiarrhythmic medications, such as metoprolol and digoxin. Unfortunately, medications used to suppress tachyarrhythmias may worsen under-lying SA node disease and bradyarrhythmias.

The patient may need anticoagulants if he develops sudden bursts, or paroxysms, of atrial fibrillation. The anticoagulants help prevent thromboembolism and stroke, a complication of the condition.

When caring for a patient with SSS, monitor and document all arrhythmias as well as signs and symptoms experienced. Note changes in heart rate and rhythm related to changes in the patient's level of activity.

Watch the patient carefully after starting beta-adrenergic blockers, calcium channel blockers, or other antiarrhythmic medications. If treatment includes anticoagulant therapy and pacemaker insertion, make sure the patient and his family receive appropriate instruction.

Atrial arrhythmias

6

Atrial arrhythmias, the most common cardiac rhythm disturbances, result from impulses originating in the atrial tissue in areas outside the sinoatrial (SA) node. These arrhythmias can affect ventricular filling time and diminish atrial kick. The term *atrial kick* refers to the complete filling of the ventricles during atrial systole and normally contributes about 25% to ventricular end-diastolic volume.

Atrial arrhythmias are thought to result from three mechanisms: altered automaticity, reentry, and afterdepolarization.

◆ *Altered automaticity.* The term *automaticity* refers to the ability of cardiac cells to initiate electrical impulses spontaneously. An increase in the automaticity of the atrial fibers can trigger abnormal impulses. Causes of increased automaticity include extracellular factors, such as hypoxia, hypocalcemia, and digoxin toxicity as well as conditions in

which the function of the heart's normal pacemaker, the SA node, is diminished. For example, increased vagal tone or hypokalemia can increase the refractory period of the SA node and allow atrial fibers to initiate impulses.

◆ *Reentry.* In reentry, an impulse is delayed along a slow conduction pathway. Despite the delay, the impulse remains active enough to produce another impulse during myocardial repolarization. Reentry may occur with coronary artery disease (CAD), cardiomyopathy, or myocardial infarction (MI).

◆ *Afterdepolarization.* Afterdepolarization can occur as a result of cell injury, digoxin toxicity, and other conditions. An injured cell sometimes only partially repolarizes. Partial repolarization can lead to repetitive ectopic firing called *triggered activity.* The depolarization produced by triggered activity, known as *afterde-*

polarization, can lead to atrial or ventricular tachycardia.

Atrial arrhythmias include premature atrial contractions, atrial tachycardia, atrial flutter, atrial fibrillation, Ashman's phenomenon, and wandering pacemaker.

Premature atrial contractions

Premature atrial contractions (PACs) originate in the atria, outside the SA node. They arise from either a single ectopic focus or from multiple atrial foci that supersede the SA node as pacemaker for one or more beats. PACs are generally caused by enhanced automaticity in the atrial tissue. (See *Recognizing PACs.*)

PACs may be conducted or nonconducted (blocked) through the atrioventricular (AV) node and the rest of the heart, depending on the status of the AV and intraventricular conduction system. If the atrial ectopic pacemaker discharges too soon after the preceding QRS complex, the AV junction or bundle branches may still be refractory from conducting the previous electrical impulse. If so, they may not be repolarized enough to conduct the premature electrical impulse into the ventricles normally.

When a PAC is conducted, ventricular conduction is usually normal. Nonconducted, or blocked, PACs aren't followed by a QRS complex. At times, it may be difficult to distinguish nonconducted PACs from SA block. (See *Distinguishing nonconducted PACs from SA block,* page 116.)

Causes

Alcohol, cigarettes, anxiety, fatigue, fever, and infectious diseases can trigger PACs, which commonly occur in a normal heart. Patients who eliminate or control these factors can usually correct the arrhythmia.

PACs may be associated with hyperthyroidism, coronary or valvular heart disease, acute respiratory failure, hypoxia, chronic pulmonary disease, digoxin toxicity, and certain electrolyte imbalances. PACs may also be caused by drugs that prolong the absolute refractory period of the SA node, including quinidine and procainamide (Procan).

Clinical significance

PACs are rarely dangerous in patients free from heart disease. They commonly cause no symptoms and can go unrecognized for years. Patients may perceive PACs as normal palpitations or skipped beats.

Recognizing PACs

To help you recognize premature atrial contractions (PACs), review this sample rhythm strip.

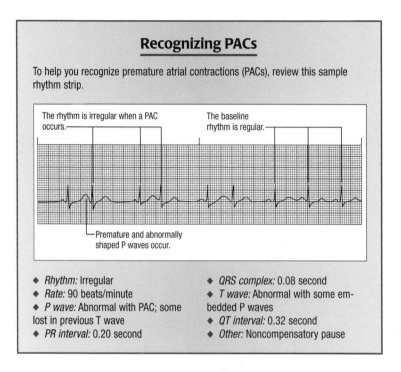

The rhythm is irregular when a PAC occurs.

The baseline rhythm is regular.

Premature and abnormally shaped P waves occur.

- ◆ *Rhythm:* Irregular
- ◆ *Rate:* 90 beats/minute
- ◆ *P wave:* Abnormal with PAC; some lost in previous T wave
- ◆ *PR interval:* 0.20 second
- ◆ *QRS complex:* 0.08 second
- ◆ *T wave:* Abnormal with some embedded P waves
- ◆ *QT interval:* 0.32 second
- ◆ *Other:* Noncompensatory pause

However, in patients with heart disease, PACs may lead to more serious arrhythmias, such as atrial fibrillation or atrial flutter. In a patient with acute MI, PACs can serve as an early sign of heart failure or electrolyte imbalance. PACs can also result from endogenous catecholamine release during episodes of pain or anxiety.

ECG characteristics

- ◆ *Rhythm:* Atrial and ventricular rhythms are irregular as a result of PACs, but the underlying rhythm may be regular.

- ◆ *Rate:* Atrial and ventricular rates vary with the underlying rhythm.
- ◆ *P wave:* The hallmark characteristic of a PAC is a premature P wave with an abnormal configuration, when compared with a sinus P wave. Varying configurations of the P wave indicate more than one ectopic site. PACs may be hidden in the preceding T wave.
- ◆ *PR interval:* Usually within normal limits but may be either shortened or slightly prolonged for the ectopic beat, depending on the origin of the ectopic focus.

LOOK-ALIKES

Distinguishing nonconducted PACs from SA block

To differentiate nonconducted prema-ture atrial contractions (PACs) from sinoatrial (SA) block, follow these in-structions:

◆ Whenever you see a pause in a rhythm, look carefully for a noncon-ducted P wave, which may occur be-fore, during, or just after the T wave preceding the pause.

◆ Compare T waves that precede a pause with the other T waves in the rhythm strip, and look for a distortion of the slope of the T wave or a difference in its height or shape. These are clues showing you where the nonconducted P wave may be hidden.

◆ If you find a P wave in the pause, check to see whether it's premature or if it occurs earlier than subsequent si-nus P waves. If it's premature (see shaded area below, top), you can be certain it's a nonconducted PAC.

◆ If there's no P wave in the pause or T wave (see shaded area below, bot-tom), the rhythm is SA block.

NONCONDUCTED PAC

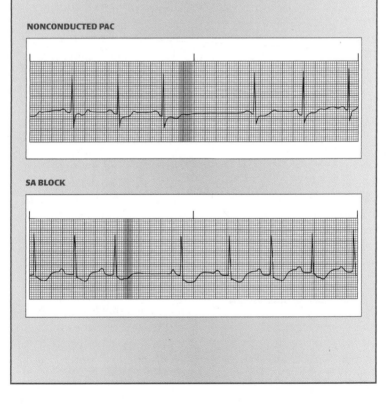

SA BLOCK

◆ *QRS complex:* Duration and configuration are usually normal when the PAC is conducted. If no QRS complex follows the PAC, the beat is called a *nonconducted PAC.*

◆ *T wave:* Usually normal; however, if the P wave is hidden in the T wave, the T wave may appear distorted.

◆ *QT interval:* Usually within normal limits.

◆ *Other:* PACs may occur as a single beat, in a bigeminal (every other beat is premature), trigeminal (every third beat), or quadrigeminal (every fourth beat) pattern, or in couplets (pairs). The presence of three or more PACs in a row is called *atrial tachycardia.*

PACs are commonly followed by a pause as the SA node resets. The PAC depolarizes the SA node early, causing it to reset itself and disrupting the normal cycle. The next sinus beat occurs sooner than it normally would, causing a P-P interval between normal beats interrupted by a PAC to be shorter than three consecutive sinus beats, an occurrence referred to as noncompensatory.

Signs and symptoms

The patient may have an irregular peripheral or apical pulse rhythm when the PACs occur.

Otherwise, the pulse rhythm and rate will reflect the underlying rhythm. Patients may complain of palpitations, skipped beats, or a fluttering sensation. In a patient with heart disease, signs and symptoms of decreased cardiac output, such as hypotension and syncope, may occur.

Interventions

Most asymptomatic patients don't need treatment. If the patient is symptomatic, however, treatment may focus on eliminating the cause, such as caffeine and alcohol. People with frequent PACs may be treated with drugs that prolong the refractory period of the atria. Such drugs include beta-adrenergic blockers and calcium channel blockers.

When caring for a patient with PACs, assess him to help determine factors that trigger ectopic beats. Tailor patient teaching to help the patient correct or avoid underlying causes. For example, the patient might need to avoid caffeine or learn stress reduction techniques to lessen anxiety.

If the patient has ischemic or valvular heart disease, monitor for signs and symptoms of heart failure, electrolyte imbalance, and more severe atrial arrhythmias.

Atrial tachycardia

Atrial tachycardia is a supraventricular tachycardia, which means that the impulses driving the rapid rhythm originate above the ventricles. Atrial tachycardia has an atrial rate of 150 to 250 beats/minute. The rapid rate shortens diastole, resulting in a loss of atrial kick, reduced cardiac output, reduced coronary perfusion, and the potential for myocardial ischemia. (See *Recognizing atrial tachycardia*.)

Three forms of atrial tachycardia—atrial tachycardia with block, multifocal atrial tachycardia (MAT, or chaotic atrial rhythm),

and paroxysmal atrial tachycardia (PAT)—are discussed here. In MAT, the tachycardia originates from multiple foci. PAT is generally a transient event in which the tachycardia appears and disappears suddenly.

Causes

Atrial tachycardia can occur in patients with a normal heart. In these cases, it's commonly related to excessive use of caffeine or other stimulants, marijuana use, electrolyte imbalance, hypoxia, or physical or psychological stress. Typically, however, atrial tachycardia is associated with

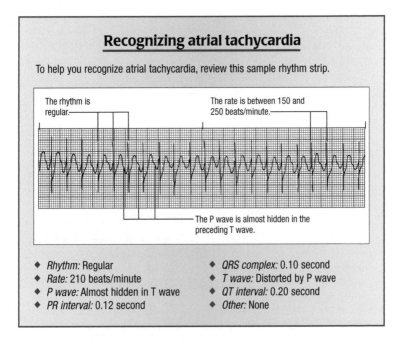

Recognizing atrial tachycardia

To help you recognize atrial tachycardia, review this sample rhythm strip.

The rhythm is regular.

The rate is between 150 and 250 beats/minute.

The P wave is almost hidden in the preceding T wave.

- ◆ *Rhythm:* Regular
- ◆ *Rate:* 210 beats/minute
- ◆ *P wave:* Almost hidden in T wave
- ◆ *PR interval:* 0.12 second
- ◆ *QRS complex:* 0.10 second
- ◆ *T wave:* Distorted by P wave
- ◆ *QT interval:* 0.20 second
- ◆ *Other:* None

primary or secondary cardiac disorders, including MI, cardiomyopathy, congenital anomalies, Wolff-Parkinson-White syndrome, and valvular heart disease.

This rhythm may be a component of sick sinus syndrome. Other problems resulting in atrial tachycardia include cor pulmonale, hyperthyroidism, systemic hypertension, and digoxin toxicity (the most common cause of atrial tachycardia). (See *Signs of digoxin toxicity*.)

Clinical significance

In a healthy person, nonsustained atrial tachycardia is usually benign. However, this rhythm may be a forerunner of more serious ventricular arrhythmias, especially if it occurs in a patient with underlying heart disease.

The increased ventricular rate that occurs in atrial tachycardia results in decreased ventricular filling time, increased myocardial oxygen consumption, and decreased oxygen supply to the myocardium. Heart failure, myocardial ischemia, and MI can result.

ECG characteristics

◆ *Rhythm:* The atrial rhythm is usually regular. The ventricular rhythm is regular or irregular, depending on the AV conduction ratio and the type of atrial tachycardia. (See *Recognizing types of atrial tachycardia,* pages 120 and 121.)

(Text continues on page 122.)

Signs of digoxin toxicity

With digoxin toxicity, atrial tachycardia isn't the only change you might see in your patient. Be alert for the following signs and symptoms, especially if the patient is taking digoxin and his potassium level is low or he's also taking amiodarone (because both combinations can increase the risk of digoxin toxicity):
◆ *Central nervous system:* fatigue, general muscle weakness, agitation, hallucinations
◆ *Eyes:* yellow-green halos around visual images, blurred vision
◆ *GI system:* anorexia, nausea, vomiting
◆ *Cardiovascular system:* arrhythmias (most commonly, conduction disturbances with or without atrioventricular block, premature ventricular contractions, and supraventricular arrhythmias), increased severity of heart failure, hypotension.
Remember: Digoxin's toxic effects on the heart may be life-threatening and always require immediate attention.

Recognizing types of atrial tachycardia

Atrial tachycardia comes in three varieties. Here's a quick rundown of each.

Atrial tachycardia with block

Atrial tachycardia with block is caused by increased automaticity of the atrial tissue. As the atrial rate speeds up and atrioventricular (AV) conduction becomes impaired, a 2:1 block typically occurs. Occasionally, a type I (Wenckebach) second-degree AV block may be seen.

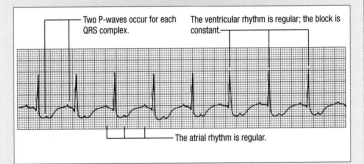

Two P-waves occur for each QRS complex.

The ventricular rhythm is regular; the block is constant.

The atrial rhythm is regular.

- ◆ *Rhythm:* Atrial—regular; ventricular—regular if block is constant, irregular if block is variable
- ◆ *Rate:* Atrial—150 to 250 beats/minute, multiple of ventricular rate; ventricular—varies with block
- ◆ *P wave:* Slightly abnormal

- ◆ *PR interval:* Usually normal; may be hidden
- ◆ *QRS complex:* Usually normal
- ◆ *T wave:* Usually indistinguishable
- ◆ *QT interval:* Indiscernible
- ◆ *Other:* More than one P wave for each QRS complex

Multifocal atrial tachycardia (MAT)

In MAT, atrial tachycardia occurs with numerous atrial foci firing intermittently. MAT produces varying P waves on the strip and occurs most commonly in patients with chronic pulmonary diseases. The irregular baseline in the strip at the top of the next page is caused by movement of the chest wall.

Recognizing types of atrial tachycardia *(continued)*

Multifocal arial tachycardia (MAT) *(continued)*

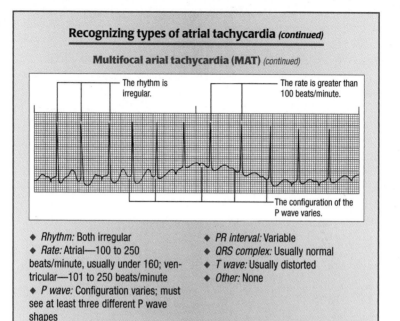

The rhythm is irregular.

The rate is greater than 100 beats/minute.

The configuration of the P wave varies.

- ◆ *Rhythm:* Both irregular
- ◆ *Rate:* Atrial—100 to 250 beats/minute, usually under 160; ventricular—101 to 250 beats/minute
- ◆ *P wave:* Configuration varies; must see at least three different P wave shapes
- ◆ *PR interval:* Variable
- ◆ *QRS complex:* Usually normal
- ◆ *T wave:* Usually distorted
- ◆ *Other:* None

Paroxysmal atrial tachycardia (PAT)

A type of paroxysmal atrial supraventricular tachycardia, PAT features brief periods of tachycardia that alternate with periods of normal sinus rhythm. PAT starts and stops suddenly as a result of rapid firing of an ectopic focus. It commonly follows frequent premature atrial contractions (PACs), one of which initiates the tachycardia.

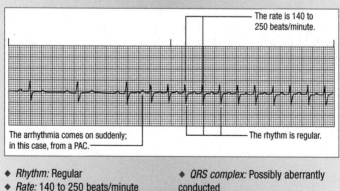

The rate is 140 to 250 beats/minute.

The arrhythmia comes on suddenly; in this case, from a PAC.

The rhythm is regular.

- ◆ *Rhythm:* Regular
- ◆ *Rate:* 140 to 250 beats/minute
- ◆ *P wave:* Abnormal; possibly hidden in previous T wave
- ◆ *PR interval:* Identical for each cycle
- ◆ *QRS complex:* Possibly aberrantly conducted
- ◆ *T wave:* Usually indistinguishable
- ◆ *Other:* One P wave for each QRS complex

◆ *Rate:* The atrial rate is characterized by three or more consecutive ectopic atrial beats occurring at a rate between 150 and 250 beats/minute. The rate rarely exceeds 250 beats/minute. The ventricular rate depends on the AV conduction ratio.

◆ *P wave:* The P wave may be aberrant (deviating from normal appearance) or hidden in the preceding T wave. If visible, it's usually upright and precedes each QRS complex.

◆ *PR interval:* The PR interval may be unmeasurable if the P wave can't be distinguished from the preceding T wave.

◆ *QRS complex:* Duration and configuration are usually normal, unless the impulses are being conducted abnormally through the ventricles.

◆ *T wave:* Usually distinguishable but may be distorted by the P wave; may be inverted if ischemia is present.

◆ *QT interval:* Usually within normal limits but may be shorter because of the rapid rate.

◆ *Other:* Sometimes it may be difficult to distinguish atrial tachycardia with block from sinus arrhythmia with U waves. (See *Distinguishing atrial tachycardia with block from sinus arrhythmia with U waves.*)

Signs and symptoms

The patient with atrial tachycardia will have a rapid apical and peripheral pulse rate. The rhythm may be regular or irregular, depending on the type of atrial tachycardia. A patient with PAT may complain that his heart suddenly starts to beat faster or that he suddenly feels palpitations. Persistent tachycardia and rapid ventricular rate cause decreased cardiac output, resulting in hypotension and syncope.

Interventions

Treatment depends on the type of tachycardia and the severity of the patient's symptoms. Because one of the most common causes of atrial tachycardia is digoxin toxicity, assess the patient for signs and symptoms of digoxin toxicity and monitor serum digoxin levels.

The Valsalva maneuver or carotid sinus massage may be used to treat PAT. (See *Understanding carotid sinus massage,* page 124.) These maneuvers increase the parasympathetic tone, which results in a slowing of the heart rate. They also allow the SA node to resume function as the primary pacemaker.

◆ **ALERT** Older adults may have undiagnosed carotid atherosclerosis and carotid bruits may be absent, even

LOOK-ALIKES

Distinguishing atrial tachycardia with block from sinus arrhythmia with U waves

Atrial tachycardia with block may appear strikingly similar to sinus arrhythmia with U waves. Always check "normal" rhythm strips carefully to make sure you haven't overlooked or misinterpreted something abnormal. Here's how to tell the difference between the two rhythms.

Atrial tachycardia with block

◆ Examine the T wave and the interval from the T wave to the next P wave for evidence of extra P waves (see shaded areas below). If you find extra P waves, map them to determine whether they occur at regular intervals with the "normal" P waves.

◆ In atrial tachycardia with block, the P-P intervals are constant.

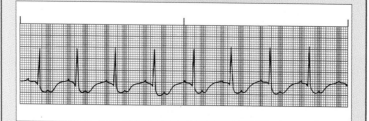

Sinus arrhythmia with U waves

◆ It's possible to mistake a U wave (see shaded areas below) for an extra P wave. The key is to determine if all of the waves occur at regular intervals. In sinus arrhythmia with U waves, the interval from a U wave to a P wave and a P wave to a U wave won't be constant.

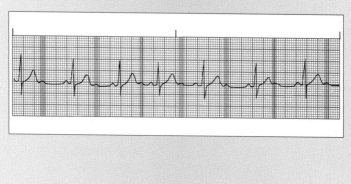

Understanding carotid sinus massage

Carotid sinus massage may be used to interrupt paroxysmal atrial tachycardia. Massaging the carotid sinus stimulates the vagus nerve, which inhibits firing of the sinoatrial (SA) node and slows atrioventricular (AV) node conduction. As a result, the SA node can resume its function as primary pacemaker.

Carotid sinus massage involves a firm massage that lasts no longer than 5 to 10 seconds. The patient's head is turned to the left to massage the right carotid sinus, as shown below. Remember that simultaneous, bilateral massage should never be attempted.

Carotid sinus massage is contraindicated in patients with carotid bruits. Risks of the procedure include decreased heart rate, syncope, sinus arrest, increased degree of AV block, cerebral emboli, stroke, and asystole.

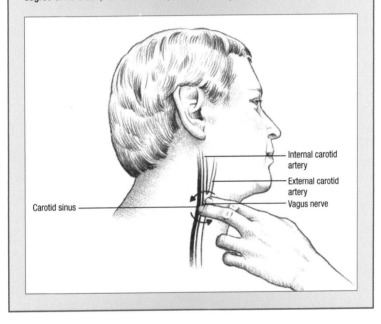

Carotid sinus

Internal carotid artery
External carotid artery
Vagus nerve

with significant disease. Cardiac sinus massage shouldn't be performed in late-middle-aged and older patients.

If vagal maneuvers are used, make sure resuscitative equipment is readily available. Keep in mind that vagal stimulation can result in bradycardia, ventricular arrhythmias, and asystole.

Drug therapy (pharmacologic cardioversion) may be used to increase the degree of AV block and decrease ventricular response rate. Appropriate drugs include adenosine, amiodarone (Cordarone), beta-adrenergic blockers, calcium channel blockers, and digoxin (Lanoxin). When other treatments fail, or if the patient is clinically unstable, synchronized electrical cardioversion may be used.

Atrial overdrive pacing (also called *rapid atrial pacing* or *overdrive suppression*) may also be used to stop the arrhythmia. This technique involves suppression of spontaneous depolarization of the ectopic pacemaker by a series of paced electrical impulses at a rate slightly higher than the intrinsic ectopic atrial rate. The pacemaker cells are depolarized prematurely and, following termination of the paced electrical impulses, the SA node resumes its normal role as the pacemaker.

Radiofrequency ablation can be used to treat PAT. After mapping the ectopic focus during electrophysiology study, the area is ablated. However, because MAT commonly occurs in patients with chronic pulmonary disease, this rhythm may not respond to ablation.

When caring for a patient with atrial tachycardia, carefully monitor the patient's rhythm strips. Doing so may provide information about the cause of atrial tachycardia, which, in turn, can facilitate treatment. Monitor the patient for chest pain, indications of decreased cardiac output, and signs and symptoms of heart failure or myocardial ischemia.

Atrial flutter

Atrial flutter, a supraventricular tachycardia, is characterized by a rapid atrial rate of 250 to 350 beats/minute, although it's generally around 300 beats/minute. Originating in a single atrial focus, this rhythm results from circus reentry and possibly increased automaticity.

On an ECG, the P waves lose their normal appearance due to the rapid atrial rate. The waves blend together in a sawtooth configuration called *flutter waves,* or F waves. These waves are the hallmark of atrial flutter. (See *Recognizing atrial flutter,* page 126.)

Causes

Atrial flutter may result from conditions that enlarge atrial tissue and elevate atrial pressures. The arrhythmia commonly occurs in patients with mitral or tricuspid valvular disease, hyperthyroidism, pericardial disease, digoxin toxicity, or primary myocardial disease. The rhythm sometimes develops in patients following cardiac surgery or in

Recognizing atrial flutter

To help you recognize atrial flutter, review this sample rhythm strip.

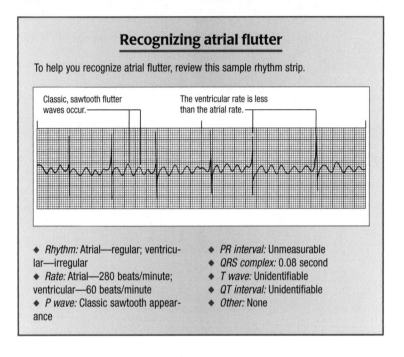

Classic, sawtooth flutter waves occur.

The ventricular rate is less than the atrial rate.

- ◆ *Rhythm:* Atrial—regular; ventricular—irregular
- ◆ *Rate:* Atrial—280 beats/minute; ventricular—60 beats/minute
- ◆ *P wave:* Classic sawtooth appearance
- ◆ *PR interval:* Unmeasurable
- ◆ *QRS complex:* 0.08 second
- ◆ *T wave:* Unidentifiable
- ◆ *QT interval:* Unidentifiable
- ◆ *Other:* None

patients with acute MI, chronic pulmonary disease, or systemic arterial hypoxia. Atrial flutter rarely occurs in healthy people. When it does, it may indicate intrinsic cardiac disease.

Clinical significance

The clinical significance of atrial flutter is determined by the number of impulses conducted through the AV node—expressed as a conduction ratio (such as 2:1 or 4:1)—and the resulting ventricular rate. If the ventricular rate is too slow (below 40 beats/ minute) or too fast (above 150

beats/minute), cardiac output can be seriously compromised.

Usually, the faster the ventricular rate, the more dangerous the arrhythmia. Rapid ventricular rates reduce ventricular filling time and coronary perfusion, which can cause angina, heart failure, pulmonary edema, hypotension, and syncope.

ECG characteristics

- ◆ *Rhythm:* Atrial rhythm is regular. Ventricular rhythm depends on the AV conduction pattern; it's typically regular, although cycles may alternate. An irregular pattern may signal atrial fibrillation or indicate development of a block.

◆ *Rate:* Atrial rate is 250 to 350 beats/minute. Ventricular rate depends on the degree of AV block; usually it's 60 to 100 beats/minute, but it may accelerate to 125 to 150 beats/minute.

Varying degrees of AV block produce ventricular rates that are usually one-half to one-fourth of the atrial rate. These are expressed as ratios, for example, 2:1 or 4:1. Usually, the AV node won't accept more than 180 impulses/minute and allows every second, third, or fourth impulse to be conducted. These impulses account for the ventricular rate. At the time atrial flutter is initially recognized, the ventricular response is typically above 100 beats/minute. One of the most common ventricular rates is 150 beats/minute with an atrial rate of 300, known as *2:1 block.*

◆ *P wave:* Atrial flutter is characterized by abnormal P waves that produce a sawtooth appearance, referred to as flutter waves, or F waves.

◆ *PR interval:* Unmeasurable.

◆ *QRS complex:* Duration is usually within normal limits, but the complex may be widened if flutter waves are buried within the complex.

◆ *T wave:* Not identifiable.

◆ *QT interval:* Unmeasurable because the T wave isn't identifiable.

◆ *Other:* The patient may develop an atrial rhythm that commonly varies between a fibrillatory line and flutter waves. This variation is referred to as atrial fib-flutter. The ventricular response is irregular. At times, it may be difficult to distinguish atrial flutter from atrial fibrillation. (See *Distinguishing atrial flutter from atrial fibrillation,* page 128.)

Signs and symptoms

When caring for a patient with atrial flutter, you may note that the peripheral and apical pulses are normal in rate and rhythm. That's because the pulse reflects the number of ventricular contractions, not the number of atrial impulses.

If the ventricular rate is normal, the patient may be asymptomatic. If the ventricular rate is rapid, the patient may experience a feeling of palpitations and may exhibit signs and symptoms of reduced cardiac output.

Interventions

If the patient is hemodynamically unstable, synchronized electrical cardioversion or countershock should be administered immedi-

LOOK-ALIKES

Distinguishing atrial flutter from atrial fibrillation

At times, you may see atrial flutter that has an irregular pattern of impulse conduction to the ventricles. In some leads, this may be confused with atrial fibrillation. Here's how to tell the two arrhythmias apart.

Atrial flutter

◆ Look for characteristic abnormal P waves that produce a sawtooth appearance, referred to as flutter waves, or F waves. These can best be identified in leads I, II, and V_1.

◆ Remember that the atrial rhythm is regular. You should be able to map the F waves across the rhythm strip. Whereas some F waves may occur within the QRS or T waves, subsequent F waves are visible and occur on time.

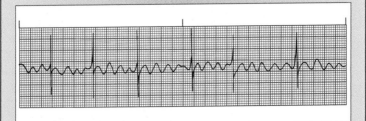

Atrial fibrillation

◆ Fibrillatory or f waves occur in an irregular pattern, making the atrial rhythm irregular.

◆ If you identify atrial activity that at times looks like flutter waves and seems to be regular for a short time, and in other places the rhythm strip contains fibrillatory waves, interpret the rhythm as atrial fibrillation. Coarse fibrillatory waves may intermittently look similar to the characteristic sawtooth appearance of flutter waves.

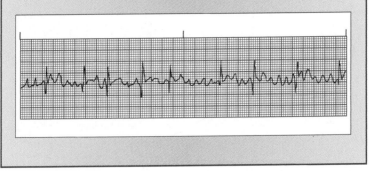

ately. Cardioversion delivers electric current to the heart to correct an arrhythmia, but unlike defibrillation, it usually uses much lower energy levels and is synchronized to discharge at the peak of the R wave. This causes immediate depolarization, interrupting reentry circuits and allowing the SA node to resume control as pacemaker. Synchronizing the energy current delivery with the R wave ensures that the current won't be delivered on the vulnerable T wave, which could initiate ventricular tachycardia or ventricular fibrillation.

The focus of treatment for hemodynamically stable patients with atrial flutter includes controlling the rate and converting the rhythm. Specific interventions depend on the patient's cardiac function, whether preexcitation syndromes are involved, and the duration of the arrhythmia. For example, in atrial flutter with normal cardiac function and a duration of less than 48 hours, electrical cardioversion may be considered. In atrial flutter existing longer than 48 hours, electrical cardioversion shouldn't be used unless the patient has been adequately anticoagulated; doing so would increase the risk of thromboembolism.

Because atrial flutter may signal intrinsic cardiac disease, monitor the patient closely for signs and symptoms of low cardiac output. Be alert to the effects of digoxin, which depresses the SA node.

If electrical cardioversion is indicated, prepare the patient for I.V. administration of a sedative or anesthetic as ordered. Keep resuscitative equipment at the bedside. Be alert for bradycardia because cardioversion can decrease the heart rate.

Atrial fibrillation

Atrial fibrillation, sometimes called *A-fib*, is defined as chaotic, asynchronous, electrical activity in atrial tissue. It results from the firing of multiple impulses from numerous ectopic pacemakers in the atria. Atrial fibrillation is characterized by the absence of P waves and an irregularly irregular ventricular response.

When a number of ectopic sites in the atria initiate impulses, depolarization can't spread in an organized manner. Small sections of the atria are depolarized individually, resulting in the atrial muscle quivering instead of contracting. On an ECG, uneven baseline fibrillatory waves, or f waves, appear rather than clearly distinguishable P waves.

The AV node protects the ventricles from the 350 to 600 erratic atrial impulses that occur each

Recognizing atrial fibrillation

To help you recognize atrial fibrillation, review this sample rhythm strip.

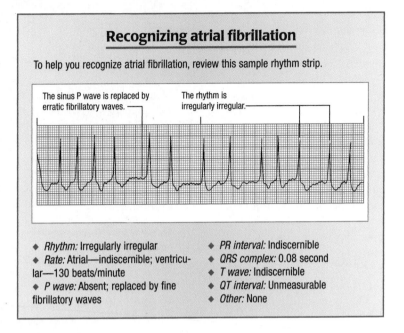

The sinus P wave is replaced by erratic fibrillatory waves.

The rhythm is irregularly irregular.

◆ *Rhythm:* Irregularly irregular
◆ *Rate:* Atrial—indiscernible; ventricular—130 beats/minute
◆ *P wave:* Absent; replaced by fine fibrillatory waves

◆ *PR interval:* Indiscernible
◆ *QRS complex:* 0.08 second
◆ *T wave:* Indiscernible
◆ *QT interval:* Unmeasurable
◆ *Other:* None

minute by acting as a filter and blocking some of the impulses. The ventricles respond only to impulses conducted through the AV node, hence the characteristic, wide variation in R-R intervals. When the ventricular response rate drops below 100, atrial fibrillation is considered controlled. When the ventricular rate exceeds 100, the rhythm is considered uncontrolled.

Like atrial flutter, atrial fibrillation results in a loss of atrial kick. The rhythm may be sustained or paroxysmal, meaning that it occurs suddenly and ends abruptly. It may be preceded by, or result from, PACs. (See *Recognizing atrial fibrillation*.)

Causes

Atrial fibrillation occurs more commonly than atrial flutter or atrial tachycardia. Atrial fibrillation can occur following cardiac surgery. Other causes of atrial fibrillation include rheumatic heart disease, valvular heart disease (especially mitral valve disease), hyperthyroidism, pericarditis, CAD, acute MI, hypertension, cardiomyopathy, atrial septal defects, and chronic obstructive pulmonary disease.

The rhythm may also occur in a healthy person who smokes or drinks coffee or alcohol or who's fatigued and under stress. Certain drugs, such as aminophylline and digoxin, may contribute to the development of atrial fibrillation. Endogenous catecholamine released during exercise may also trigger the arrhythmia.

Clinical significance

The loss of atrial kick from atrial fibrillation can result in the loss of approximately 20% of normal end-diastolic volume. Combined with the decreased diastolic filling time associated with a rapid heart rate, clinically significant reductions in cardiac output can result. In uncontrolled atrial fibrillation, the patient may develop heart failure, myocardial ischemia, or syncope.

Patients with preexisting cardiac disease, such as hypertrophic cardiomyopathy, mitral stenosis, rheumatic heart disease, or those with mitral prosthetic valves, tend to tolerate atrial fibrillation poorly and may develop severe heart failure.

Left untreated, atrial fibrillation can lead to cardiovascular collapse, thrombus formation, and systemic arterial or pulmonary embolism. (See *Risk of restoring sinus rhythm*.)

Risk of restoring sinus rhythm

A patient with atrial fibrillation is at increased risk for developing atrial thrombus and subsequent systemic arterial embolism. In atrial fibrillation, neither atrium contracts as a whole. As a result, blood may pool on the atrial wall, and thrombi may form. Thrombus formation places the patient at higher risk for emboli and stroke.

If normal sinus rhythm is restored and the atria contract normally, clots may break away from the atrial wall and travel through the pulmonary or systemic circulation with potentially disastrous results, such as stroke, pulmonary embolism, or arterial occlusion.

ECG characteristics

◆ *Rhythm:* Atrial and ventricular rhythms are grossly irregular, typically described as irregularly irregular.
◆ *Rate:* The atrial rate is almost indiscernible and usually exceeds 350 beats/minute. The atrial rate far exceeds the ventricular rate because most impulses aren't conducted through the AV junction. The ventricular rate usually varies, typically from 100 to 150 beats/minute but can be below 100 beats/minute.
◆ *P wave:* The P wave is absent. Erratic baseline F waves appear

in place of P waves. These chaotic waves represent atrial tetanization from rapid atrial depolarizations.

◆ *PR interval:* Indiscernible.

◆ *QRS complex:* Duration and configuration are usually normal.

◆ *T wave:* Indiscernible.

◆ *QT interval:* Unmeasurable.

◆ *Other:* The patient may develop an atrial rhythm that commonly varies between a fibrillatory line and flutter waves, a phenomenon called *atrial fib-flutter.* At times, it may be difficult to distinguish atrial fibrillation from multifocal atrial tachycardia and from junctional rhythm. (See *Distinguishing atrial fibrillation from MAT.* Also see *Distinguishing atrial fibrillation from junctional rhythm,* page 134.)

Signs and symptoms

When caring for a patient with atrial fibrillation, you may find that the radial pulse rate is slower than the apical rate. The weaker contractions that occur in atrial fibrillation don't produce a palpable peripheral pulse; only the stronger ones do.

The pulse rhythm will be irregularly irregular, with a normal or abnormal heart rate. Patients with a new onset of atrial fibrillation and a rapid ventricular rate may demonstrate signs and symptoms of decreased cardiac output, including hypotension and light-headedness. Patients with chronic atrial fibrillation may be able to compensate for the decreased cardiac output. Although these patients may be asymptomatic, they face a greater-than-normal risk of pulmonary, cerebral, or other thromboembolic events.

Interventions

Treatment for atrial fibrillation aims to reduce the ventricular response rate to below 100 beats/minute. This reduction may be accomplished either by giving drugs that control the ventricular response or by a combination of electrical cardioversion and drug therapy, which convert the arrhythmia to normal sinus rhythm. When the onset of atrial fibrillation is acute and the patient can cooperate, vagal maneuvers or carotid sinus massage may slow the ventricular response but won't convert the arrhythmia.

If the patient is hemodynamically unstable, synchronized electrical cardioversion should be administered immediately. Electrical cardioversion is most successful if used within the first 48 hours after onset and less successful the longer the duration of the arrhythmia. Conversion to normal sinus rhythm will cause forceful atrial contractions to re-

LOOK-ALIKES

Distinguishing atrial fibrillation from MAT

To help you determine whether a rhythm is atrial fibrillation or the similar multifocal atrial tachycardia (MAT), focus on the presence of P waves as well as the atrial and ventricular rhythms. You may find it helpful to look at a longer (greater than 6 seconds) rhythm strip.

Atrial fibrillation

◆ Carefully look for discernible P waves before each QRS complex.
◆ If you can't clearly identify P waves, and fibrillatory waves, or f waves, appear in the place of P waves, then the rhythm is probably atrial fibrillation.
◆ Carefully look at the rhythm, focusing on the R-R intervals. Remember that one of the hallmarks of atrial fibrillation is an irregularly irregular rhythm.

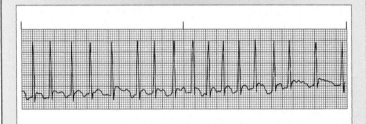

MAT

◆ P waves are present in MAT. Keep in mind, though, that the shape of the P waves varies, with at least three different P-wave shapes visible in a single rhythm strip.
◆ You should be able to see most, if not all, the various P-wave shapes repeat.
◆ Although the atrial and ventricular rhythms are irregular, the irregularity generally isn't as pronounced as in atrial fibrillation.

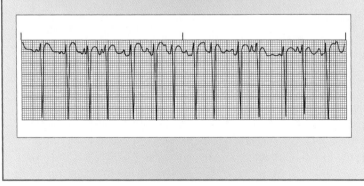

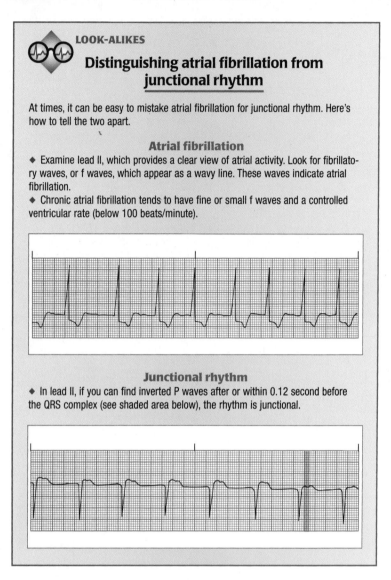

LOOK-ALIKES

Distinguishing atrial fibrillation from junctional rhythm

At times, it can be easy to mistake atrial fibrillation for junctional rhythm. Here's how to tell the two apart.

Atrial fibrillation

◆ Examine lead II, which provides a clear view of atrial activity. Look for fibrillatory waves, or f waves, which appear as a wavy line. These waves indicate atrial fibrillation.

◆ Chronic atrial fibrillation tends to have fine or small f waves and a controlled ventricular rate (below 100 beats/minute).

Junctional rhythm

◆ In lead II, if you can find inverted P waves after or within 0.12 second before the QRS complex (see shaded area below), the rhythm is junctional.

sume abruptly. If a thrombus has formed in the atria, the resumption of contractions can result in systemic emboli. (See *How synchronized cardioversion works*.)

The focus of treatment for hemodynamically stable patients with atrial fibrillation includes controlling the rate, converting the rhythm, and providing anti-

How synchronized cardioversion works

A patient experiencing an arrhythmia that leads to reduced cardiac output may be a candidate for synchronized cardioversion. This procedure may be done electively or as an emergency. For example, it may be an elective procedure in a patient with recurrent atrial fibrillation or an emergency procedure in a patient with ventricular tachycardia and a pulse.

Synchronized cardioversion is similar to defibrillation, also called *unsynchronized cardioversion,* except that synchronized cardioversion generally requires lower energy levels. Synchronizing the energy delivered to the patient reduces the risk that the current will strike during the relative refractory period of a cardiac cycle and induce ventricular fibrillation (VF).

In synchronized cardioversion, the R wave on the patient's electrocardiogram is synchronized with the cardioverter (defibrillator). After the firing buttons have been pressed, the cardioverter discharges energy when it senses the next R wave.

Keep in mind that a slight delay occurs between the time the discharge buttons are depressed and the moment the energy is discharged. When using handheld paddles, continue to hold the paddles on the patient's chest until the energy is delivered.

Remember to reset the "sync mode" on the defibrillator after each synchronized cardioversion. Resetting this switch is necessary because most defibrillators automatically reset to an unsynchronized mode.

If VF occurs during the procedure, turn off the SYNC button and immediately deliver an unsynchronized defibrillation to terminate the arrhythmia. Be aware that synchronized cardioversion carries the risk of lethal arrhythmia when used in patients with digoxin toxicity.

coagulation if indicated. Specific interventions depend on the patient's cardiac function, whether preexcitation syndromes are involved, and the duration of the arrhythmia.

Beta-adrenergic blockers and calcium channel blockers are the drugs of choice to control the ventricular rate. Patients with reduced left ventricular function typically receive digoxin. Anticoagulation is crucial in reducing the risk of thromboembolism. Heparin and warfarin (Coumadin) are used for anticoagulation and to prepare the patient for electrical cardioversion. Symptomatic atrial fibrillation that doesn't respond to routine treatment may be treated with radiofrequency ablation therapy.

When assessing a patient with atrial fibrillation, assess the peripheral and apical pulses. If the patient isn't on a cardiac monitor, be alert for an irregular pulse and differences in the radial and apical pulse rates.

Assess for symptoms of decreased cardiac output and heart failure. If drug therapy is used, monitor serum drug levels and observe the patient for evidence of toxicity. Tell the patient to report pulse rate changes, syncope or dizziness, chest pain, and signs of heart failure, such as dyspnea and peripheral edema.

Ashman's phenomenon

Ashman's phenomenon refers to the aberrant conduction of premature supraventricular beats to the ventricles. (See *Recognizing Ashman's phenomenon.*) This benign phenomenon is frequently associated with atrial fibrillation but can occur with any arrhythmia that affects the R-R interval.

Causes

Ashman's phenomenon is caused by a prolonged refractory period associated with slower rhythms. In theory, a conduction aberration occurs when a short cycle follows a long cycle because the refractory period varies with the length of the cycle. An impulse that ends a short cycle preceded by a long one is more likely to reach refractory tissue.

The normal refractory period for the right bundle branch is slightly longer than the left one, so premature beats frequently reach the right bundle when it's partially or completely refractory. Because of this tendency, the abnormal beat is usually seen as a right bundle-branch block (RBBB).

Clinical significance

The importance of recognizing aberrantly conducted beats is primarily to prevent misdiagnosis and subsequent mistaken treatment of ventricular ectopy.

ECG characteristics

◆ *Rhythm:* Atrial and ventricular rhythms are irregular.
◆ *Rate:* Atrial and ventricular rates reflect the underlying rhythm.
◆ *P wave:* The P wave has an abnormal configuration. It may be visible. If present in the underlying rhythm, the P wave is unchanged.
◆ *PR interval:* If measurable, the interval often changes on the premature beat.
◆ *QRS complex:* Configuration is usually altered, revealing an RBBB pattern.
◆ *T wave:* Deflection opposite that of the QRS complex occurs in most leads as a result of RBBB.

Recognizing Ashman's phenomenon

To help you recognize Ashman's phenomenon, review this sample rhythm strip.

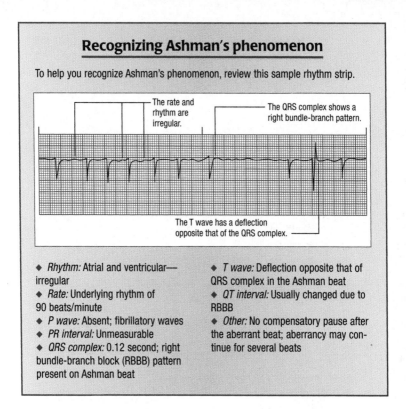

The rate and rhythm are irregular.

The QRS complex shows a right bundle-branch pattern.

The T wave has a deflection opposite that of the QRS complex.

◆ *Rhythm:* Atrial and ventricular—irregular

◆ *Rate:* Underlying rhythm of 90 beats/minute

◆ *P wave:* Absent; fibrillatory waves

◆ *PR interval:* Unmeasurable

◆ *QRS complex:* 0.12 second; right bundle-branch block (RBBB) pattern present on Ashman beat

◆ *T wave:* Deflection opposite that of QRS complex in the Ashman beat

◆ *QT interval:* Usually changed due to RBBB

◆ *Other:* No compensatory pause after the aberrant beat; aberrancy may continue for several beats

◆ *QT interval:* Usually has changed as a result of the RBBB.

◆ *Other:* There's no compensatory pause after an aberrant beat. The aberrancy may continue for several beats and typically ends a short cycle preceded by a long cycle.

Signs and symptoms

Patients with Ashman's phenomenon are usually asymptomatic.

Interventions

No interventions are necessary.

Wandering pacemaker

Wandering pacemaker, also called *wandering atrial pacemaker,* is an atrial arrhythmia that results when the site of impulse formation shifts from the SA node to another area above the ventricles. The origin of the impulse may wander beat to beat from the SA node to ectopic sites

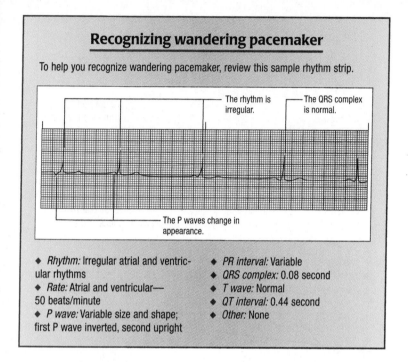

Recognizing wandering pacemaker

To help you recognize wandering pacemaker, review this sample rhythm strip.

The rhythm is irregular.

The QRS complex is normal.

The P waves change in appearance.

- ◆ *Rhythm:* Irregular atrial and ventricular rhythms
- ◆ *Rate:* Atrial and ventricular— 50 beats/minute
- ◆ *P wave:* Variable size and shape; first P wave inverted, second upright
- ◆ *PR interval:* Variable
- ◆ *QRS complex:* 0.08 second
- ◆ *T wave:* Normal
- ◆ *QT interval:* 0.44 second
- ◆ *Other:* None

in the atria or to the AV junctional tissue. The P wave and PR interval vary from beat to beat as the pacemaker site changes. (See *Recognizing wandering pacemaker.*)

Causes

In most cases, wandering pacemaker occurs because of increased parasympathetic (vagal) influences on the SA node or AV junction. It may also result from chronic pulmonary disease, valvular heart disease, digoxin toxicity, and inflammation of the atrial tissue.

Clinical significance

The arrhythmia may be normal in young patients and commonly occurs in athletes who have slow heart rates. The arrhythmia may be difficult to identify because it's commonly transient. Although wandering pacemaker is rarely serious, chronic arrhythmias are a sign of heart disease and should be monitored.

ECG characteristics

◆ *Rhythm:* The atrial rhythm varies slightly, with an irregular P-P interval. The ventricular

LOOK-ALIKES
Distinguishing wandering pacemaker from PACs

Because premature atrial contractions (PACs) are commonly encountered, it's possible to mistake wandering pacemaker for PACs unless the rhythm strip is carefully examined. In such cases, you may find it helpful to look at a longer (greater than 6 seconds) rhythm strip.

Wandering pacemaker

◆ Carefully examine the P waves. You must be able to identify at least three different shapes of P waves (see shaded areas below) in wandering pacemaker.
◆ Atrial rhythm varies slightly, with an irregular P-P interval. Ventricular rhythm varies slightly, with an irregular R-R interval. These slight variations in rhythm result from the changing site of impulse formation.

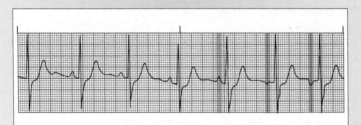

PAC

◆ The PAC occurs earlier than the sinus P wave, with an abnormal configuration when compared with a sinus P wave (see shaded area below). It's possible, but rare, to see multifocal PACs, which originate from multiple ectopic pacemaker sites in the atria. In this setting, the P waves may have different shapes.
◆ With the exception of the irregular atrial and ventricular rhythms as a result of the PAC, the underlying rhythm is usually regular.

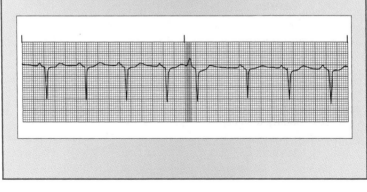

rhythm varies slightly, with an irregular R-R interval.

◆ *Rate:* Atrial and ventricular rates vary but are usually within normal limits, or below 60 beats/ minute.

◆ *P wave:* Altered size and configuration are due to the changing pacemaker site (SA node, atria, or AV junction). The P wave may also be absent, inverted, or may follow the QRS complex if the impulse originates in the AV junction. A combination of these variations may appear, with at least three different P-wave shapes visible.

◆ *PR interval:* The PR interval varies from beat to beat as the pacemaker site changes but is usually less than 0.20 second. If the impulse originates in the AV junction, the PR interval will be less than 0.12 second. This variation in PR interval will cause a slightly irregular R-R interval. When the P wave is present, the PR interval may be normal or shortened.

◆ *QRS complex:* Ventricular depolarization is normal, so duration of the QRS complex is usually within normal limits and is of normal configuration.

◆ *T wave:* Normal size and configuration.

◆ *QT interval:* Usually within normal limits, but may vary.

◆ *Other:* At times it may be difficult to distinguish wandering pacemaker from PACs. (See *Distinguishing wandering pacemaker from PACs,* page 139.)

Signs and symptoms

Patients are generally asymptomatic and unaware of the arrhythmia. The pulse rate may be normal or below 60 beats/ minute, and the rhythm may be regular or slightly irregular.

Interventions

Usually, no treatment is needed for asymptomatic patients. If the patient is symptomatic, however, his medications should be reviewed and the underlying cause investigated and treated. Monitor the patient's heart rhythm and assess for signs of hemodynamic instability, such as hypotension and changes in mental status.

Junctional arrhythmias

7

Junctional arrhythmias originate in the atrioventricular (AV) junction—the area in and around the AV node and the bundle of His. The specialized pacemaker cells in the AV junction take over as the heart's pacemaker if the sinoatrial (SA) node fails to function properly or if the electrical impulses originating in the SA node are blocked. These junctional pacemaker cells have an inherent firing rate of 40 to 60 beats/minute.

In normal impulse conduction, the AV node slows transmission of the impulse from the atria to the ventricles, which allows the ventricles to fill as much as possible before they contract. However, these impulses don't always follow the normal conduction pathway. (See *Conduction in Wolff-Parkinson-White syndrome,* page 142.)

Because of the location of the AV junction within the conduction pathway, electrical impulses originating in this area cause abnormal depolarization of the heart. The impulse is conducted in a retrograde (backward) fashion to depolarize the atria, and antegrade (forward) to depolarize the ventricles.

Depolarization of the atria can precede depolarization of the ventricles, or the ventricles can be depolarized before the atria. Depolarization of the atria and ventricles can also occur simultaneously. Retrograde depolarization of the atria results in inverted P waves in leads II, III, and aV_F, leads in which you would normally see upright P waves. (See *Locating the P wave,* page 143.)

Keep in mind that arrhythmias causing inverted P waves on an ECG may originate in the atria or AV junction. Atrial arrhythmias are sometimes mistaken for junctional arrhythmias because impulses are generated so low in the atria that they cause retro-

◆

Conduction in Wolff-Parkinson-White syndrome

Electrical impulses in the heart don't always follow normal conduction pathways. In preexcitation syndromes, electrical impulses enter the ventricles from the atria through an accessory pathway that bypasses the atrioventricular junction. Wolff-Parkinson-White (WPW) syndrome is a common type of preexcitation syndrome.

WPW syndrome commonly occurs in young children and in adults ages 20 to 35. The syndrome causes the PR interval to shorten and the QRS complex to lengthen as a result of a delta wave. Delta waves, which in WPW occur just before normal ventricular depolarization, are produced as a result of the premature depolarization or preexcitation of a portion of the ventricles.

WPW is clinically significant because the accessory pathway—in this case, Kent's bundle—may result in paroxysmal tachyarrhythmias by reentry and rapid conduction mechanisms.

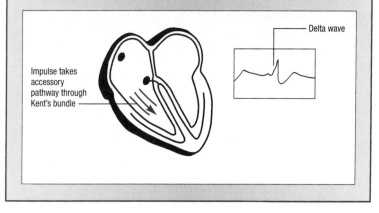

Delta wave

Impulse takes accessory pathway through Kent's bundle

grade depolarization and inverted P waves. Looking at the PR interval will help you determine whether an arrhythmia is atrial or junctional. An arrhythmia with an inverted P wave before the QRS complex and with a normal PR interval (0.12 to 0.20 second) originates in the atria. An arrhythmia with a PR interval less than 0.12 second originates in the AV junction.

Junctional arrhythmias include premature junctional contractions, junctional escape rhythm, accelerated junctional rhythm, and junctional tachycardia.

Premature junctional contractions

A premature junctional contraction (PJC) is a junctional beat

Locating the P wave

When the specialized pacemaker cells in the atrioventricular junction take over as the dominant pacemaker of the heart:
◆ depolarization of the atria can precede depolarization of the ventricles
◆ the ventricles can be depolarized before the atria
◆ simultaneous depolarization of the atria and ventricles can occur.
   The rhythm strips shown here demonstrate the various locations of the P waves in junctional arrhythmias, depending on the direction of depolarization.

Inverted P wave
If the atria are depolarized first, the P wave occurs before the QRS complex.

Inverted P wave
If the ventricles are depolarized first, the P wave occurs after the QRS complex.

Inverted P wave (hidden)
If the ventricles and atria are depolarized simultaneously, the P wave is hidden in the QRS complex.

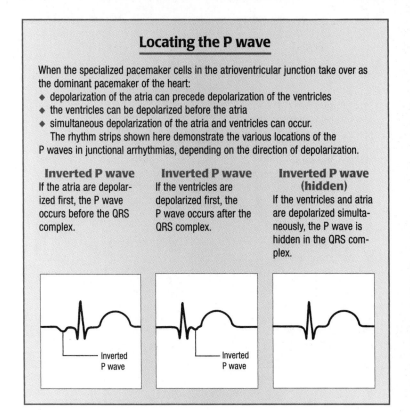

Inverted P wave

Inverted P wave

that comes from the AV junction before the next expected sinus beat; it interrupts the underlying rhythm and causes an irregular rhythm. These ectopic beats commonly occur as a result of enhanced automaticity in the junctional tissue or bundle of His. As with all impulses generated in the AV junction, the atria are depolarized in a retrograde fashion, causing an inverted P wave. The ventricles are depo-larized normally. (See *Recognizing a PJC,* page 144.)

Causes

PJCs may be caused by digoxin (Lanoxin) toxicity, excessive caffeine intake, amphetamine ingestion, excessive alcohol intake, excessive nicotine intake, stress, coronary artery disease, myocardial ischemia, valvular heart disease, pericarditis, heart failure, chronic obstructive pulmonary

Recognizing a PJC

To help you recognize a premature junctional contraction (PJC), review this sample rhythm strip.

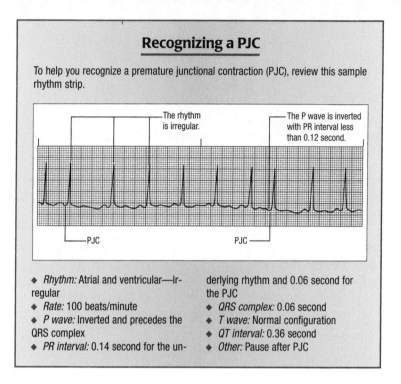

The rhythm is irregular.

The P wave is inverted with PR interval less than 0.12 second.

PJC   PJC

◆ *Rhythm:* Atrial and ventricular—Irregular
◆ *Rate:* 100 beats/minute
◆ *P wave:* Inverted and precedes the QRS complex
◆ *PR interval:* 0.14 second for the underlying rhythm and 0.06 second for the PJC
◆ *QRS complex:* 0.06 second
◆ *T wave:* Normal configuration
◆ *QT interval:* 0.36 second
◆ *Other:* Pause after PJC

disease, hyperthyroidism, electrolyte imbalances, or inflammatory changes in the AV junction after heart surgery.

Clinical significance

PJCs are generally considered harmless unless they occur frequently—typically defined as more than six per minute. Frequent PJCs indicate junctional irritability and can precipitate a more serious arrhythmia, such as junctional tachycardia. In patients taking digoxin, PJCs are a common early sign of toxicity.

ECG characteristics

◆ *Rhythm:* Atrial and ventricular rhythms are irregular during PJCs; the underlying rhythm may be regular.
◆ *Rate:* Atrial and ventricular rates reflect the underlying rhythm.
◆ *P wave:* The P wave is usually inverted. It may occur before or after the QRS complex or may appear absent when hidden in the QRS complex. Look for an inverted P wave in leads II, III, and aV$_F$. Depending on the initial direction of depolarization, the

P wave may fall before, during, or after the QRS complex.

◆ *PR interval:* If the P wave precedes the QRS complex, the PR interval is shortened (less than 0.12 second); otherwise, it can't be measured.

◆ *QRS complex:* Because the ventricles are usually depolarized normally, the QRS complex usually has a normal configuration and a normal duration of less than 0.12 second.

◆ *T wave:* Usually has a normal configuration.

◆ *QT interval:* Usually within normal limits.

◆ *Other:* A compensatory pause reflecting retrograde atrial conduction may follow the PJC.

Signs and symptoms

The patient is usually asymptomatic. He may complain of palpitations or a feeling of "skipped heart beats." You may be able to palpate an irregular pulse when PJCs occur. If PJCs are frequent enough, the patient may experience hypotension from a transient decrease in cardiac output.

Interventions

PJCs don't usually require treatment unless the patient is symptomatic. In those cases, the underlying cause should be treated. For example, in digoxin toxicity,

the medication should be discontinued and serum digoxin levels monitored.

Monitor the patient for hemodynamic instability as well. If ectopic beats occur frequently, the patient should decrease or eliminate his caffeine intake.

Junctional escape rhythm

A junctional escape rhythm, also referred to as *junctional rhythm,* is an arrhythmia originating in AV junction. In this arrhythmia, the AV junction takes over as a secondary, or "escape" pacemaker. This usually occurs only when a higher pacemaker site in the atria, usually the SA node, fails as the heart's dominant pacemaker.

Remember that the AV junction can take over as the heart's dominant pacemaker if the firing rate of the higher pacemaker sites falls below the AV junction's intrinsic firing rate, if the pacemaker fails to generate an impulse, or if the conduction of the impulses is blocked.

In a junctional escape rhythm, as in all junctional arrhythmias, the atria are depolarized by means of retrograde conduction. The P waves are inverted, and impulse conduction through the ventricles is normal. The normal

Recognizing junctional escape rhythm

To help you recognize junctional escape rhythm, review this sample rhythm strip.

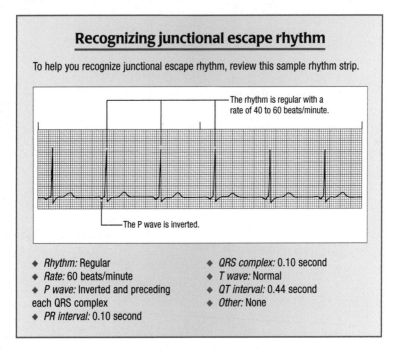

The rhythm is regular with a rate of 40 to 60 beats/minute.

The P wave is inverted.

- ◆ *Rhythm:* Regular
- ◆ *Rate:* 60 beats/minute
- ◆ *P wave:* Inverted and preceding each QRS complex
- ◆ *PR interval:* 0.10 second

- ◆ *QRS complex:* 0.10 second
- ◆ *T wave:* Normal
- ◆ *QT interval:* 0.44 second
- ◆ *Other:* None

intrinsic firing rate for cells in the AV junction is 40 to 60 beats/minute. (See *Recognizing junctional escape rhythm.*)

Causes

A junctional escape rhythm can be caused by a condition that disturbs normal SA node function or impulse conduction. Causes of the arrhythmia include SA node ischemia, hypoxia, electrolyte imbalances, valvular heart disease, heart failure, cardiomyopathy, myocarditis, sick sinus syndrome, and increased parasympathetic (vagal) tone. Drugs,

such as digoxin, calcium channel blockers, and beta-adrenergic blockers, can also cause a junctional escape rhythm.

Clinical significance

The clinical significance of junctional escape rhythm depends on how well the patient tolerates a decreased heart rate (40 to 60 beats/minute) and associated decrease in cardiac output. In addition to a decreased cardiac output from a slower heart rate, depolarization of the atria either after or simultaneously with ventricular depolarization results in loss of atrial kick. Remember that junctional escape rhythms protect the heart from potentially life-threatening ventricular escape rhythms.

ECG characteristics

◆ *Rhythm:* Atrial and ventricular rhythms are regular.
◆ *Rate:* The atrial and ventricular rates are 40 to 60 beats/minute.
◆ *P wave:* The P wave is inverted (look for inverted P waves in leads II, III, and aV$_F$). The P wave may occur before or after the QRS complex or may appear absent when hidden within QRS complex.
◆ *PR interval:* If the P wave precedes the QRS complex, the PR interval is shortened (less than 0.12 second); otherwise, it can't be measured.
◆ *QRS complex:* Duration is usually within normal limits; configuration is usually normal.
◆ *T wave:* Usually normal configuration.
◆ *QT interval:* Usually within normal limits.
◆ *Other:* None.

Signs and symptoms

A patient with a junctional escape rhythm will have a slow, regular pulse rate of 40 to 60 beats/minute. The patient may be asymptomatic. However, pulse rates under 60 beats/minute may lead to inadequate cardiac output, causing hypotension, syncope, or blurred vision.

Interventions

Treatment for a junctional escape rhythm involves identification and correction of the underlying cause, whenever possible. If the patient is symptomatic, atropine may be used to increase the heart rate, or a temporary (transcutaneous or transvenous) or permanent pacemaker may be inserted. Because junctional escape rhythm can prevent ventricular standstill, it should never be suppressed.

Monitor the patient's serum digoxin and electrolyte levels and watch for signs of decreased cardiac output, such as hypotension, syncope, and blurred vision.

Accelerated junctional rhythm

An accelerated junctional rhythm is an arrhythmia that originates in the AV junction and is usually caused by enhanced automaticity of the AV junctional tissue. It's called accelerated because it occurs at a rate of 60 to 100 beats/minute, exceeding the inherent

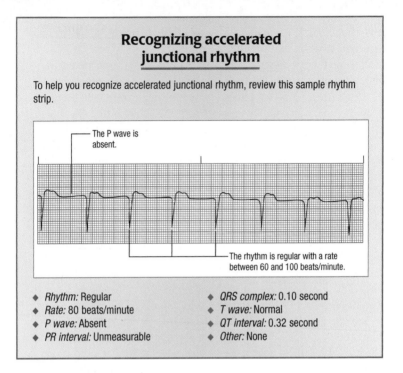

Recognizing accelerated junctional rhythm

To help you recognize accelerated junctional rhythm, review this sample rhythm strip.

The P wave is absent.

The rhythm is regular with a rate between 60 and 100 beats/minute.

◆ *Rhythm:* Regular
◆ *Rate:* 80 beats/minute
◆ *P wave:* Absent
◆ *PR interval:* Unmeasurable

◆ *QRS complex:* 0.10 second
◆ *T wave:* Normal
◆ *QT interval:* 0.32 second
◆ *Other:* None

junctional escape rate of 40 to 60 beats/minute.

Because the rate is below 100 beats/minute, the arrhythmia isn't classified as junctional tachycardia. The atria are depolarized by means of retrograde conduction, and the ventricles are depolarized normally. (See *Recognizing accelerated junctional rhythm.*)

Causes

Digoxin toxicity is a common cause of accelerated junctional rhythm. Other causes include electrolyte disturbances, valvular heart disease, rheumatic heart disease, heart failure, myocarditis, cardiac surgery, and inferior- or posterior-wall myocardial infarction.

Clinical significance

Patients experiencing accelerated junctional rhythm are generally asymptomatic because the rate corresponds to the normal inherent firing rate of the SA node (60 to 100 beats/minute). However, symptoms of decreased cardiac output, including hypotension and syncope, can occur if atrial depolarization occurs after or simultaneously with ventricular depolarization, which causes the subsequent loss of atrial kick.

ECG characteristics

◆ *Rhythm:* Atrial and ventricular rhythms are regular.
◆ *Rate:* Atrial and ventricular rates range from 60 to 100 beats/ minute.
◆ *P wave:* If the P wave is present, it will be inverted in leads II, III, and aV$_F$. It may precede, follow, or be hidden in the QRS complex.
◆ *PR interval:* If the P wave occurs before the QRS complex, the PR interval is shortened (less than 0.12 second). Otherwise, it can't be measured.
◆ *QRS complex:* Duration is usually within normal limits. Configuration is usually normal.
◆ *T wave:* Usually within normal limits.
◆ *QT interval:* Usually within normal limits.
◆ *Other:* None.
  Accelerated junctional rhythm can sometimes be difficult to distinguish from accelerated idioventricular rhythm. (See *Distinguishing accelerated idioventricular rhythm from accelerated junctional rhythm*, page 150.)

Signs and symptoms

The pulse rate will be normal with a regular rhythm. The patient may be asymptomatic because accelerated junctional rhythm has the same rate as sinus rhythm. However, if cardiac output is decreased, the patient may exhibit symptoms, such as hypotension, changes in mental status, and weak peripheral pulses.

Interventions

Treatment for accelerated junctional rhythm involves identifying and correcting the underlying cause. Assessing the patient for signs and symptoms related to decreased cardiac output and hemodynamic instability is key, as is monitoring serum digoxin and electrolyte levels.

Junctional tachycardia

In junctional tachycardia, three or more PJCs occur in a row. This supraventricular tachycardia generally occurs as a result of enhanced automaticity of the AV junction, which causes the AV junction to override the SA node as the dominant pacemaker.
  In junctional tachycardia, the atria are depolarized by retrograde conduction. Conduction through the ventricles is normal.

LOOK-ALIKES

Distinguishing accelerated idioventricular rhythm from accelerated junctional rhythm

Accelerated idioventricular rhythm and accelerated junctional rhythm appear similar but have different causes. To distinguish between the two, closely examine the duration of the QRS complex and then look for P waves.

Accelerated idioventricular rhythm

◆ The QRS duration is greater than 0.12 second.
◆ The QRS has a wide and bizarre configuration.
◆ P waves are usually absent.
◆ The ventricular rate is generally between 40 and 100 beats/minute.

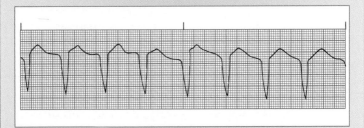

Accelerated junctional rhythm

◆ The QRS duration and configuration are usually normal.
◆ Inverted P waves generally occur before or after the QRS complex. However, remember that the P waves may also appear absent when hidden within the QRS complex.
◆ The ventricular rate is typically between 60 and 100 beats/minute.

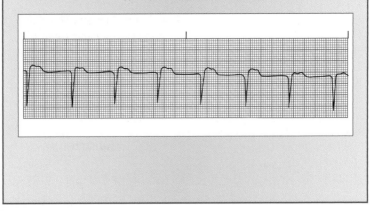

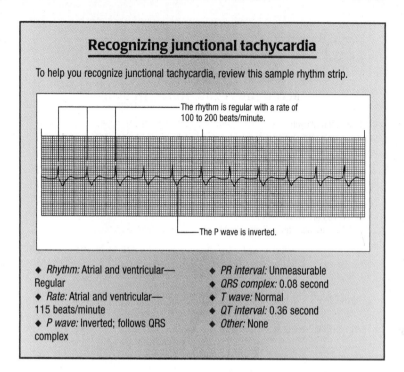

Recognizing junctional tachycardia

To help you recognize junctional tachycardia, review this sample rhythm strip.

The rhythm is regular with a rate of 100 to 200 beats/minute.

The P wave is inverted.

◆ *Rhythm:* Atrial and ventricular—Regular
◆ *Rate:* Atrial and ventricular—115 beats/minute
◆ *P wave:* Inverted; follows QRS complex

◆ *PR interval:* Unmeasurable
◆ *QRS complex:* 0.08 second
◆ *T wave:* Normal
◆ *QT interval:* 0.36 second
◆ *Other:* None

(See *Recognizing junctional tachycardia.*)

Causes

Digoxin toxicity is the most common cause of junctional tachycardia. In such cases, the arrhythmia can be aggravated by hypokalemia. Other causes of junctional tachycardia include inferior- or posterior-wall myocardial infarction or ischemia, inflammation of the AV junction after heart surgery, heart failure, electrolyte imbalances, and valvular heart disease.

Clinical significance

The clinical significance of junctional tachycardia depends on the rate and underlying cause. At higher ventricular rates, junctional tachycardia may reduce cardiac output by decreasing ventricular filling time. A loss of atrial kick also occurs with atrial depolarization that follows or occurs simultaneously with ventricular depolarization.

ECG characteristics

◆ *Rhythm:* Atrial and ventricular rhythms are usually regular. The atrial rhythm may be difficult to determine if the P wave is hidden in the QRS complex or preceding T wave.

◆ *Rate:* Atrial and ventricular rates exceed 100 beats/minute (usually between 100 and 200 beats/minute). The atrial rate may be difficult to determine if the P wave is hidden in the QRS complex or the preceding T wave.

◆ *P wave:* The P wave is usually inverted in leads II, III, and aV_F. It may occur before or after the QRS complex or be hidden in the QRS complex.

◆ *PR interval:* If the P wave precedes the QRS complex, the PR interval is shortened (less than 0.12 second); otherwise, the PR interval can't be measured.

◆ *QRS complex:* Duration is within normal limits; configuration is usually normal.

◆ *T wave:* Configuration is usually normal but may be abnormal if the P wave is hidden in the T wave. The fast rate may make T waves indiscernible.

◆ *QT interval:* Usually within normal limits.

◆ *Other:* None.

Signs and symptoms

The patient's pulse rate will be above 100 beats/minute and have a regular rhythm. Patients with a rapid heart rate may experience signs and symptoms of decreased cardiac output and hemodynamic instability including hypotension.

Interventions

The underlying cause should be identified and treated. If the cause is digoxin toxicity, the drug should be discontinued. In some cases of digoxin toxicity, a digoxin-binding drug may be used to reduce serum digoxin levels. Vagal maneuvers and drugs, such as adenosine, may slow the heart rate for symptomatic patients. Patients with recurrent junctional tachycardia may be treated with ablation therapy, followed by permanent pacemaker insertion.

Monitor patients with junctional tachycardia for signs of decreased cardiac output. In addition, check digoxin and potassium levels and administer potassium supplements as ordered.

Ventricular arrhythmias

8

Ventricular arrhythmias originate in the ventricles below the bifurcation of the bundle of His. These arrhythmias occur when electrical impulses depolarize the myocardium using a different pathway from normal impulse conduction.

Ventricular arrhythmias appear on an ECG in characteristic ways. The QRS complex in most of these arrhythmias is wider than normal because of the prolonged conduction time through, and abnormal depolarization of, the ventricles. The deflections of the T wave and the QRS complex are in opposite directions because ventricular repolarization, as well as ventricular depolarization, is abnormal. The P wave in many ventricular arrhythmias is absent because atrial depolarization doesn't occur. If the P wave does occur, it usually doesn't have any relationship to the QRS complex.

When electrical impulses come from the ventricles instead of the atria, atrial kick is lost and cardiac output can decrease by as much as 30%. This decrease is one reason why patients with ventricular arrhythmias may show signs and symptoms of heart failure, including hypotension, angina, syncope, and respiratory distress.

Although ventricular arrhythmias may be benign, they're generally considered the most serious arrhythmias because the ventricles are ultimately responsible for cardiac output. Rapid recognition and treatment of ventricular arrhythmias increases the chances of successful resuscitation. Ventricular arrhythmias include premature ventricular contractions, idioventricular rhythm, ventricular tachycardia, ventricular fibrillation, and asystole.

◆

◼**LIFE-THREATENING**

Premature ventricular contractions

Premature ventricular contractions (PVCs) are ectopic beats that originate in the ventricles and occur earlier than expected. PVCs may occur in healthy people without being clinically significant. When PVCs occur in patients with underlying heart disease, however, they may herald the development of lethal ventricular arrhythmias, including ventricular tachycardia (VT) and ventricular fibrillation (VF).

PVCs may occur singly, in pairs (couplets), or in clusters. PVCs may also appear in patterns, such as bigeminy or trigeminy. (See *Recognizing PVCs*.) In many cases, PVCs are followed by a compensatory pause. (See *Compensatory pause*.)

PVCs may be uniform in appearance, arising from a single ectopic ventricular pacemaker site, or multiform, originating

---

Recognizing PVCs

To help you recognize premature ventricular contraction (PVC), review this sample rhythm strip. On this strip, PVC occurs on beats 1, 6, and 11.

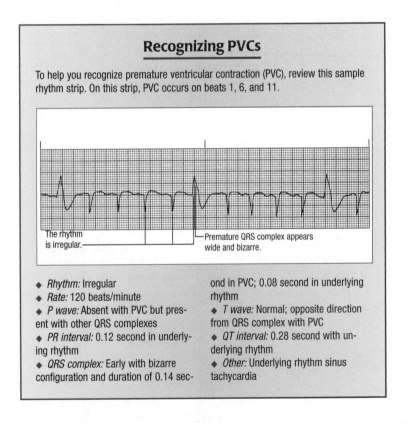

The rhythm is irregular.

Premature QRS complex appears wide and bizarre.

◆ *Rhythm:* Irregular
◆ *Rate:* 120 beats/minute
◆ *P wave:* Absent with PVC but present with other QRS complexes
◆ *PR interval:* 0.12 second in underlying rhythm
◆ *QRS complex:* Early with bizarre configuration and duration of 0.14 second in PVC; 0.08 second in underlying rhythm
◆ *T wave:* Normal; opposite direction from QRS complex with PVC
◆ *QT interval:* 0.28 second with underlying rhythm
◆ *Other:* Underlying rhythm sinus tachycardia

Compensatory pause

You can determine if a compensatory pause exists by using calipers to mark off two normal P-P intervals. Place one leg of the calipers on the sinus P wave that comes just before the PVC. If the pause is compensatory, the other leg of the calipers will fall precisely on the P wave that comes after the pause.

from different sites or originating from a single pacemaker site but having QRS complexes that differ in size, shape, and direction. PVCs may also be described as unifocal or multifocal. Unifocal PVCs originate from the same ventricular ectopic pacemaker site, whereas multifocal PVCs originate from different ectopic pacemaker sites in the ventricles.

Causes

PVCs are usually caused by enhanced automaticity in the ventricular conduction system or muscle tissue. The irritable focus results from a disruption of the normal electrolyte shifts during cellular depolarization and repolarization. Possible causes of PVCs include:
◆ anesthetics
◆ electrolyte imbalances, such as hypokalemia, hyperkalemia, hypomagnesemia, and hypocalcemia
◆ enlargement or hypertrophy of the ventricular chambers
◆ hypoxia

◆ increased sympathetic stimulation
◆ infection
◆ irritation of the ventricles by pacemaker electrodes or a pulmonary artery catheter
◆ metabolic acidosis
◆ mitral valve prolapse
◆ myocardial ischemia and infarction
◆ myocarditis
◆ sympathomimetic drugs, such as epinephrine and isoproterenol
◆ tobacco use
◆ caffeine or alcohol ingestion
◆ drug intoxication, particularly with cocaine, amphetamines, digoxin (Lanoxin), phenothiazines, and tricyclic antidepressants.

Clinical significance

PVCs are significant for two reasons. First, they can lead to more serious arrhythmias, such as VT or VF. The risk of developing a more serious arrhythmia increases in patients with ischemic or damaged hearts.

PVCs also decrease cardiac output, especially if ectopic beats are frequent or sustained. The decrease in cardiac output with a PVC stems from reduced ventricular diastolic filling time and the loss of atrial kick for that beat. The clinical impact of PVCs hinges on the body's ability to maintain adequate perfusion and the duration of the abnormal rhythm.

To help determine the seriousness of PVCs, ask these questions:

◆ How often do they occur? In patients with chronic PVCs, an increase in frequency or a change in the pattern of PVCs from the baseline rhythm may signal a more serious condition.

◆ What's the pattern of PVCs? If the ECG shows a dangerous pattern—such as paired PVCs, PVCs with more than one focus, a bigeminal rhythm, or R-on-T phenomenon (when a PVC strikes on the down slope of the preceding normal T wave)—the patient may require immediate treatment. (See *Patterns of potentially dangerous PVCs*.)

◆ Are they really PVCs? Make sure the complex is a PVC, not another, less dangerous arrhythmia. PVCs may be mistaken for ventricular escape beats or normal impulses with aberrant ventricular conduction. Ventricular escape beats serve as a safety

mechanism to protect the heart from ventricular standstill. Some supraventricular impulses may follow an abnormal (aberrant) conduction pathway causing an abnormal appearance to the QRS complex. In any event, never delay treatment if the patient is unstable.

ECG characteristics

◆ *Rhythm:* Atrial and ventricular rhythms are irregular during PVCs; the underlying rhythm may be regular.

◆ *Rate:* Atrial and ventricular rates reflect the underlying rhythm.

◆ *P wave:* Usually absent in the ectopic beat, but with retrograde conduction to the atria, the P wave may appear after the QRS complex. It's usually normal if present in the underlying rhythm.

◆ *PR interval:* Not measurable except in the underlying rhythm.

◆ *QRS complex:* Occurrence is earlier than expected. Duration exceeds 0.12 second, with a bizarre and wide configuration. Configuration of the QRS complex is usually normal in the underlying rhythm.

◆ *T wave:* Occurrence is in opposite direction to the QRS complex. When a PVC strikes on the downslope of the preceding normal T wave—the R-on-T phe-

Patterns of potentially dangerous PVCs

Some premature ventricular contractions (PVCs) are more dangerous than others. Here are examples of patterns of potentially dangerous PVCs.

Paired PVCs
Two PVCs in a row, called *paired PVCs* or a *ventricular couplet* (see shaded areas), can produce ventricular tachycardia (VT). That's because the second contraction usually meets refractory tissue. A burst, or a *salvo*, of three or more PVCs in a row is considered a run of VT.

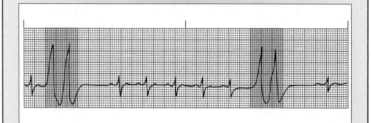

Multiform PVCs
Multiform PVCs, which look different from one another, arise from different sites or from the same site with abnormal conduction (see shaded areas). Multiform PVCs may indicate severe heart disease or digoxin toxicity.

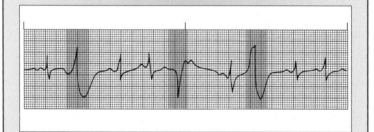

Bigeminy and trigeminy
PVCs that occur every other beat (*bigeminy*) or every third beat (*trigeminy*) may indicate increased ventricular irritability, which can result in VT or ventricular fibrillation (see shaded areas). The rhythm strip shown at the top of the next page illustrates ventricular bigeminy.

(continued)

Patterns of potentially dangerous PVCs *(continued)*

Bigeminy and trigeminy *(continued)*

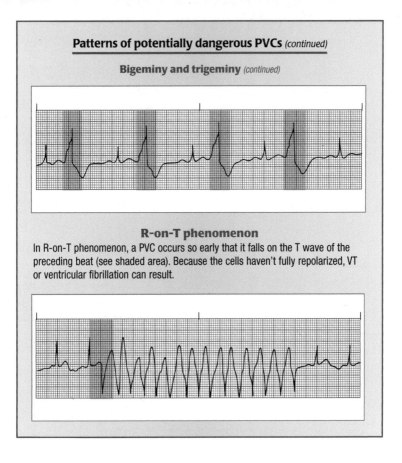

R-on-T phenomenon

In R-on-T phenomenon, a PVC occurs so early that it falls on the T wave of the preceding beat (see shaded area). Because the cells haven't fully repolarized, VT or ventricular fibrillation can result.

nomenon—it can trigger more serious rhythm disturbances such as ventricular fibrillation.

◆ *QT interval:* Not usually measured, except in the underlying rhythm.

◆ *Other:* A PVC may be followed by a compensatory pause, which can be full or incomplete. The sum of a full compensatory pause and the preceding R-R interval is equal to the sum of two R-R intervals of the underlying rhythm. If the sinoatrial (SA) node is depolarized by the PVC, the timing of the SA node is reset, and the compensatory pause is called incomplete. In this case, the sum of an incomplete compensatory pause and the preceding R-R interval is less than the sum of two R-R intervals of the underlying rhythm. A PVC occurring between two normally conducted QRS complexes without greatly disturbing the underlying rhythm is referred to as interpolated. A full compensatory pause, usually accompanying PVCs, is absent with interpolated PVCs.

Sometimes it's difficult to distinguish PVCs from aberrant ventricular conduction. (See *Distinguishing PVCs from ventricular aberrancy,* pages 160 and 161.)

Signs and symptoms

The patient experiencing PVCs usually has a normal pulse rate with a momentarily irregular pulse rhythm when a PVC occurs.

With PVCs, the patient has a weaker pulse wave after the premature beat and a longer-than-normal pause between pulse waves. If the carotid pulse is visible, however, you may see a weaker arterial wave after the premature beat. When auscultating for heart sounds, you hear an abnormally early heart sound with each PVC.

A patient with PVCs may be asymptomatic; however, patients with frequent PVCs may complain of palpitations. The patient may also exhibit signs and symptoms of decreased cardiac output, including hypotension and syncope.

Interventions

If the PVCs are infrequent and the patient has normal heart function and is asymptomatic, the arrhythmia probably doesn't require treatment. If symptoms or a dangerous form of PVCs occur, the type of treatment given depends on the cause of the problem.

If PVCs have a purely cardiac origin, drugs to suppress ventricular irritability, such as procainamide (Procan), amiodarone (Cordarone), or lidocaine, may be used. When PVCs have a noncardiac origin, treatment is aimed at correcting the cause. For example, drug therapy may be adjusted or the patient's acidosis or electrolyte imbalance may be corrected.

Patients who have recently developed PVCs need prompt assessment, especially if they have underlying heart disease or complex medical problems. Patients with chronic PVCs should be closely observed for the development of more frequent PVCs or more dangerous PVC patterns.

Until effective treatment is begun, patients with PVCs accompanied by serious symptoms should have continuous ECG monitoring and ambulate only with assistance. If the patient is discharged on antiarrhythmic medications, family members should know how to contact the

(Text continues on page 162.)

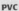 **LOOK-ALIKES**

Distinguishing PVCs from ventricular aberrancy

Perhaps one of the most challenging look-alikes—premature ventricular contractions (PVCs) versus ventricular aberrancy—can sometimes be distinguished with complete confidence only in the electrophysiology laboratory. Ventricular aberrancy, or aberrant ventricular conduction, occurs when an electrical impulse originating in the sinoatrial node, atria, or atrioventricular junction is temporarily conducted abnormally through the bundle branches.

The abnormal conduction results in a bundle-branch block and usually stems from the arrival of electrical impulses at the bundle branches before the branches have been sufficiently repolarized.

To distinguish between PVCs and ventricular aberrancy, examine the deflection of the QRS complex in lead V_1. Determine whether the QRS complex is primarily positive or negative. Based on this information, follow these clues to guide your analysis.

Mostly positive QRS

◆ Right bundle-branch aberrancy has a triphasic rSR′ configuration in V_1 and a triphasic qRS configuration in V_6.
◆ If there are two positive peaks in V_1 and the left peak is taller, the beat is probably a PVC.
◆ PVCs are monophasic or biphasic in V_1, and biphasic in V_6, with a deep S wave.

Comparing PVC with right bundle-branch aberrancy

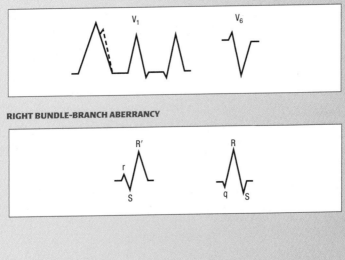

PVC

RIGHT BUNDLE-BRANCH ABERRANCY

Mostly negative QRS

◆ Left bundle-branch aberrancy has a narrow R wave with a quick downstroke in leads V_1 and V_2, with no Q wave in V_6.

◆ PVCs have a wide R wave (> 0.03 second) and a notched or slurred S-wave downstroke in leads V_1 and V_2, with a duration of > 0.06 second from the onset of the R wave to the deepest point of the S wave in V_1 and V_2, with a Q wave in V_6.

◆ P waves commonly precede aberrancies, but don't generally precede PVCs.

◆ Aberrancies usually have a QRS duration of 0.12 second. PVCs are more likely to have a QRS duration of 0.14 second or more.

Comparing PVC with left bundle-branch aberrancy

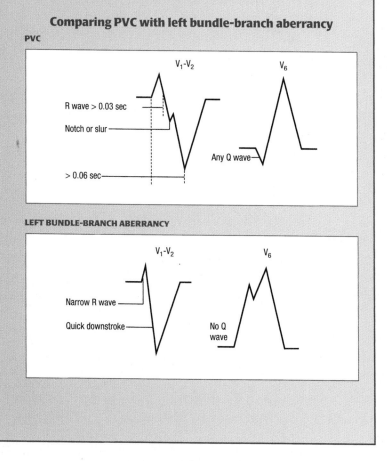

PVC

V₁-V₂   V₆

R wave > 0.03 sec

Notch or slur

Any Q wave

> 0.06 sec

LEFT BUNDLE-BRANCH ABERRANCY

V₁-V₂   V₆

Narrow R wave

Quick downstroke

No Q wave

emergency medical system and perform cardiopulmonary resuscitation (CPR).

⧅LIFE-THREATENING

Idioventricular rhythm

Idioventricular rhythm, also referred to as *ventricular escape rhythm,* originates in an escape pacemaker site in the ventricles. The inherent firing rate of this ectopic pacemaker is usually 20 to 40 beats/minute. The rhythm acts as a safety mechanism by preventing ventricular standstill, or asystole—the absence of electrical activity in the ventricles. When fewer than three QRS complexes arising from the escape pacemaker occur, they're called *ventricular escape beats* or *complexes.* (See *Recognizing idioventricular rhythm.*)

When the rate of an ectopic pacemaker site in the ventricles is less than 100 beats/minute but exceeds the inherent ventricular escape rate of 20 to 40 beats/minute, it's called *accelerated idioventricular rhythm* (AIVR). (See *Recognizing AIVR.*) The rate of AIVR isn't fast enough to be considered VT. The rhythm is usually related to enhanced automaticity of the ventricular tissue. AIVR and idioventricular rhythm share the same ECG characteristics, differing only in heart rate.

Causes

Idioventricular rhythms occur when all of the heart's higher pacemakers fail to function or when supraventricular impulses can't reach the ventricles because of a block in the conduction system. Idioventricular rhythms may accompany third-degree heart block. Possible causes of the rhythm include:
◆ myocardial ischemia
◆ myocardial infarction (MI)
◆ digoxin toxicity, beta-adrenergic blockers, calcium antagonists, and tricyclic antidepressants
◆ pacemaker failure
◆ metabolic imbalances
◆ sick sinus syndrome
◆ successful reperfusion therapy.

Clinical significance

Idioventricular rhythm may be transient or continuous. Transient ventricular escape rhythm is usually related to increased parasympathetic effect on the higher pacemaker sites and isn't generally clinically significant. Although idioventricular rhythms act to protect the heart from ventricular standstill, a continuous idioventricular rhythm presents a clinically serious situation.

The slow ventricular rate of this arrhythmia and the associated loss of atrial kick markedly reduce cardiac output. If not rapidly identified and appropriately

Recognizing idioventricular rhythm

To help you recognize idioventricular rhythm, review this sample rhythm strip.

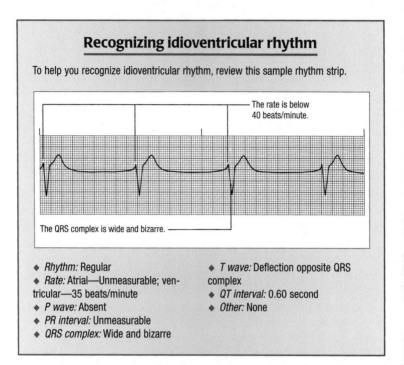

The rate is below 40 beats/minute.

The QRS complex is wide and bizarre.

- *Rhythm:* Regular
- *Rate:* Atrial—Unmeasurable; ventricular—35 beats/minute
- *P wave:* Absent
- *PR interval:* Unmeasurable
- *QRS complex:* Wide and bizarre

- *T wave:* Deflection opposite QRS complex
- *QT interval:* 0.60 second
- *Other:* None

Recognizing AIVR

An accelerated idioventricular rhythm (AIVR) has the same characteristics as an idioventricular rhythm except that it's faster. The rate shown here varies between 40 and 100 beats/minute.

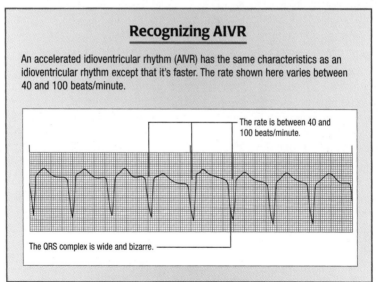

The rate is between 40 and 100 beats/minute.

The QRS complex is wide and bizarre.

managed, idioventricular arrhythmias can cause death.

ECG characteristics

◆ *Rhythm:* Usually, atrial rhythm can't be determined. Ventricular rhythm is usually regular.
◆ *Rate:* Usually, atrial rate can't be determined. Ventricular rate is 20 to 40 beats/minute.
◆ *P wave:* Absent.
◆ *PR interval:* Not measurable because of the absent P wave.
◆ *QRS complex:* Because of abnormal ventricular depolarization, the QRS complex has a duration longer than 0.12 second, with a wide and bizarre configuration.
◆ *T wave:* The T wave is abnormal. Deflection usually occurs in the opposite direction from that of the QRS complex.
◆ *QT interval:* Usually prolonged.
◆ *Other:* Idioventricular rhythm commonly occurs with third-degree atrioventricular block.

Signs and symptoms

The patient with continuous idioventricular rhythm is generally symptomatic because of the marked reduction in cardiac output that occurs with the arrhythmia. Blood pressure may be difficult or impossible to auscultate or palpate. The patient may experience dizziness, light-headedness, syncope, or loss of consciousness.

Interventions

Treatment should be initiated immediately to increase the patient's heart rate, improve cardiac output, and establish a normal rhythm. Atropine may be administered to increase the heart rate.

If atropine isn't effective or if the patient develops hypotension or other signs of clinical instability, a pacemaker may be needed to reestablish a heart rate that provides enough cardiac output to perfuse organs properly. A transcutaneous pacemaker may be used in an emergency until a temporary or transvenous pacemaker can be inserted. (See *Transcutaneous pacemaker.*)

Remember that the goal of treatment doesn't include suppressing the idioventricular rhythm because it acts as a safety mechanism to protect the heart from ventricular standstill. Idioventricular rhythm should never be treated with lidocaine or other antiarrhythmics that would suppress the escape beats.

Patients with idioventricular rhythm need continuous ECG monitoring and constant assessment until treatment restores hemodynamic stability. Keep atropine and pacemaker equipment

Transcutaneous pacemaker

Transcutaneous pacing, also referred to as *external pacing* or *noninvasive pacing*, involves the delivery of electrical impulses through externally applied cutaneous electrodes. The electrical impulses are conducted through an intact chest wall using skin electrodes placed either in anterior-posterior or sternal-apex positions. (An anterior-posterior placement is shown here.)

Transcutaneous pacing is the initial pacing method of choice in emergency situations because it's the least invasive technique and can be instituted quickly.

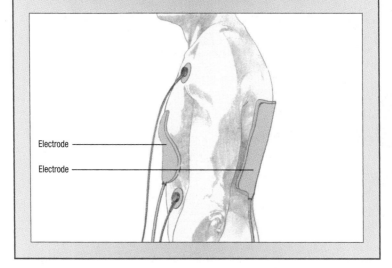

Electrode

Electrode

available at the bedside. Enforce bed rest until an effective heart rate has been maintained and the patient is clinically stable.

Tell the patient and his family about the serious nature of this arrhythmia and the treatment it requires. If the patient needs a permanent pacemaker, teach the patient and his family how it works, how to recognize problems, when to contact the practitioner, and how pacemaker function is monitored.

⧰ LIFE-THREATENING

Ventricular tachycardia

Ventricular tachycardia, also called *V-tach* or *VT,* occurs when three or more PVCs strike in a row and the ventricular rate exceeds 100 beats/minute. This life-threatening arrhythmia may precede VF and sudden cardiac death, especially in patients who aren't in a health care facility.

Recognizing VT

To help you recognize ventricular tachycardia (VT), review this sample rhythm strip.

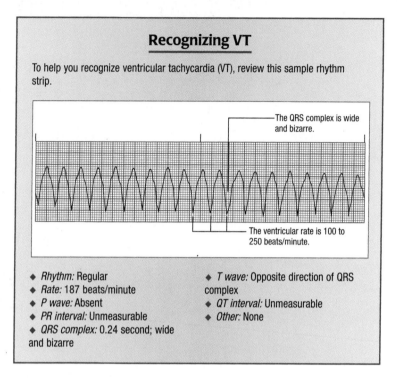

The QRS complex is wide and bizarre.

The ventricular rate is 100 to 250 beats/minute.

◆ *Rhythm:* Regular
◆ *Rate:* 187 beats/minute
◆ *P wave:* Absent
◆ *PR interval:* Unmeasurable
◆ *QRS complex:* 0.24 second; wide and bizarre

◆ *T wave:* Opposite direction of QRS complex
◆ *QT interval:* Unmeasurable
◆ *Other:* None

VT is an extremely unstable rhythm and may be sustained or nonsustained. When it occurs in short, paroxysmal bursts lasting less than 30 seconds and causing few or no symptoms, it's called *nonsustained.* When the rhythm is sustained, however, it requires immediate treatment to prevent death, even in patients initially able to maintain adequate cardiac output. (See *Recognizing VT.*)

Causes

This arrhythmia usually results from increased myocardial irritability, which may be triggered by enhanced automaticity, reentry within the Purkinje system, or by PVCs occurring during the downstroke of the preceding T wave.

Other causes of VT include:
◆ myocardial ischemia
◆ MI
◆ coronary artery disease (CAD)

◆ valvular heart disease
◆ heart failure
◆ cardiomyopathy
◆ electrolyte imbalances such as hypokalemia
◆ drug intoxication from digoxin, procainamide, quinidine, or cocaine
◆ proarrhythmic effects of some antiarrhythmics.

Clinical significance

VT is significant because of its unpredictability and potential for causing death. A patient may be hemodynamically stable, with a normal pulse and blood pressure; clinically unstable, with hypotension and poor peripheral pulses; or unconscious, without respirations or pulse.

Because of the reduced ventricular filling time and the drop in cardiac output that occurs with this arrhythmia, the patient's condition can quickly deteriorate to VF and complete cardiovascular collapse.

ECG characteristics

◆ *Rhythm:* Atrial rhythm can't be determined. Ventricular rhythm is usually regular but may be slightly irregular.

◆ *Rate:* Atrial rate can't be determined. Ventricular rate is usually rapid (100 to 250 beats/minute).
◆ *P wave:* The P wave is usually absent. It may be obscured by the QRS complex; P waves are dissociated from the QRS complexes. Retrograde P waves may be present.
◆ *PR interval:* Not measurable because the P wave can't be seen in most cases.
◆ *QRS complex:* Duration is greater than 0.12 second; it usually has a bizarre appearance with increased amplitude. QRS complexes in monomorphic VT have a uniform shape. In polymorphic VT, the shape of the QRS complex constantly changes.
◆ *T wave:* If the T wave is visible, it occurs in the opposite direction of the QRS complex.
◆ *QT interval:* Not measurable.
◆ *Other:* Ventricular flutter and torsades de pointes are two variations of this arrhythmia. Torsades de pointes is a special variation of polymorphic VT. (See *Recognizing torsades de pointes,* page 168.) Although a relatively rare occurrence, torsades de pointes is sometimes difficult to distinguish from ventricular flutter. (See *Distinguishing ventricular flutter from torsades de pointes,* page 169.)

Recognizing torsades de pointes

Torsades de pointes, which means "twisting about the points," is a special form of polymorphic ventricular tachycardia (VT). The hallmark characteristics of this rhythm, shown below, are QRS complexes that rotate about the baseline, deflecting downward and upward for several beats.

The rate is 150 to 250 beats/minute, usually with an irregular rhythm, and the QRS complexes are wide with changing amplitude. The P wave is usually absent.

Paroxysmal rhythm

This arrhythmia may be paroxysmal, starting and stopping suddenly, and may deteriorate into ventricular fibrillation. It should be considered when VT doesn't respond to antiarrhythmic therapy or other treatments.

Reversible causes

The cause of this form of VT is usually reversible. The most common causes are drugs that lengthen the QT interval, such as amiodarone, ibutilide, erythromycin, haloperidol, droperidol, and sotalol. Other causes include myocardial ischemia and electrolyte abnormalities, such as hypokalemia, hypomagnesemia, and hypocalcemia.

Going into overdrive

Torsades de pointes is treated by correcting the underlying cause, especially if the cause is related to specific drug therapy. The practitioner may order mechanical overdrive pacing, which overrides the ventricular rate and breaks the triggered mechanism for the arrhythmia. Magnesium sulfate may also be effective. Electrical cardioversion may be used when torsades de pointes doesn't respond to other treatment.

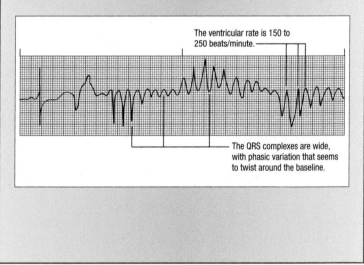

The ventricular rate is 150 to 250 beats/minute.

The QRS complexes are wide, with phasic variation that seems to twist around the baseline.

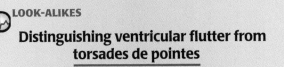

LOOK-ALIKES

Distinguishing ventricular flutter from torsades de pointes

Torsades de pointes is a variant form of ventricular tachycardia, with a rapid ventricular rate that varies between 250 and 350 beats/minute. It's characterized by QRS complexes that gradually change back and forth, with the amplitude of each successive complex gradually increasing and decreasing. These changes result in an overall outline of the rhythm commonly described as *spindle-shaped*.

Ventricular flutter, although rarely recognized, results from the rapid, regular, repetitive beating of the ventricles. It's produced by a single ventricular focus firing at a rapid rate of 250 to 350 beats/minute. The hallmark of this arrhythmia is its smooth sine-wave appearance.

The illustrations shown here highlight key differences in the two arrhythmias.

Ventricular flutter

◆ Smooth, sine-wave appearance

Torsades de pointes

◆ Spindle-shaped appearance

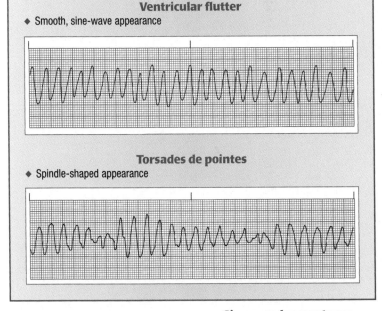

Sometimes distinguishing VT from supraventricular tachycardia (SVT) can be extremely challenging, especially in the setting of aberrant ventricular conduction. (See *Distinguishing VT from SVT*, pages 170 and 171.)

Signs and symptoms

Although some patients have only minor symptoms initially, they still require rapid intervention to prevent cardiovascular collapse. Most patients with VT

(Text continues on page 172.)

LOOK-ALIKES

Distinguishing VT from SVT

Differentiating ventricular tachycardia (VT) from supraventricular tachycardia (SVT) with aberrancy is difficult. Careful assessment of a 12-lead ECG or rhythm strip can help you differentiate the arrhythmia with 90% accuracy.

Begin by looking at the deflection—negative or positive. Then use these illustrations to guide your assessment. If the QRS complex is wide and mostly negative in deflection in V_1 or MCL_1, use these clues.

VENTRICULAR TACHYCARDIA
◆ If the QRS complex has an R wave $\geq$ 0.04 second, a slurred S (shown below, shaded), or a notched S (shown at right) on the downstroke, suspect VT.

SUPRAVENTRICULAR TACHYCARDIA
◆ If the QRS complex has an R wave $\leq$ 0.04 second and a swift, straight S on the downstroke (shown below, shaded, and at right), suspect SVT with aberrancy.

If the QRS complex is wide and mostly positive in deflection in V_1 or MCL_1, use these clues.

VENTRICULAR TACHYCARDIA
◆ If the QRS complex is biphasic, suspect VT.

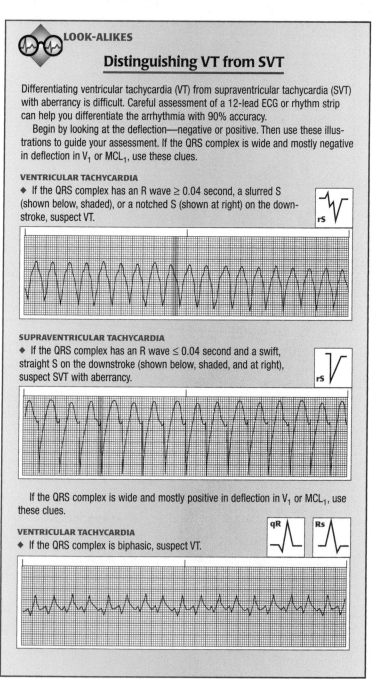

Distinguishing VT from SVT *(continued)*

SUPRAVENTRICULAR TACHYCARDIA
◆ If the beat is triphasic, similar to a right bundle-branch block, suspect SVT with aberrancy.

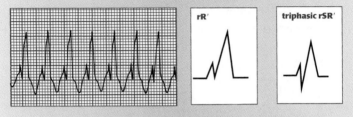

Here are additional clues you can use if the QRS complex is wide and mostly positive in deflection in lead V_1 or MCL_1.

If the QRS complex is tall and shaped like rabbit ears, with the left peak taller than the right, suspect VT.	If the QRS complex is monophasic, suspect VT.	If you still have difficulty differentiating the rhythm, look at V_6 or MCL_6. If the S wave is larger than the R wave, suspect VT.	If any Q wave is present, suspect VT.

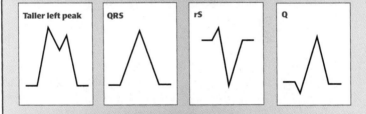

Other general criteria can also help you differentiate VT from SVT with aberrancy.
◆ A QRS complex > 0.14 second suggests VT.
◆ A regular, wide, complex rhythm suggests VT.
◆ An irregular, wide, complex rhythm suggests SVT with aberrancy.
◆ Concordant V leads (the QRS complex either mainly positive or mainly negative in all V leads) suggest VT.
◆ Atrioventricular dissociation suggests VT.

have weak or absent pulses. Low cardiac output causes hypotension and a decreased level of consciousness (LOC), quickly leading to unresponsiveness if left untreated. VT may prompt angina, heart failure, or a substantial decrease in organ perfusion.

Interventions

Treatment depends on the patient's clinical status. Is the patient conscious? Does the patient have spontaneous respirations? Is a palpable carotid pulse present?

Patients with pulseless VT are treated the same as those with VF and require immediate defibrillation and CPR. Treatment for patients with a detectable pulse depends on whether they're unstable or stable.

Unstable patients generally have ventricular rates greater than 150 beats/minute and have serious signs and symptoms related to the tachycardia, which may include hypotension, shortness of breath, chest pain, or altered LOC. These patients are usually treated with immediate synchronized cardioversion.

Treatment for a clinically stable patient with VT and no signs of heart failure depends on whether the rhythm is regular or irregular. If the rhythm is regular (monomorphic), the patient is

treated with amiodarone and possible synchronized cardioversion. If the rate is irregular (polymorphic), look at the length of the T interval during periods of normal sinus rhythm. If the QT interval is long, the polymorphic rhythm is most likely torsades de pointes. The treatment for polymorphic VT is to stop medications that may cause a long QT, correct electrolyte imbalances, and administer antiarrhythmics, such as magnesium or amiodarone. If at any point the patient becomes clinically unstable, immediate synchronized cardioversion is the best treatment.

Patients with VT or VF that doesn't result from a transient or reversible cause may need an implanted cardioverter-defibrillator (ICD). This device is a permanent solution to recurrent episodes of VT.

A 12-lead ECG and all other available clinical information are critical for establishing a specific diagnosis in a stable patient with wide QRS complex tachycardia of unknown type but regular rate. If a definitive diagnosis of SVT or VT can't be established, use amiodarone to control the rate and elective synchronized cardioversion.

Teach the patient and his family about the serious nature of this arrhythmia and the need for prompt treatment. If the patient is stable and is undergoing electrical cardioversion, inform him that he'll receive a sedative, and possibly an analgesic, before the procedure.

If a patient will be discharged with an ICD or a prescription for long-term antiarrhythmics, make sure family members know when and how to seek emergency medical care and how to perform CPR.

⚡LIFE-THREATENING

Ventricular fibrillation

Ventricular fibrillation, commonly called *V-fib* or *VF,* is characterized by a chaotic, disorganized pattern of electrical activity. The pattern arises from electrical impulses coming from multiple ectopic pacemakers in the ventricles.

The arrhythmia produces no effective ventricular mechanical activity or contractions and no cardiac output. Untreated VF is the most common cause of sudden cardiac death in people outside of a health care facility. (See *Recognizing VF,* page 174.)

Causes

Causes of VF include:
◆ CAD
◆ myocardial ischemia
◆ MI

◆ untreated VT
◆ underlying heart disease such as dilated cardiomyopathy
◆ acid-base imbalance
◆ electric shock
◆ severe hypothermia
◆ drug toxicity, including digoxin, quinidine, and procainamide
◆ electrolyte imbalances, such as hypokalemia, hyperkalemia, and hypercalcemia
◆ severe hypoxia.

Clinical significance

With VF, the ventricular muscle quivers, replacing effective muscular contraction with completely ineffective contraction. Cardiac output falls to zero and, if allowed to continue, leads to ventricular standstill and death.

ECG characteristics

◆ *Rhythm:* Atrial rhythm can't be determined. Ventricular rhythm has no pattern or regularity. Ventricular electrical activity appears as fibrillatory waves with no recognizable pattern.
◆ *Rate:* Atrial and ventricular rates can't be determined.
◆ *P wave:* Can't be determined.
◆ *PR interval:* Can't be determined.
◆ *QRS complex:* Duration can't be determined.
◆ *T wave:* Can't be determined.
◆ *QT interval*: Not applicable.

Recognizing VF

To help you recognize ventricular fibrillation (VF), review these sample rhythm strips. The first strip illustrates coarse VF. The second strip illustrates fine VF.

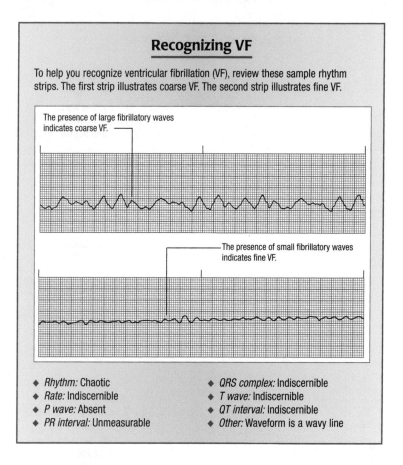

The presence of large fibrillatory waves indicates coarse VF.

The presence of small fibrillatory waves indicates fine VF.

- ◆ *Rhythm:* Chaotic
- ◆ *Rate:* Indiscernible
- ◆ *P wave:* Absent
- ◆ *PR interval:* Unmeasurable
- ◆ *QRS complex:* Indiscernible
- ◆ *T wave:* Indiscernible
- ◆ *QT interval:* Indiscernible
- ◆ *Other:* Waveform is a wavy line

◆ *Other:* Coarse fibrillatory waves are generally associated with greater chances of successful electrical defibrillation than smaller amplitude waves. Fibrillatory waves become finer as hypoxemia and acidosis progress, making the VF more resistant to defibrillation.

Signs and symptoms

The patient in VF is in full cardiac arrest, unresponsive, and without a detectable blood pressure or central pulses. Whenever you see an ECG pattern resembling VF, check the patient immediately and initiate definitive treatment.

Understanding defibrillation

In defibrillation, two electrode pads are applied to the chest wall: one to the right of the upper sternum and one over the fifth or sixth intercostal space at the left anterior axillary line. Current is then directed through the pads and, subsequently, the patient's chest and heart. (During cardiac surgery, internal paddles are placed directly on the myocardium.) The current causes the myocardium to completely depolarize, which, in turn, encourages the sinoatrial node to resume normal control of the heart's electrical activity.

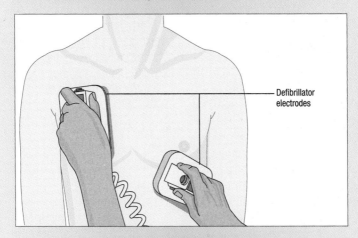

Defibrillator electrodes

Automated external defibrillators

Automated external defibrillators (AEDs) are typically used outside of the hospital setting to provide early defibrillation. AEDs vary with the manufacturer, but the basic components of each device are similar. After a patient is confirmed to be unresponsive, breathless, and pulseless, the AED power is turned on and the electrode pads and cables are attached. The AED can analyze the patient's cardiac rhythm and provide the caregiver with step-by-step instructions on how to proceed. These defibrillators can be used by people without medical training as long as they're instructed in the proper use of the device.

Interventions

When faced with a rhythm that appears to be VF, always assess the patient first. Other events can mimic VF on an ECG strip, including interference from an elec-tric razor, shivering, or seizure activity.

For the patient in VF, successful resuscitation requires rapid recognition of the problem and prompt defibrillation. Many health care facilities and emergency medical systems have established protocols allowing health care workers to initiate prompt treatment. Make sure you know the location of your facility's emergency equipment, and that you know how to use it. Keep in mind that CPR must be performed until the defibrillator arrives to preserve oxygen supply to the brain and other vital organs. (See *Understanding defibrillation,* page 175.)

Drugs such as epinephrine and vasopressin may be used for persistent VF if the first two attempts at electrical defibrillation fail to correct the arrhythmia. Antiarrhythmic agents, such as amiodarone, lidocaine, and magnesium, may also be considered.

Teach the patient and his family how to use the emergency medical system following discharge from the facility. Family members may need instruction in CPR and in how to use an automated external defibrillator. Teach them about long-term therapies that help prevent recurrent episodes of VF, including antiarrhythmic drug therapy and ICDs.

LIFE-THREATENING

Asystole

Ventricular asystole, also called *asystole* and *ventricular standstill,* is the absence of discernible electrical activity in the ventricles. Although some electrical activity may be evident in the atria, these impulses aren't conducted to the ventricles. (See *Recognizing asystole.*)

Asystole usually results from a prolonged period of cardiac arrest without effective resuscitation. It's important to distinguish asystole from fine ventricular fibrillation, which is managed differently. Therefore, asystole must be confirmed in more than one ECG lead.

Causes

Possible reversible causes of asystole include:
◆ hypovolemia
◆ MI (coronary thrombosis)
◆ severe electrolyte disturbances, especially hyperkalemia and hypokalemia
◆ massive pulmonary embolism
◆ hypoxia
◆ severe, uncorrected acid-base disturbances, especially metabolic acidosis
◆ drug overdose
◆ hypothermia
◆ cardiac tamponade
◆ tension pneumothorax.

Clinical significance

Without ventricular electrical activity, ventricular contractions can't occur. As a result, cardiac

Recognizing asystole

To help you recognize asystole—the absence of electrical activity in the ventricles—review this sample rhythm strip. Except for a few P waves or pacer spikes, nothing appears on the waveform and the line is almost flat.

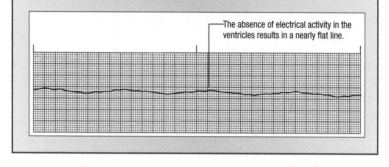

The absence of electrical activity in the ventricles results in a nearly flat line.

output drops to zero and vital organs are no longer perfused. Asystole has been called the *arrhythmia of death* and is typically considered to be a confirmation of death, rather than an arrhythmia to be treated.

The patient with asystole is completely unresponsive, without spontaneous respirations or a pulse (cardiopulmonary arrest). Without immediate initiation of CPR and rapid identification and treatment of the underlying cause, the condition quickly becomes irreversible.

ECG characteristics

◆ *Rhythm:* Atrial rhythm is usually indiscernible; no ventricular rhythm is present.

◆ *Rate:* Atrial rate is usually indiscernible; no ventricular rate is present.
◆ *P wave:* May be present.
◆ *PR interval:* Not measurable.
◆ *QRS complex:* Absent or occasional escape beats.
◆ *T wave:* Absent.
◆ *QT interval:* Not measurable.
◆ *Other:* On a rhythm strip, asystole looks like a nearly flat line (except for changes caused by chest compressions during CPR). In a patient with a pacemaker, pacer spikes may be evident on the strip but no P wave or QRS complex occurs in response to the stimulus.

Signs and symptoms

The patient is unresponsive and has no spontaneous respirations,

Understanding pulseless electrical activity

Pulseless electrical activity (PEA) defines a group of arrhythmias characterized by the presence of some type of electrical activity without a detectable pulse. Although organized electrical depolarization occurs, no synchronous shortening of the myocardial fibers occurs. As a result, no mechanical activity or contractions take place.

Causes

The most common causes of PEA include hypovolemia, hypoxia, acidosis, tension pneumothorax, cardiac tamponade, massive pulmonary embolism, hypothermia, hyperkalemia and hypokalemia, massive acute myocardial infarction, and overdoses of drugs such as tricyclic antidepressants.

Treatment

Rapid identification and treatment of underlying reversible causes is critical for treating PEA. For example, hypovolemia is treated with volume expansion. Tension pneumothorax is treated with needle decompression.

Institute cardiopulmonary resuscitation, tracheal intubation, and I.V. administration of epinephrine or atropine.

---

discernible pulse, or blood pressure.

Interventions

Immediate treatment includes CPR along with the administration of supplemental oxygen. I.V. or intraosseous epinephrine, or a onetime dose of vasopressin and atropine, may also be given. Resuscitation should be attempted unless otherwise indicated, such as when a do-not-resuscitate order is in effect.

Always verify asystole in more than one ECG lead. Priority must also be given to searching for and treating potentially reversible causes of asystole, such as hypovolemia, cardiac tamponade, and tension pneumothorax.

 ALERT Be aware that pulseless electrical activity can appear as any cardiac rhythm, including asystole. Know how to recognize this problem and treat it. (See Understanding pulseless electrical activity.)

If asystole persists despite appropriate interventions, consider terminating resuscitation.

Atrioventricular blocks

9

Atrioventricular (AV) heart block refers to an interruption or delay in the conduction of electrical impulses between the atria and the ventricles. The block can occur at the AV node, the bundle of His, or the bundle branches. When the site of the block is the bundle of His or the bundle branches, the block is referred to as *infranodal AV block*. AV block can be partial, where some or all of the P waves are conducted to the ventricle (first or second degree), or complete, where no P waves conduct to the ventricle (third degree).

The heart's electrical impulses normally originate in the sino-atrial (SA) node, so when those impulses are blocked at the AV node, atrial rates are usually normal (60 to 100 beats/minute). The clinical significance of the block depends on the number of impulses completely blocked and the resulting ventricular rate. A slow ventricular rate can decrease cardiac output and cause symptoms such as light-headedness, hypotension, and confusion.

Various factors may lead to AV block. Typical causes include:

◆ myocardial ischemia, which impairs cellular function and causes cells to conduct impulses slowly or inconsistently

◆ myocardial infarction (MI)

◆ excessive serum levels of, or an exaggerated response to, a drug (such as digoxin [Lanoxin], amiodarone [Cordarone], beta-adrenergic blockers, and calcium channel blockers), which may increase the refractory period of a portion of the conduction system

◆ lesions along the conduction pathway

◆ congenital anomalies that affect the conduction system (such as ventricular septal defects) as well as anomalies of the conduction system

◆ inadvertent damage to the heart's conduction system during cardiac surgery

◆ inadvertent damage to the conduction system during radiofrequency ablation.

AV blocks are classified according to the site of the block and the severity of the conduction abnormality. The sites of AV block include the AV node, bundle of His, and bundle branches. Severity of AV block is classified in degrees: first-degree AV block; second-degree AV block, type I (Wenckebach or Mobitz I); second-degree AV block, type II (Mobitz II) AV block; and third-degree (complete) AV block. The classification system for AV blocks aids in the determination of the patient's treatment and prognosis.

First-degree atrioventricular block

First-degree AV block occurs when the conduction of electrical impulses from the atria to the ventricles is delayed. This delay usually occurs at the level of the AV node, or bundle of His. After being delayed, the impulse is conducted through the normal conduction pathway.

First-degree AV block is characterized by a PR interval greater than 0.20 second. This interval remains constant beat to beat.

Causes

First-degree AV block may result from myocardial ischemia or MI, myocarditis, hyperkalemia, rheumatic fever, or degenerative changes in the heart associated with aging. The condition may also result from the toxic effects of drugs, such as digoxin, calcium channel blockers, and beta-adrenergic blockers.

Clinical significance

First-degree block, the least dangerous type of AV block, indicates a delay in the conduction of electrical impulses through the normal conduction pathway. In general, a rhythm strip with this block looks like normal sinus rhythm except that the PR interval is longer than normal.

First-degree AV block may cause no symptoms in a healthy person. The arrhythmia may be transient, especially if it occurs secondary to drugs or ischemia early in the course of an MI.

Because first-degree AV block can progress to a more severe type of AV block, the patient's cardiac rhythm should be monitored for changes. (See *Recognizing first-degree AV block*.)

Recognizing first-degree AV block

To help you recognize first-degree atrioventricular (AV) block, review this sample rhythm strip.

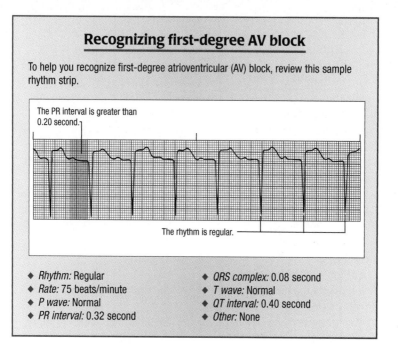

The PR interval is greater than 0.20 second.

The rhythm is regular.

◆ *Rhythm:* Regular
◆ *Rate:* 75 beats/minute
◆ *P wave:* Normal
◆ *PR interval:* 0.32 second

◆ *QRS complex:* 0.08 second
◆ *T wave:* Normal
◆ *QT interval:* 0.40 second
◆ *Other:* None

ECG characteristics

◆ *Rhythm:* Atrial and ventricular rhythms are regular.
◆ *Rate:* Atrial and ventricular rates are the same and within normal limits.
◆ *P wave:* Normal size and configuration; each P wave followed by a QRS complex.
◆ *PR interval:* Prolonged (greater than 0.20 second) but constant.
◆ *QRS complex:* Duration usually remains within normal limits if the conduction delay occurs in the AV node. If the QRS duration exceeds 0.12 second, the conduction delay may be in the His-Purkinje system.

◆ *T wave:* Normal size and configuration unless the QRS complex is prolonged.
◆ *QT interval:* Usually within normal limits.
◆ *Other:* None.

Signs and symptoms

The patient's pulse rate is usually normal and the rhythm is regular. Most patients with first-degree AV block are asymptomatic because cardiac output isn't significantly affected. If the PR interval is extremely long, a longer interval between the first heart sound and the second heart sound may be noted on cardiac auscultation.

Interventions

Treatment generally focuses on identification and correction of the underlying cause. For example, if a drug is causing the AV block, the dosage may be reduced or the drug discontinued. Close monitoring can help detect progression of first-degree AV block to a more serious form of block.

Evaluate a patient with first-degree AV block for underlying causes that can be corrected, such as drugs or myocardial ischemia. Observe the ECG for progression of the block to a more severe form. Administer digoxin, calcium channel blockers, and beta-adrenergic blockers cautiously.

Type I second-degree AV block

Also called *Wenckebach* or *Mobitz I block,* type I second-degree AV block occurs when each successive impulse from the SA node is delayed slightly longer than the previous impulse. This pattern of progressive prolongation of the PR interval continues until an impulse fails to be conducted to the ventricles. (See *Recognizing type I second-degree AV block.*)

Usually, only a single impulse is blocked from reaching the ventricles. Following this nonconducted P wave or dropped beat, the pattern is repeated. This repetitive sequence of two or more consecutive beats followed by a dropped beat results in "group beating." Type I second-degree AV block generally occurs at the level of the AV node.

Causes

Type I second-degree AV block commonly results from increased parasympathetic tone or the effects of certain drugs. Coronary artery disease (CAD), inferior-wall MI, and rheumatic fever may increase parasympathetic tone and result in the arrhythmia. It may also be caused by cardiac medications, such as beta-adrenergic blockers, digoxin, and calcium channel blockers.

Clinical significance

Type I second-degree AV block may occur normally in an otherwise healthy person. Almost always transient, this type of block usually resolves when the underlying condition is corrected. Although an asymptomatic patient with this block has a good prognosis, the block may progress to

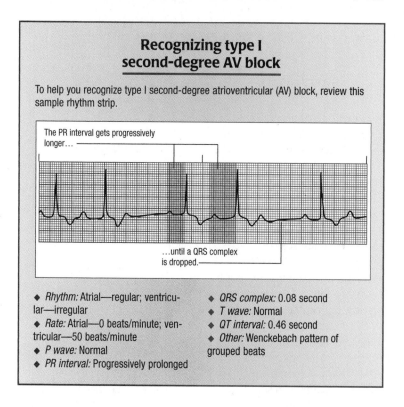

Recognizing type I second-degree AV block

To help you recognize type I second-degree atrioventricular (AV) block, review this sample rhythm strip.

The PR interval gets progressively longer...

...until a QRS complex is dropped.

◆ *Rhythm:* Atrial—regular; ventricular—irregular
◆ *Rate:* Atrial—0 beats/minute; ventricular—50 beats/minute
◆ *P wave:* Normal
◆ *PR interval:* Progressively prolonged

◆ *QRS complex:* 0.08 second
◆ *T wave:* Normal
◆ *QT interval:* 0.46 second
◆ *Other:* Wenckebach pattern of grouped beats

a more serious form, especially if it occurs early in an MI.

ECG characteristics

When you're trying to identify type I second-degree AV block, think of the phrase "long, longer, dropped," which describes the progressively prolonged PR intervals and the missing QRS complexes. The QRS complexes are usually normal because the delays occur in the AV node. (See *Rhythm strip patterns,* page 184.)

◆ *Rhythm:* Atrial rhythm is regular, and the ventricular rhythm is irregular. The R-R interval shortens progressively until a P wave appears without a QRS complex. The cycle is then repeated.
◆ *Rate:* The atrial rate exceeds the ventricular rate because of the nonconducted beats, but both usually remain within normal limits.
◆ *P wave:* Normal size and configuration; each P wave is followed by a QRS complex except for the blocked P wave.

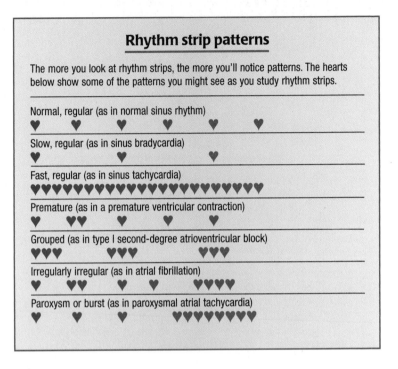

Rhythm strip patterns

The more you look at rhythm strips, the more you'll notice patterns. The hearts below show some of the patterns you might see as you study rhythm strips.

Normal, regular (as in normal sinus rhythm)

Slow, regular (as in sinus bradycardia)

Fast, regular (as in sinus tachycardia)

Premature (as in a premature ventricular contraction)

Grouped (as in type I second-degree atrioventricular block)

Irregularly irregular (as in atrial fibrillation)

Paroxysm or burst (as in paroxysmal atrial tachycardia)

◆ *PR interval:* The PR interval is progressively longer with each cycle until a P wave appears without a QRS complex. The variation in delay from cycle to cycle is typically slight. The PR interval after the nonconducted beat is shorter than the interval preceding it. The phrase commonly used to describe this pattern is long, longer, dropped.

◆ *QRS complex:* Duration usually remains within normal limits because the block commonly occurs at the level of the AV node. The complex is absent when the impulse isn't conducted.

◆ *T wave:* Normal size and configuration.

◆ *QT interval:* Usually within normal limits.

◆ *Other:* The pattern of group beating is sometimes referred to as the footprints of Wenckebach (named for the Dutch internist K. Frederik Wenckebach, who first described the two forms of what's now known as second-degree AV block).

Signs and symptoms

Usually asymptomatic, a patient with type I second-degree AV block may show signs and symptoms of decreased cardiac output, such as light-headedness or hypotension. Symptoms may be especially pronounced if the ventricular rate is slow.

Interventions

Treatment is rarely needed because the patient is generally asymptomatic. A transcutaneous pacemaker may be required for a symptomatic patient until the arrhythmia resolves. For a patient with serious signs and symptoms related to a low heart rate, atropine may be used to improve AV node conduction.

When caring for a patient with this block, assess his tolerance for the rhythm and evaluate whether treatment is needed to improve cardiac output. Evaluate the patient for possible causes of the block, including the use of certain medications or the presence of myocardial ischemia.

Check the ECG frequently to see if a more severe type of AV block develops. Make sure the patient has a patent I.V. line. Provide patient teaching about a temporary pacemaker, if indicated.

◢ LIFE-THREATENING

Type II second-degree AV block

Type II second-degree AV block (also known as *Mobitz II block*) is less common than type I, but more serious. It occurs when impulses from the SA node occasionally fail to conduct to the ventricles. This form of second-degree AV block occurs below the level of the AV node, either at the bundle of His or, more commonly, at the bundle branches.

One of the hallmarks of this type of block is that, unlike type I second-degree AV block, the PR interval doesn't lengthen before a dropped beat. In addition, more than one nonconducted beat can occur in succession. (See *2:1 AV block*, page 186, and *Recognizing type II second-degree AV block*, page 187.)

Causes

Unlike type I second-degree AV block, type II second-degree AV block rarely results from increased parasympathetic tone or drug effect. Because the arrhythmia is usually associated with organic heart disease, it's usually associated with a poorer prognosis, and complete heart block may develop.

Type II second-degree AV block is commonly caused by an

2:1 AV block

In 2:1 second-degree atrioventricular (AV) block, every other QRS complex is dropped, so there are always two P waves for every QRS complex. The resulting ventricular rhythm is regular.

Type I or type II?

To help determine whether a rhythm is type I or type II block, look at the width of the QRS complexes. If they're wide and a short PR interval is present, the block is probably type II.

Type II block is more likely to impair cardiac output, lead to symptoms such as syncope, and progress to a more severe form of block. Be sure to monitor the patient carefully.

anterior-wall MI, degenerative changes in the conduction system, or severe CAD. The arrhythmia indicates a conduction disturbance at the level of the bundle of His or bundle branches.

Clinical significance

Type II second-degree AV block is more severe than type I. The ventricular rate tends to be slower than in type I, leading to decreased cardiac output. Cardiac output is further diminished if the sinus rhythm is slow and the ratio of conducted beats to dropped beats is low, such as 2:1. If the block develops following an anterior-wall MI, it indicates damage to the conduction system. In this instance, the block will most likely be permanent.

ECG characteristics

◆ *Rhythm:* The atrial rhythm is regular. The ventricular rhythm can be regular or irregular. Pauses correspond to the dropped beat. When the block is intermittent or when the conduction ratio is variable, the rhythm is commonly irregular. When a constant conduction ratio occurs, for example, 2:1 or 3:1, the rhythm is regular.

◆ *Rate:* The atrial rate is usually within normal limits. The ventricular rate, slower than the atrial rate, may be within normal limits.

◆ *P wave:* The P wave is normal in size and configuration, but some P waves aren't followed by a QRS complex. The R-R interval containing a nonconducted P wave equals two normal R-R intervals.

◆ *PR interval:* The PR interval is within normal limits or prolonged but generally always constant for the conducted beats.

◆ *QRS complex:* Duration is within normal limits if the block occurs at the bundle of His. If

Recognizing type II second-degree AV block

To help you recognize type II second-degree atrioventricular (AV) block, review this sample rhythm strip.

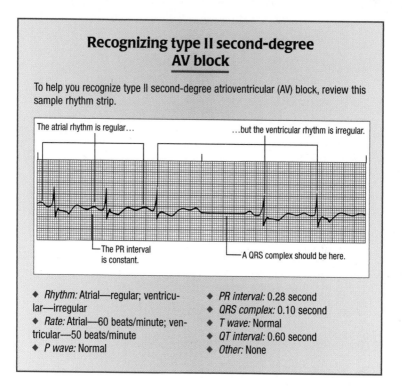

The atrial rhythm is regular... ...but the ventricular rhythm is irregular.

The PR interval is constant.

A QRS complex should be here.

- ◆ *Rhythm:* Atrial—regular; ventricular—irregular
- ◆ *Rate:* Atrial—60 beats/minute; ventricular—50 beats/minute
- ◆ *P wave:* Normal

- ◆ *PR interval:* 0.28 second
- ◆ *QRS complex:* 0.10 second
- ◆ *T wave:* Normal
- ◆ *QT interval:* 0.60 second
- ◆ *Other:* None

the block occurs at the bundle branches, however, the QRS is widened and displays the features of bundle-branch block. The complex is absent periodically.

◆ *T wave:* Usually of normal size and configuration.

◆ *QT interval:* Usually within normal limits.

◆ *Other:* The PR and R-R intervals don't vary before a dropped beat, so no warning occurs. For a dropped beat to occur, there must be complete block in one bundle branch with intermittent interruption in conduction in the other bundle as well. As a result, this type of second-degree AV block is commonly associated with a wide QRS complex. However, when the block occurs at the bundle of His, the QRS may be narrow because ventricular conduction is undisturbed in beats that aren't blocked.

It may be difficult to distinguish nonconducted premature atrial contractions (PACs) from type II second-degree AV block. (See *Distinguishing nonconduct-*

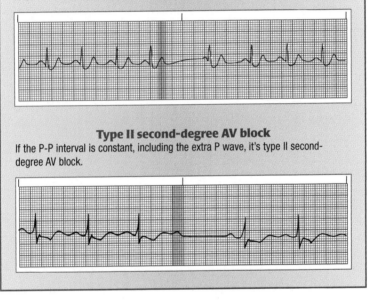

LOOK-ALIKES

Distinguishing nonconducted PACs from type II second-degree AV block

An isolated P wave that doesn't conduct through to the ventricle (P wave without a QRS complex following it; see shaded areas) may occur with a nonconducted premature atrial contraction (PAC) or may indicate type II second-degree atrioventricular (AV) block. Mistakenly identifying AV block as nonconducted PACs may have serious consequences. The latter is generally benign; the former can be life-threatening.

Nonconducted PAC
If the P-P interval, including the extra P wave, isn't constant, it's a nonconducted PAC.

Type II second-degree AV block
If the P-P interval is constant, including the extra P wave, it's type II second-degree AV block.

ed PACs from type II second-degree AV block.)

Signs and symptoms

Most patients who experience occasional dropped beats remain asymptomatic as long as cardiac output is maintained. As the number of dropped beats increases, the patient may experience signs and symptoms of decreased cardiac output, including fatigue, dyspnea, chest pain, or light-headedness. On physical examination, you may note hypotension and a slow pulse, with a regular or irregular rhythm.

Interventions

Because this form of second-degree AV block occurs below the level of the AV node—either at the bundle of His or, more commonly, at the bundle branches—transcutaneous pacing should be initiated quickly, when indicated. For this reason, type II second-degree AV block may also require placement of a permanent pacemaker. A temporary pacemaker may be used until a permanent pacemaker can be inserted.

When caring for a patient with type II second-degree block, assess tolerance for the rhythm and the need for treatment to improve cardiac output. Besides transcutaneous pacing, I.V. dopamine, I.V. epinephrine, or I.V. atropine may be used to increase cardiac output. Use atropine cautiously because it can worsen ischemia during an MI. It may also induce ventricular tachycardia or fibrillation in patients with this form of second-degree AV block.

Keep the patient on bed rest, if indicated, to reduce myocardial oxygen demands. Evaluate for possible correctable causes of the arrhythmia such as ischemia. Administer oxygen therapy as or-

dered. Observe the patient's cardiac rhythm for progression to a more severe form of AV block. Teach the patient and his family about the use of pacemakers if the patient requires one.

■ LIFE-THREATENING

Third-degree atrioventricular block

Also called *complete heart block,* third-degree AV block indicates the complete absence of impulse conduction between the atria and ventricles. There's no correlation between the conduction of the P waves and the QRS complex. In complete heart block, the atrial rate is generally faster than the ventricular rate.

Third-degree AV block may occur at the level of the AV node, the bundle of His, or the bundle branches. The patient's treatment and prognosis vary depending on the anatomic level of the block.

When third-degree AV block occurs at the level of the AV node, ventricular depolarization is typically initiated by a junctional escape pacemaker. This pacemaker is usually stable with a rate of 40 to 60 beats/minute. The sequence of ventricular depolarization is usually normal because the block is located above the bifurcation of the bundle of His, which results in a normal-

Recognizing third-degree AV block

To help you recognize third-degree atrioventricular (AV) block, review this sample rhythm strip.

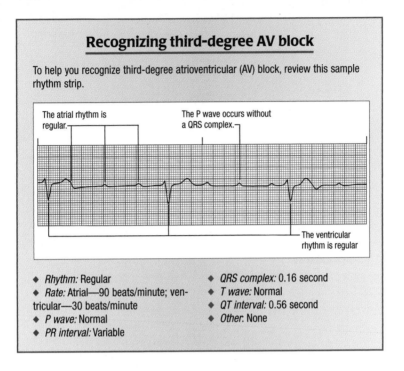

The atrial rhythm is regular.

The P wave occurs without a QRS complex.

The ventricular rhythm is regular

- *Rhythm:* Regular
- *Rate:* Atrial—90 beats/minute; ventricular—30 beats/minute
- *P wave:* Normal
- *PR interval:* Variable
- *QRS complex:* 0.16 second
- *T wave:* Normal
- *QT interval:* 0.56 second
- *Other:* None

appearing QRS complex. (*See Recognizing third-degree AV block.*)

On the other hand, when third-degree AV block occurs at the infranodal level, a block involving the right and left bundle branches is most commonly the cause. In this case, extensive disease exists in the infranodal conduction system, and the only available escape mechanism is located distal to the site of block in the ventricle. This unstable, ventricular escape pacemaker has a slow intrinsic rate of less than 40 beats/minute. Because these depolarizations originate in the ventricle, the QRS complex has a wide and bizarre appearance.

Causes

Third-degree AV block occurring at the anatomic level of the AV node can result from increased parasympathetic tone associated with inferior-wall MI, AV node damage, or toxic effects of such drugs as digoxin and propranolol.

Third-degree AV block occurring at the infranodal level is commonly associated with extensive anterior MI. It generally isn't the result of increases in parasympathetic tone or drug effect.

Clinical significance

Third-degree AV block occurring at the AV node, with a junctional escape rhythm, is usually transient and generally associated with a favorable prognosis. In third-degree AV block at the infranodal level, however, the pacemaker is unstable and episodes of ventricular asystole are common. Third-degree AV block at this level is generally associated with a less favorable prognosis.

Because the ventricular rate in third-degree AV block can be slow and the decrease in cardiac output so significant, the arrhythmia usually results in a life-threatening situation. In addition, the loss of AV synchrony results in the loss of atrial kick, which further decreases cardiac output.

ECG characteristics

◆ *Rhythm:* Atrial and ventricular rhythms are usually regular.
◆ *Rate:* Acting independently, the atria, generally under the control of the SA node, tend to maintain a regular rate of 60 to 100 beats/minute. The atrial rate exceeds the ventricular rate. With intranodal block, the ventricular rate is usually 40 to 60 beats/minute (a junctional escape

rhythm). With infranodal block, the ventricular rate is usually below 40 beats/minute (a ventricular escape rhythm).
◆ *P wave:* The P wave is normal in size and configuration. Some P waves may be buried in QRS complexes or T waves.
◆ *PR interval:* Not applicable or measurable because the atria and ventricles are depolarized from different pacemakers and beat independently of each other.
◆ *QRS complex:* Configuration depends on the location of the escape mechanism and origin of ventricular depolarization. When the block occurs at the level of the AV node or bundle of His, the QRS complex appears normal. When the block occurs at the level of the bundle branches, the QRS is widened.
◆ *T wave:* Normal size and configuration unless the QRS complex originates in the ventricle.
◆ *QT interval:* May be within normal limits.
◆ *Other:* None.

Signs and symptoms

Most patients with third-degree AV block experience significant signs and symptoms, including severe fatigue, dyspnea, chest pain, light-headedness, changes in mental status, and changes in the level of consciousness. Hypotension, pallor, and diaphoresis may also occur. The peripheral pulse rate is slow, but the rhythm is regular.

A few patients are relatively free from symptoms, complaining only that they can't tolerate exercise and that they're typically tired for no apparent reason. The severity of symptoms depends to a large extent on the resulting ventricular rate and the patient's ability to compensate for decreased cardiac output.

Interventions

If the patient is experiencing serious signs and symptoms related to the low heart rate, or if the patient's condition seems to be deteriorating, interventions may include transcutaneous pacing or I.V. atropine, dopamine, or epinephrine. Atropine isn't indicated for third-degree AV block with new wide QRS complexes. In such cases, a permanent pacemaker is indicated because atropine rarely increases sinus rate and AV node conduction when AV block is at the His-Purkinje level.

Asymptomatic patients with third-degree AV block should be prepared for insertion of a transvenous temporary pacemaker until a decision is made about the need for a permanent pacemaker. If symptoms develop, a transcutaneous pacemaker should be used until the transvenous pacemaker is placed.

Because third-degree AV block occurring at the infranodal level is usually associated with extensive anterior MI, patients are more likely to have permanent third-degree AV block, which most likely requires insertion of a permanent pacemaker.

Third-degree AV block occurring at the anatomic level of the AV node can result from increased parasympathetic tone associated with an inferior-wall MI. As a result, the block is more likely to be short-lived. In these patients, the decision to insert a permanent pacemaker is commonly delayed to assess how well the conduction system recovers.

When caring for a patient with third-degree AV block, immediately assess the patient's tolerance of the rhythm and the need for interventions to support cardiac output and relieve symptoms. Make sure that the patient has a patent I.V. line. Administer oxygen therapy as ordered. Evaluate for possible correctable causes of the arrhythmia, such as drugs or myocardial ischemia. Minimize the patient's activity and maintain bed rest.

Electrolyte imbalances and drugs

10

Patients with electrolyte imbalances—such as hyperkalemia, hypokalemia, hypercalcemia, and hypocalcemia—frequently show distinctive rhythm changes on electrocardiograms (ECGs). Likewise, patients taking such drugs as digoxin (Lanoxin) may also exhibit characteristic ECG patterns that can provide early warnings of drug toxicity. Learning to recognize these variations early will help you identify and treat potentially dangerous conditions before they become serious.

Keep in mind, however, that the patient's ECG is only part of the clinical picture. Additional information, such as the patient's medical history, findings on physical examination, and additional diagnostic studies, are necessary to confirm an initial diagnosis based on ECG analysis.

ELECTROLYTE IMBALANCES

Potassium and calcium ions play a major role in the heart's electrical activity. Depolarization results from the exchange of these ions across the cell membrane. Changes in ion concentration can affect the heart's electrical activity and, as a result, the patient's ECG. This section discusses the effects of high and low potassium and calcium levels on an ECG.

Hyperkalemia

Potassium, the most plentiful intracellular cation (positively charged electrolyte), contributes to many important cellular functions. Most of the body's potassium content is located in the cells. The intracellular fluid (ICF) concentration of potassium is 150 to 160 mEq/L; the extracellular fluid (ECF) concentration, 3.5 to 5.0 mEq/L. Many symptoms associated with potassium imbalance result from changes in this ratio of ICF to ECF potassium concentration. Hyperkalemia is generally defined as serum potassium level greater than 5 mEq/L. It's most commonly seen in people with renal insufficiency.

Causes

Increased intake of potassium—from excessive dietary intake, I.V. administration of penicillin G (Pfizerpen), potassium supplements, or banked whole blood—is one factor contributing to the development of hyperkalemia. Also, changes in cell membrane permeability or damage to cells from surgery, burns, massive crush injuries, cell hypoxia, acidosis, and insulin deficiency may cause potassium to shift from the intracellular space to the extracellular space. Increased serum levels of potassium may also stem from decreased renal excretion of potassium. This excretion may occur because of renal failure, decreased production and secretion of aldosterone, Addison's disease, and the use of potassium-sparing diuretics.

Clinical significance

When extracellular potassium concentrations increase without a significant change in intracellular potassium concentrations, the cell becomes less negative, or partially depolarized, and the resting cell membrane potential decreases. Mild elevations in extracellular potassium result in cells that repolarize faster and are more irritable. More critical elevations in extracellular potassium result in an inability of cells to repolarize and respond to electrical stimuli. Cardiac standstill, or asystole, is the most serious consequence of severe hyperkalemia.

ECG characteristics

◆ *Rhythm:* Atrial and ventricular rhythms are regular.
◆ *Rate:* Atrial and ventricular rates are within normal limits.
◆ *P wave:* In mild hyperkalemia, the amplitude is low; in moderate hyperkalemia, P waves are wide and flattened; in severe hyperkalemia, the P wave may be indiscernible.
◆ *PR interval:* Normal or prolonged; not measurable if P wave can't be detected.
◆ *QRS complex:* Widened because ventricular depolarization takes longer.
◆ *ST segment:* May be elevated in severe hyperkalemia.

ECG effects of hyperkalemia

The classic and most striking electrocardiogram (ECG) feature of hyperkalemia is tall, peaked T waves. This rhythm strip shows a typical peaked T wave (shaded area).

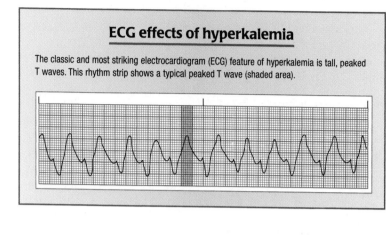

◆ *T wave:* Tall, peaked; the classic and most striking feature of hyperkalemia.
◆ *QT interval:* Shortened.
◆ *Other:* Intraventricular conduction disturbances commonly occur. (See *ECG effects of hyperkalemia.*)

Signs and symptoms

Mild hyperkalemia may cause neuromuscular irritability, including restlessness, intestinal cramping, diarrhea, and tingling lips and fingers. Severe hyperkalemia may cause loss of muscle tone, muscle weakness, and paralysis.

Interventions

Treatment depends upon the severity of hyperkalemia and the patient's signs and symptoms. The underlying cause must be identified and the extracellular potassium concentration brought back to normal. Drug therapy to normalize potassium levels includes calcium gluconate to decrease neuromuscular irritability, insulin and glucose to facilitate the entry of potassium into the cell, and sodium bicarbonate to correct metabolic acidosis.

Oral or rectal administration of cation exchange resins, such as sodium polystyrene sulfonate (Kayexalate), may be used to exchange sodium for potassium in the intestine. In the setting of renal failure or severe hyperkalemia, dialysis may be necessary to remove excess potassium. The patient's serum potassium levels should be monitored closely until they return to normal, and arrhythmias should be identified and managed appropriately.

Cell lysis resulting from chemotherapy can be prevented with adequate hydration before, during, and after the administration of the chemotherapy. If the patient isn't able to tolerate oral fluids, I.V. fluids may be given.

Hypokalemia

Hypokalemia, or potassium deficiency, occurs when the ECF concentration of potassium drops below 3.5 mEq/L, usually indicating a loss of total body potassium. The concentration of ECF potassium is so small that even minor changes in ECF potassium affect resting membrane potential.

Causes

Factors contributing to hypokalemia include increased loss of body potassium, increased entry of potassium into cells, and reduced potassium intake. Shifts in potassium from the extracellular space to the intracellular space may be caused by alkalosis, especially respiratory alkalosis. Intracellular uptake of potassium is also increased by catecholamines. Although rare, a dietary deficiency may contribute to hypokalemia in an elderly person. The condition is also seen in patients with alcoholism, hepatic disease, and anorexia nervosa. Potassium is also lost during diabetic ketoacidosis because of osmotic diuresis.

GI and renal disorders are the most common causes of potassium loss from body stores. GI losses of potassium are associated with laxative abuse, intestinal fistulae or drainage tubes, diarrhea, vomiting, and continuous nasogastric drainage.

Renal loss of potassium is related to increased secretion of potassium by the distal tubule. Diuretics, a low serum magnesium concentration, and excessive aldosterone secretion may cause urinary loss of potassium. In addition, several antibiotics, including gentamicin (Garamycin) and amphotericin B (Fungizone), are known to cause hypokalemia.

Clinical significance

When extracellular potassium levels decrease rapidly and intracellular potassium concentration doesn't change, the resting membrane potential becomes more negative and the cell membrane becomes hyperpolarized. The cardiac effects of hypokalemia are related to these changes in membrane excitability. Ventricular repolarization is delayed because potassium contributes to the repolarization phase of the action potential. Hypokalemia can cause dangerous ventricular

ECG effects of hypokalemia

As the serum potassium concentration drops, the T wave becomes flat and a U wave appears as shown (shaded area) in this electrocardiogram (ECG) rhythm strip.

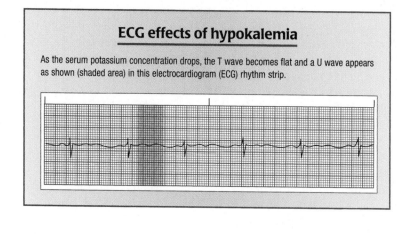

arrhythmias and increases the risk of digoxin toxicity.

ECG characteristics

◆ *Rhythm:* Atrial and ventricular rhythms are regular.
◆ *Rate:* Atrial and ventricular rates are within normal limits.
◆ *P wave:* Usually normal size and configuration but may become peaked in severe hypokalemia.
◆ *PR interval:* May be prolonged.
◆ *QRS complex:* Within normal limits or possibly widened; prolonged in severe hypokalemia.
◆ *QT interval:* Usually indiscernible as the T wave flattens.
◆ *ST segment:* Depressed.
◆ *T wave:* Amplitude is decreased. The T wave becomes flat as the potassium level drops. In severe hypokalemia, it flattens completely and may become inverted. The T wave may also fuse with an increasingly prominent U wave.
◆ *Other:* Amplitude of the U wave is increased, becoming more prominent as hypokalemia worsens and fusing with the T wave. (See *ECG effects of hypokalemia.*)

Signs and symptoms

The most common symptoms of hypokalemia are caused by neuromuscular and cardiac effects, including smooth muscle atony, skeletal muscle weakness, and cardiac arrhythmias. Loss of smooth muscle tone results in constipation, intestinal distention, nausea, vomiting, anorexia, and paralytic ileus. Skeletal muscle weakness occurs first in the larger muscles of the arms and legs and eventually affects the diaphragm, causing respiratory arrest.

Cardiac effects of hypokalemia include arrhythmias, such as bradycardia, atrioventricular (AV) block, and paroxysmal atrial tachycardia. Delayed depolarization results in characteristic changes on the ECG.

Interventions

The underlying causes of hypokalemia should be identified and corrected. Acid-base imbalances should be corrected, potassium losses replaced, and further losses prevented. Encourage intake of foods and fluids rich in potassium. Oral or I.V. potassium supplements may be administered. The patient's serum potassium levels should be monitored closely until they return to normal, and cardiac arrhythmias should be identified and managed appropriately.

Hypercalcemia

Most of the body's calcium stores (99%) are located in bone. The remainder is found in the plasma and body cells. Approximately 50% of plasma calcium is bound to plasma proteins. About 40% is found in the ionized or free form.

Calcium plays an important role in myocardial contractility. Ionized calcium is more important than plasma-bound calcium in physiologic functions. Hypercalcemia is usually defined as a serum calcium concentration greater than 10.5 mg/dl.

Causes

The most common causes of hypercalcemia include excess vitamin D intake; bone metastasis and calcium resorption associated with cancers of the breast, prostate, and cervix; hyperparathyroidism; sarcoidosis; thyrotoxicosis; thiazide diuretic therapy; and many parathyroid hormone–producing tumors.

Clinical significance

In hypercalcemia, calcium is found inside cells in greater abundance than normal. The cell membrane becomes refractory to depolarization as a result of a more positive action potential, and a stronger stimulus is needed to cause a response in the cell membrane. This loss of cell membrane excitability causes many of the cardiac symptoms seen in patients with hypercalcemia.

Both ventricular depolarization and repolarization are accelerated. The patient may experience bradyarrhythmias and varying degrees of AV block.

ECG effects of hypercalcemia

Increased serum concentrations of calcium cause shortening of the QT interval as shown (shaded area) in this electrocardiogram (ECG) rhythm strip.

ECG characteristics

◆ *Rhythm:* Atrial and ventricular rhythms are regular.
◆ *Rate:* Atrial and ventricular rates are within normal limits, but bradycardia can occur.
◆ *P wave:* Normal size and configuration.
◆ *PR interval:* May be prolonged.
◆ *QRS complex:* Within normal limits, but may be prolonged.
◆ *QT interval:* Shortened.
◆ *ST segment:* Shortened.
◆ *T wave:* Normal size and configuration; may be depressed.
◆ *Other:* None. (See *ECG effects of hypercalcemia.*)

Signs and symptoms

Common signs and symptoms of hypercalcemia include anorexia, nausea, constipation, lethargy, fatigue, polyuria, and weakness. Behavioral changes may also occur. Renal calculi may form as precipitates of calcium salts. Impaired renal function commonly occurs. A reciprocal decrease in serum phosphate levels commonly accompanies elevated levels of serum calcium.

Interventions

Treatment of hypercalcemia focuses on identifying and managing the underlying cause. Treatment measures are guided by the severity of the patient's symptoms. Administering oral phosphate is usually effective as long as renal function is normal. In more critical situations, I.V. administration of large volumes of normal saline solution may enhance renal excretion of calcium. Patients in renal failure may need dialysis. Corticosteroids and calcitonin (Miacalcin) may be used in severe hypercalcemia.

Hypocalcemia

Low calcium levels also affect myocardial contractility. Hypocalcemia occurs when the total serum calcium level is less than 8.5 mg/dl or when the ionized calcium level falls below 4.5 mg/dl.

Causes

Hypocalcemia may be related to decreases in parathyroid hormone and vitamin D, inadequate intestinal absorption, blood administration, or deposition of ionized calcium into soft tissue or bone.

Inadequate dietary intake of green, leafy vegetables or dairy products may result in a nutritional deficiency of calcium. Excessive dietary intake of phosphorus binds with calcium and prevents calcium absorption. The citrate solution used in storing whole blood binds with calcium, commonly resulting in hypocalcemia. Pancreatitis decreases ionized calcium, and neoplastic bone metastases decrease serum calcium levels.

Decreased intestinal absorption of calcium is caused by vitamin D deficiency, either from inadequate vitamin D intake or insufficient exposure to sunlight. Other causes of hypocalcemia include malabsorption of fats, removal of the parathyroid glands, metabolic or respiratory alkalosis, and hypoalbuminemia. Medications associated with hypocalcemia include magnesium sulfate, colchicine, anticonvulsants, aspirin, steroids, loop diuretics, and antacids.

Clinical significance

Hypocalcemia causes an increase in neuromuscular excitability. Partial depolarization of nerves and muscle cells result from a decrease in threshold potential. Consequently, a smaller stimulus is needed to initiate an action potential. Characteristic ECG changes result from prolonged ventricular depolarization and decreased cardiac contractility.

ECG characteristics

◆ *Rhythm:* Atrial and ventricular rhythms are regular.
◆ *Rate:* Atrial and ventricular rates are within normal limits.
◆ *P wave:* Normal size and configuration.
◆ *PR interval:* Within normal limits.
◆ *QRS complex:* Within normal limits.
◆ *QT interval:* Prolonged.
◆ *ST segment:* Prolonged.
◆ *T wave:* Normal size and configuration, but may become flat or inverted.

ECG effects of hypocalcemia

Decreased serum concentrations of calcium prolong the QT interval, as shown (shaded area) in this electrocardiogram (ECG) rhythm strip.

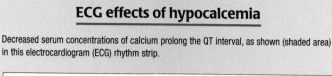

◆ *Other:* None. (See *ECG effects of hypocalcemia*.)

Signs and symptoms

Symptoms of hypocalcemia include hyperreflexia, carpopedal spasm, confusion, and circumoral and digital paresthesia. Hyperactive bowel sounds and intestinal cramping may also occur. Severe symptoms include tetany, seizures, respiratory arrest, and death. Clinical signs indicating hypocalcemia include Trousseau's sign and Chvostek's sign.

Interventions

Treatment should focus on identifying and managing the underlying causes of hypocalcemia. Severe symptoms require emergency treatment with I.V. calcium gluconate. Serum calcium levels should be monitored and oral calcium replacement initiated when possible. Cardiac arrhythmias need to be identified and managed appropriately. Long-term management of hypocalcemia includes decreasing phosphate intake.

CARDIAC DRUGS

Almost 500,000 U.S. residents die each year from cardiac arrhythmias; countless others experience symptoms and require lifestyle modifications. Along with other treatments, cardiac drugs can help alleviate symptoms, control heart rate and rhythm, decrease preload and afterload, and prolong life.

Antiarrhythmics affect ion movement across the cell membrane and alter the electrophysiology of the cardiac cell. These drugs are classified according to their effect on the cell's electrical activity (action potential) and their mechanism of action. Because the drugs can alter the myocardial action potential, characteristic ECG changes can occur.

The classification system divides antiarrhythmic drugs into four major classes based on their dominant mechanism of action: class I, class II, class III, and class IV. Class I antiarrhythmics are further divided into class IA, class IB, and class IC.

Certain antiarrhythmics can't be classified specifically into one group. For example, sotalol possesses characteristics of both class II and class III drugs. Still other drugs, such as adenosine (Adenocard), digoxin (Lanoxin), atropine, epinephrine, and magnesium, don't fit into the classification system at all. Despite its limitations, the classification system is helpful in understanding how antiarrhythmics prevent and treat arrhythmias.

This section reviews ECG changes that result when patients take therapeutic doses of antiarrhythmics (separated by classification), digoxin, adenosine, atropine, and epinephrine. When drug levels are toxic, ECG changes are typically exaggerated.

Class I antiarrhythmics

Class I antiarrhythmics block the influx of sodium into the cell during phase 0 of the action potential. Because phase 0 is also referred to as the *sodium channel,* these drugs may also be called *sodium channel blockers.* Class I antiarrhythmics are subdivided into three groups—A, B, and C—according to their interactions with cardiac sodium channels or the drug's effects on the duration of the action potential.

Class IA

Class IA antiarrhythmics include disopyramide (Norpace), procainamide (Procan), and quinidine (Quinidex). These drugs lengthen the duration of the action potential, and their interaction with the sodium channels is classified as intermediate. As a result, conductivity is reduced and repolarization is prolonged. With the introduction of many new drugs, class IA antiarrhythmics commonly aren't used.

ECG characteristics
◆ *QRS complex:* Slightly widened; increased widening is an early sign of toxicity.
◆ *T wave:* May be flattened or inverted.

ECG effects of class IA antiarrhythmics

Class IA antiarrhythmics—such as quinidine and procainamide—affect the cardiac cycle in specific ways and lead to specific electrocardiogram (ECG) changes, as shown here. Class IA antiarrhythmics:

◆ block sodium influx during phase 0, which depresses the rate of depolarization
◆ prolong repolarization and the duration of the action potential
◆ lengthen the refractory period
◆ decrease contractility.

ECG characteristics of class IA antiarrhythmics

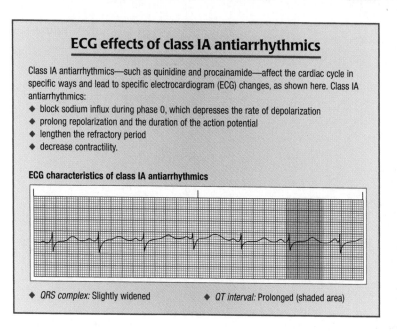

◆ *QRS complex:* Slightly widened   ◆ *QT interval:* Prolonged (shaded area)

◆ *U wave:* May be present.
◆ *QT interval:* Prolonged.
◆ Because these drugs prolong the QT interval, the patient is prone to polymorphic ventricular tachycardia. (See *ECG effects of class IA antiarrhythmics.*)

Class IB

Class IB antiarrhythmics include phenytoin (Dilantin), lidocaine, and mexiletine (Mexitil). These drugs interact rapidly with sodium channels, slowing phase 0 of the action potential and shortening phase 3. The drugs in this class are effective in suppressing ventricular ectopy.

ECG characteristics

◆ *PR interval:* May be slightly shortened.
◆ *QRS complex:* May be slightly widened.
◆ *QT interval:* Shortened. (See *ECG effects of class IB antiarrhythmics,* page 204.)

Class IC

Class IC antiarrhythmics, including flecainide (Tambocor), propafenone (Rythmol), and moricizine (Ethmozine), may minimally increase or have no effect on the action potential duration. Class IC drugs interact slowly with sodium channels.

ECG effects of class IB antiarrhythmics

Class IB antiarrhythmics such as lidocaine may affect the QRS complex, as shown in this electrocardiogram (ECG) rhythm strip. The drugs may also:
◆ block sodium influx during phase 0, which depresses the rate of depolarization
◆ shorten repolarization and the duration of the action potential
◆ suppress ventricular automaticity in ischemic tissue.

ECG characteristics of class IB antiarrhythmics

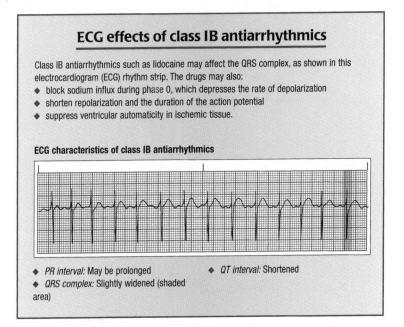

◆ *PR interval:* May be prolonged
◆ *QRS complex:* Slightly widened (shaded area)

◆ *QT interval:* Shortened

ECG effects of class IC antiarrhythmics

Class IC antiarrhythmics—such as flecainide, propafenone, and moricizine—exert particular actions on the cardiac cycle and lead to specific electrocardiogram (ECG) changes, as shown here. Class IC antiarrhythmics block sodium influx during phase 0, which depresses the rate of depolarization. The drugs exert no effect on repolarization or the duration of the action potential.

ECG characteristics of class IC antiarrhythmics

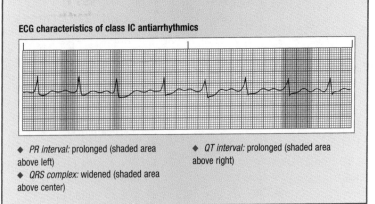

◆ *PR interval:* prolonged (shaded area above left)
◆ *QRS complex:* widened (shaded area above center)

◆ *QT interval:* prolonged (shaded area above right)

Phase 0 is markedly slowed and conduction is decreased.

These drugs are usually reserved for refractory arrhythmias because they may cause or worsen arrhythmias.

ECG characteristics

◆ *PR interval:* Prolonged.
◆ *QRS complex:* Widened.
◆ *QT interval:* Prolonged. (See *ECG effects of class IC antiarrhythmics.*)

Class II antiarrhythmics

Class II antiarrhythmics include drugs that reduce adrenergic activity in the heart. Beta-adrenergic antagonists, also called *beta-adrenergic blockers,* are class II antiarrhythmics and include such drugs as acebutolol (Sectral), esmolol (Brevibloc), and propranolol (Inderal). Beta-adrenergic antagonists block beta receptors in the sympathetic nervous system. As a result, phase 4 depolarization is diminished, which leads to depressed automaticity of the sinoatrial (SA) node and increased atrial and AV node refractory periods.

Class II antiarrhythmics are used to treat supraventricular and ventricular arrhythmias, especially those caused by excess circulating catecholamines. Beta-adrenergic blockers are classified according to their effects. $Beta_1$-adrenergic blockers decrease heart rate, contractility, and conductivity. $Beta_2$-adrenergic blockers may cause vasoconstriction and bronchospasm because $beta_2$ receptors relax smooth muscle in the bronchi and blood vessels.

Beta-adrenergic blockers that block only $beta_1$ receptors are referred to as cardioselective. Those that block both $beta_1$- and $beta_2$-receptor activity are referred to as noncardioselective.

ECG characteristics

◆ *Rate:* Atrial and ventricular rates are decreased.
◆ *PR interval:* Slightly prolonged.
◆ *QT interval:* Slightly shortened. (See *ECG effects of class II antiarrhythmics,* page 206.)

Class III antiarrhythmics

Class III antiarrhythmics prolong the action potential duration, which, in turn, prolongs the effective refractory period. Class III antiarrhythmics are called potassium channel blockers because they block the movement of potassium during phase 3 of the action potential. Drugs in this class include amiodarone (Cordarone), ibutilide (Corvert), and

ECG effects of class II antiarrhythmics

Class II antiarrhythmics—including such beta-adrenergic blockers as propranolol, esmolol, and acebutolol—exert particular actions on the cardiac cycle and lead to specific electrocardiogram (ECG) changes, as shown here. Class II antiarrhythmics:
◆ depress sinoatrial node automaticity
◆ shorten the duration of the action potential
◆ increase the refractory period of atrial and atrioventricular junctional tissues, which slows conduction
◆ inhibit sympathetic activity.

ECG characteristics of class II antiarrhythmics

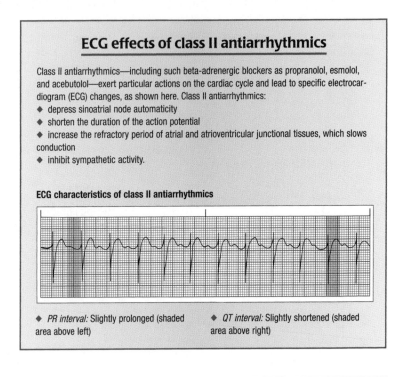

◆ *PR interval:* Slightly prolonged (shaded area above left)
◆ *QT interval:* Slightly shortened (shaded area above right)

sotalol (Betapace) (a nonselective beta-adrenergic blocker with mainly class III properties). All class III antiarrhythmics have proarrhythmic potential.

ECG characteristics

◆ *PR interval:* Prolonged.
◆ *QRS complex:* Widened.
◆ *QT interval:* Prolonged. (See *ECG effects of class III antiarrhythmics.*)

Class IV antiarrhythmics

Class IV antiarrhythmics block the movement of calcium during phase 2 of the action potential. Because phase 2 is also called the *calcium channel,* drugs that affect phase 2 are also known as *calcium channel blockers.* These drugs slow conduction and increase the refractory period of calcium-dependent tissues, including the AV node. Drugs in this class include verapamil (Calan) and diltiazem (Cardizem).

ECG effects of class III antiarrhythmics

Class III antiarrhythmics—such as amiodarone, sotalol, and ibutilide—affect the cardiac cycle and cause the changes shown in this electrocardiogram (ECG) rhythm strip. Class III antiarrhythmics:

◆ block potassium movement during phase 3
◆ increase the duration of the action potential
◆ prolong the effective refractory period.

ECG characteristics of class III antiarrhythmics

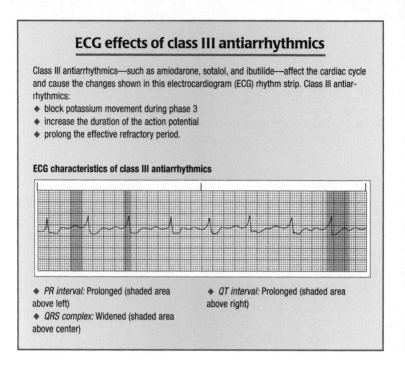

◆ *PR interval:* Prolonged (shaded area above left)
◆ *QRS complex:* Widened (shaded area above center)

◆ *QT interval:* Prolonged (shaded area above right)

Administer diltiazem cautiously in the older adult because the drug's half-life may be prolonged. Be especially careful if the older adult also has heart failure or impaired hepatic or renal function.

ECG characteristics

◆ *Rate:* Atrial and ventricular rates are decreased.
◆ *PR interval:* Prolonged. (See *ECG effects of class IV antiarrhythmics,* page 208.)

Digoxin

Digoxin (Lanoxin), the most commonly used cardiac glycoside, works by inhibiting the enzyme adenosine triphosphatase. This enzyme is found in the plasma membrane and acts as a pump to exchange sodium ions for potassium ions. Inhibition of sodium-potassium–activated adenosine triphosphatase results in enhanced movement of calcium from the extracellular space to the intracellular space, thereby strengthening myocardial contractions.

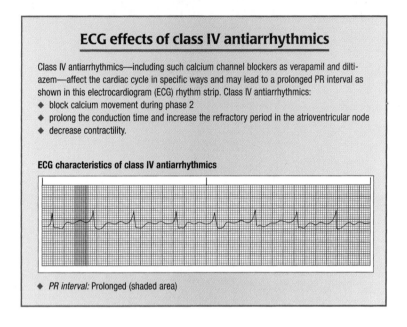

ECG effects of class IV antiarrhythmics

Class IV antiarrhythmics—including such calcium channel blockers as verapamil and diltiazem—affect the cardiac cycle in specific ways and may lead to a prolonged PR interval as shown in this electrocardiogram (ECG) rhythm strip. Class IV antiarrhythmics:

◆ block calcium movement during phase 2
◆ prolong the conduction time and increase the refractory period in the atrioventricular node
◆ decrease contractility.

ECG characteristics of class IV antiarrhythmics

◆ *PR interval:* Prolonged (shaded area)

The effects of digoxin on the electrical properties of the heart include direct and autonomic effects. Direct effects result in shortening of the action potential, which contributes to the shortening of atrial and ventricular refractoriness. Autonomic effects involve the sympathetic and parasympathetic systems. Vagal tone is enhanced, and conduction through the SA and AV nodes is slowed. The drug also exerts an antiarrhythmic effect.

Digoxin is indicated in the treatment of heart failure, paroxysmal supraventricular tachycardia, atrial fibrillation, and atrial flutter.

ECG characteristics

◆ *Rate:* Atrial and ventricular rates are decreased.
◆ *PR interval:* Shortened.
◆ *T wave:* Decreased.
◆ *ST segment:* Shortened and depressed. Sagging (scooping or sloping) of the segment is characteristic.
◆ *QT interval:* Shortened due to the shortened ST segment.
◆ Digoxin has a very narrow window of therapeutic effectiveness and, at toxic levels, may cause numerous arrhythmias, including paroxysmal atrial tachycardia with block, AV block, atrial and junctional tachyarrhythmias, and ventricular

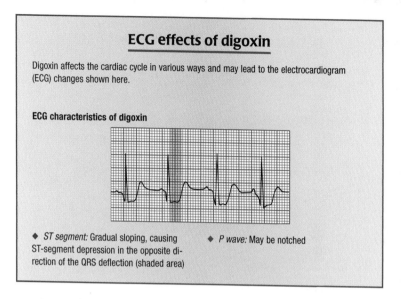

ECG effects of digoxin

Digoxin affects the cardiac cycle in various ways and may lead to the electrocardiogram (ECG) changes shown here.

ECG characteristics of digoxin

◆ *ST segment:* Gradual sloping, causing ST-segment depression in the opposite direction of the QRS deflection (shaded area)

◆ *P wave:* May be notched

arrhythmias. (See *ECG effects of digoxin.*)

Adenosine

Adenosine (Adenocard) is a naturally occurring nucleoside that's most commonly used to slow the heart rate and restore normal conduction. It depresses the SA node's pacemaker activity, reducing the heart rate and the AV node's ability to conduct impulses from the atria to the ventricles. Adenosine isn't chemically related to other antiarrhythmic drugs.

Adenosine is most effective in treating reentry tachycardias that involve the AV node. It's also effective with more than 90% of paroxysmal supraventricular tachycardias. In addition, adenosine is useful in treating arrhythmias related to accessory bypass tracts, such as in Wolff-Parkinson-White syndrome.

Adenosine has a very short half-life, and must be given by rapid I.V. push followed by an immediate flush of 20 ml of normal saline.

◆ **ALERT** Because adenosine administration carries a risk of heart block, the patient must be on a monitor while receiving this drug.

ECG characteristics

◆ *Rate:* Varies; initially tachycardic and then becomes normal.

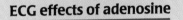

ECG effects of adenosine

Adenosine affects the conduction through the atrioventricular node and may lead to the electrocardiogram (ECG) changes shown here.

ECG characteristics of adenosine

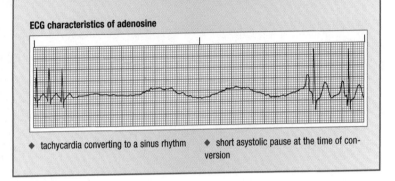

◆ tachycardia converting to a sinus rhythm   ◆ short asystolic pause at the time of conversion

◆ *PR interval:* Difficult to determine initially; later becomes normal or, occasionally, exhibits a first-degree block.

◆ *QT interval:* Shortened because of the increased heart rate; becomes normal when the heart rate slows.

◆ *Other:* Adenosine commonly causes an asystolic pause that lasts a few seconds at the time of conversion. (See *ECG effects of adenosine.*)

Atropine

Atropine is an anticholinergic that works by blocking the neurotransmitter acetylcholine. When the cholinergic receptors are stimulated by acetylcholine,

it causes increased vagal stimulation, which decreases the heart rate. When atropine is given, it competes with acetylcholine to bind to the cholinergic receptors on the SA and the AV nodes. By blocking acetylcholine from these receptors, atropine causes the heart rate to increase. Atropine may need to be given more than once because the effects wear off.

Atropine is indicated for the treatment of symptomatic bradycardia, including second- and third-degree heart blocks and idioventricular rhythms.

◆ **ALERT** Because an increased heart rate increases myocardial oxygen consumption, atropine shouldn't be given to treat bradycardia in patients with acute myocardial infarction to avoid worsening the infarction.

ECG characteristics

◆ *Rate:* Atrial and ventricular rates are increased.
◆ *PR interval:* Varies depending on underlying rhythm.
◆ *QT interval:* Decreases as the rate increases.
◆ *Other:* The rate will gradually increase after the administration of atropine.

ECG characteristics

◆ *Rate:* Atrial and ventricular rates are increased.
◆ *PR interval:* Varies depending on underlying rhythm.
◆ *QT interval:* Decreases as the rate increases.
◆ *Other:* The rate will gradually increase after administering epinephrine.

Epinephrine

Epinephrine is a catecholamine that works on the alpha- and beta-adrenergic receptor sites of the sympathetic nervous system. Epinephrine increases the force of the heart's contraction, increasing the heart's workload and oxygen demand. It can also stimulate the pacemaker cells in the SA node to depolarize at a faster rate, producing a positive chronotropic effect. This effect leads to an increase in the heart rate and blood pressure.

Epinephrine is indicated to help restore cardiac rhythm in cardiac arrest and to treat symptom-producing bradycardia.

Nonpharmacologic treatment

11

Nonpharmacologic treatments for arrhythmias—including pacemakers, implantable cardioverter-defibrillators (ICDs), and radio-frequency ablation—produce distinctive electrocardiogram (ECG) tracings. By understanding how these devices work, and the ECG changes they produce, you'll be better able to evaluate whether the devices are functioning properly, and you'll know what to do if they malfunction.

Pacemakers

A pacemaker is an artificial device that electrically stimulates the myocardium to depolarize, initiating mechanical contractions. It works by generating an impulse from a power source and transmitting that impulse to the heart muscle. The impulse flows throughout the heart and causes the heart muscle to depolarize. Pacemakers may be used as a temporary measure or a perma-

nent one, depending on the patient's condition.

A pacemaker may be used to treat arrhythmias—such as certain bradyarrhythmias and tachyarrhythmias, sick sinus syndrome (SSS), or an atrioventricular (AV) block—as well as following myocardial infarction or cardiac surgery.

Pacemaker fundamentals

Pacemakers consist of three main components: a pulse generator, pacing leads or wires, and one or more electrodes at the distal ends of leadwires. The pulse generator contains the pacemaker's power source and circuitry. It creates an electrical impulse that moves through the pacing leads to the electrodes, transmitting that impulse to the heart muscle and causing the heart to depolarize.

In a permanent or implanted pacemaker, a lithium battery serves as its power source and lasts between 5 and 10 years. A

◆

microchip in the device guides heart pacing. A temporary pacemaker, which isn't implanted, is about the size of a small radio or telemetry box and is powered by alkaline batteries. These units also contain a microchip and are programmed by a touch pad or dials.

In temporary and permanent pacemakers, an electrical stimulus from the pulse generator moves through wires, or pacing leads, to the electrode tips. The leads for a pacemaker, designed to stimulate a single heart chamber, are placed in either the atrium or the ventricle. For dual-chamber (AV) pacing, the leads are placed in both chambers, usually on the right side of the heart. (See *Pacing leads,* page 214.)

The electrodes—one on a unipolar lead or two on a bipolar lead—send information about electrical impulses in the myocardium back to the pulse generator. The pulse generator senses the heart's electrical activity and responds according to how it was programmed.

A unipolar lead system is more sensitive to the heart's intrinsic electrical activity than a bipolar system. A bipolar system isn't as easily affected by electrical activity, such as skeletal muscle contraction or magnetic fields, originating outside the heart and the generator. A bipolar system is more difficult to implant, however.

Permanent pacemakers

A permanent pacemaker is used to treat chronic heart conditions such as AV block. It's surgically implanted, usually under local anesthesia. The leads are placed transvenously, positioned in the appropriate chambers, and then anchored to the endocardium. The generator is then implanted in a pocket made from subcutaneous tissue, usually under the clavicle. (See *Placing a permanent pacemaker,* page 215.)

Most permanent pacemakers are programmed before implantation. The programming sets the conditions under which the pacemaker functions and can be adjusted externally if necessary.

The biventricular pacemaker, a type of permanent pacemaker, uses three leads—one in the right atrium and one in each ventricle. Unlike traditional lead placement, the electrode tip for the left ventricle is placed in the coronary sinus to a branch of the inferior cardiac vein. Because this electrode tip isn't anchored in place, lead displacement may occur. (See *Understanding biventricular pacemakers,* page 216, and *Biventricular lead placement,* page 217.)

Pacing leads

Pacing leads have either one electrode (unipolar) or two (bipolar). These illustrations show the difference between the two leads.

Unipolar lead

In a unipolar system, electric current moves from the pulse generator through the leadwire to the negative pole. From there, it stimulates the heart and returns to the pulse generator's metal surface (the positive pole) to complete the circuit.

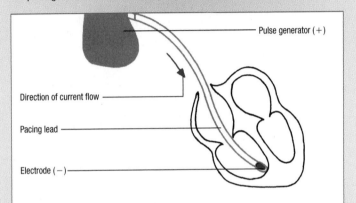

Pulse generator (+)

Direction of current flow

Pacing lead

Electrode (−)

Bipolar lead

In a bipolar system, current flows from the pulse generator through the leadwire to the negative pole at the tip. At that point, it stimulates the heart and then flows to the positive pole in the tip to complete the circuit.

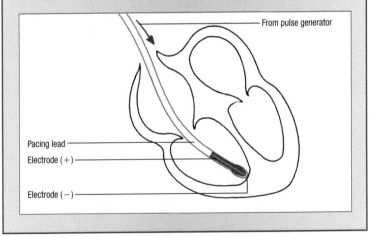

From pulse generator

Pacing lead

Electrode (+)

Electrode (−)

Placing a permanent pacemaker

Implanting a pacemaker is a simple surgical procedure performed with local anesthesia and conscious sedation. To implant an endocardial pacemaker, the cardiologist usually selects a transvenous route and begins lead placement by inserting a catheter percutaneously or by venous cutdown. Then, using fluoroscopic guidance, the cardiologist threads the catheter through the vein until the tip reaches the endocardium.

Lead placement

For lead placement in the atrium, the tip must lodge in the right atrium or coronary sinus, as shown below. For placement in the ventricle, it must lodge in the right ventricular apex in one of the interior muscular ridges, or trabeculae.

Implanting the generator

When the lead is in proper position, the cardiologist secures the pulse generator in a subcutaneous pocket of tissue just below the patient's clavicle. Changing the generator's battery or microchip circuitry requires only a shallow incision over the site and a quick exchange of components.

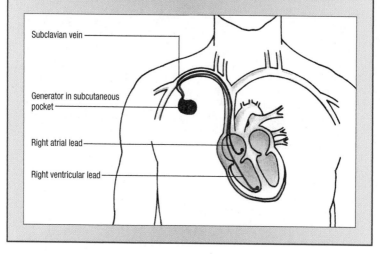

Subclavian vein

Generator in subcutaneous pocket

Right atrial lead

Right ventricular lead

Temporary pacemakers

A temporary pacemaker is commonly inserted in an emergency. The patient may show signs of decreased cardiac output, such as hypotension or syncope. The temporary pacemaker supports the patient until the condition resolves.

A temporary pacemaker can also serve as a bridge until a per-

Understanding biventricular pacemakers

Biventricular pacing (referred to as cardiac resynchronization therapy) is used to treat patients with moderate to severe heart failure who have left ventricular dyssynchrony.

What happens in heart failure

Under normal conditions, the right and left ventricles contract simultaneously to pump blood to the lungs and body, respectively. However, in heart failure, the damaged ventricles can't pump as forcefully, and the amount of blood ejected with each contraction is reduced. If the ventricular conduction pathways are also damaged, electrical impulses reach the ventricles at different times, producing asynchronous contractions (intraventricular conduction defect), which further reduces the amount of blood that the heart pumps, worsening the patient's symptoms.

To compensate for this reduced cardiac output, the sympathetic nervous system releases neurohormones, such as aldosterone, norepinephrine, and vasopressin, to boost the amount of blood ejected with each contraction. The resultant tachycardia and vasoconstriction increase the heart's demand for oxygen, reduce diastolic filling time, promote sodium and water retention, and increase the pressure that the heart must pump against.

How biventricular pacemakers help

Biventricular pacemakers pace both ventricles at the same time, causing them to contract simultaneously. This coordinates ventricular contractions, which increases cardiac output and improves hemodynamic status. This produces an immediate improvement in the patient's symptoms and activity tolerance.

Moreover, biventricular pacing improves left ventricular remodeling and diastolic function and reduces sympathetic stimulation. This, in turn, slows the progression of heart failure and improves the patient's quality of life.

Who are candidates for biventricular pacing?

Not all patients with heart failure benefit from biventricular pacing. Candidates should have systolic heart failure and ventricular dyssynchrony along with the following characteristics:
◆ symptom-producing heart failure despite maximal medical therapy
◆ moderate to severe heart failure (New York Heart Association class III or IV)
◆ QRS complex greater than 0.13 second
◆ left ventricular ejection fraction of 35% or less.

manent pacemaker is inserted. These pacemakers are used for patients with high-grade heart block, bradycardia, or low cardiac output.

Types of temporary pacemakers

Several types of temporary pacemakers are available, including transvenous, transcutaneous, transthoracic, and epicardial.

Biventricular lead placement

The biventricular pacemaker uses three leads: one to pace the right atrium, one to pace the right ventricle, and one to pace the left ventricle. The left ventricular lead is placed in the coronary sinus. Both ventricles are paced at the same time, causing them to contract simultaneously, improving cardiac output.

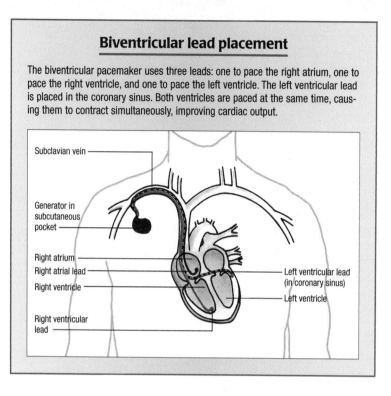

Subclavian vein

Generator in subcutaneous pocket

Right atrium

Right atrial lead

Right ventricle

Right ventricular lead

Left ventricular lead (in coronary sinus)

Left ventricle

Transvenous pacemakers

The transvenous pacemaker is probably the most common and reliable type of temporary pacemaker. It's inserted through a vein, such as the subclavian or internal jugular vein, at the bedside or in a fluoroscopy suite. The leadwires are advanced through a catheter into the right ventricle or atrium and then connected to the pulse generator.

Transcutaneous pacemakers

Use of an external or transcutaneous pacemaker has become commonplace in the past several years. In this noninvasive method, one electrode is placed on the patient's anterior chest wall to the right of the upper sternum below the clavicles and a second electrode is applied to his back (anterior-posterior electrodes). An electrode may also be placed to the left of the left nipple with the center of the electrode in the midaxillary line (also called the anterior-apex position). An external pulse generator then emits pacing impulses that travel through the skin to the heart muscle. Transcutaneous pacing is built into many defibrillators for use in emergencies. In this case, the electrodes are built into the same pads used for defibrillation.

Transcutaneous pacing is a quick, effective method of pacing heart rhythm and is commonly used in emergencies until a transvenous pacemaker can be inserted. However, some patients can't tolerate the irritating sensations produced from prolonged pacing at the levels needed to pace the heart externally. If hemodynamically stable, these patients may require sedation.

Transthoracic pacemakers
A transthoracic pacemaker is a type of temporary ventricular pacemaker only used during cardiac emergencies as a last resort. Transthoracic pacing requires insertion of a long needle into the right ventricle, using a subxiphoid approach. A pacing wire is then guided directly into the endocardium.

Epicardial pacemakers
Epicardial pacemakers are commonly used for patients undergoing cardiac surgery. The tips of the leadwires are attached to the heart's surface and then the wires are brought through the chest wall, below the incision. Finally, they're attached to the pulse generator. The leadwires are usually removed several days after surgery or when the patient no longer requires them.

Temporary pacemaker settings
A temporary pacemaker has several types of settings on the pulse generator. The rate control regulates how many impulses are generated in 1 minute and is measured in pulses per minute (ppm). The rate is usually set at 60 to 80 ppm. (See *Temporary pulse generator*.) The pacemaker fires if the patient's heart rate falls below the preset rate. The rate may be set higher if the patient has a tachyarrhythmia being treated with overdrive pacing.

A pacemaker's energy output is measured in milliamperes (mA), a measurement that represents the stimulation threshold, or how much energy is required to stimulate the cardiac muscle to depolarize. The stimulation threshold is sometimes referred to as energy required for capture.

You can also program the pacemaker's sensitivity, measured in millivolts. Most pacemakers allow the heart to function naturally and assist only when necessary. The sensing threshold allows the pacemaker to do this by sensing the heart's normal activity.

Temporary pulse generator

The settings on a temporary pulse generator may be changed in several ways to meet the patient's specific needs. The illustration below shows a single-chamber temporary pulse generator and brief descriptions of its various parts.

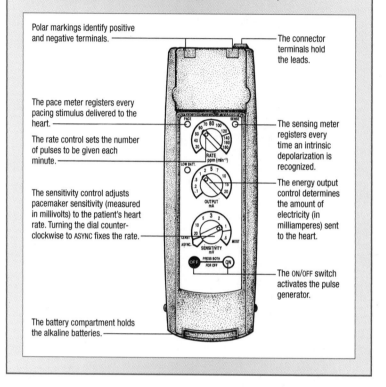

Polar markings identify positive and negative terminals.

The connector terminals hold the leads.

The pace meter registers every pacing stimulus delivered to the heart.

The rate control sets the number of pulses to be given each minute.

The sensing meter registers every time an intrinsic depolarization is recognized.

The sensitivity control adjusts pacemaker sensitivity (measured in millivolts) to the patient's heart rate. Turning the dial counter-clockwise to ASYNC fixes the rate.

The energy output control determines the amount of electricity (in milliamperes) sent to the heart.

The ON/OFF switch activates the pulse generator.

The battery compartment holds the alkaline batteries.

ECG characteristics

The most prominent characteristic of a pacemaker on an ECG is the pacemaker spike that occurs when the pacemaker sends an electrical impulse to the heart muscle. (See *Pacemaker spikes,* page 220.) The impulse appears as a vertical line, or spike. The collective group of spikes on an ECG is called pacemaker artifact.

Depending on the electrode's position in the heart, the spike appears in different locations on the waveform:

◆ When the pacemaker stimulates the atria, the spike is followed by a P wave and the patient's baseline QRS complex and

Pacemaker spikes

Pacemaker impulses—the stimuli that travel from the pacemaker to the heart—are visible on an electrocardiogram tracing as spikes. Large or small, pacemaker spikes appear above or below the isoelectric line. This ECG complex shows an atrial and a ventricular pacemaker spike.

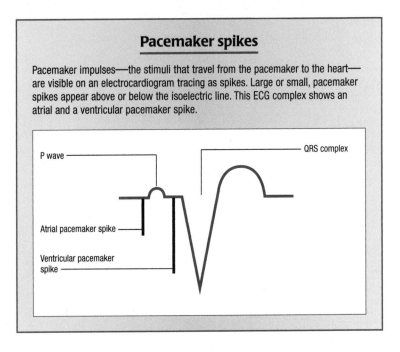

T wave. This series of waveforms represents successful pacing, or capture, of the myocardium. The P wave appears different from the patient's normal P wave.

◆ When the ventricles are stimulated by a pacemaker, the spike is followed by a QRS complex and a T wave. The QRS complex appears wider than the patient's own QRS complex because of how the pacemaker depolarizes the ventricles.

◆ When the pacemaker stimulates the atria and ventricles, the spike is followed by a P wave, then a spike, and then a QRS complex. Be aware that the type of pacemaker used and the patient's condition may affect whether every beat is paced.

Knowing your patient's medical history and whether a pacemaker has been implanted also helps you to determine whether your patient is experiencing ventricular ectopy or paced activity on the ECG. (See *Distinguishing intermittent ventricular pacing from PVCs.*)

Pacemaker modes

Pacemakers have two basic modes for pacing: synchronous and asynchronous. In synchronous, or demand, pacing, the pacemaker initiates electrical im-

LOOK-ALIKES

Distinguishing intermittent ventricular pacing from PVCs

Knowing whether your patient has an artificial pacemaker helps you avoid mistaking a ventricular paced beat for a premature ventricular contraction (PVC). If your facility uses a monitoring system that eliminates artifact, make sure the monitor is set up correctly for a patient with a pacemaker. Otherwise, the pacemaker spikes may be eliminated as well.

If your patient has intermittent ventricular pacing, the paced ventricular complex will have a pacemaker spike preceding it, as shown in the shaded area of the top electrocardiogram (ECG) strip. You may need to look in different leads for a bipolar pacemaker spike because it's small and may be difficult to see. What's more, the paced ventricular complex of a properly functioning pacemaker won't occur early or prematurely, it will occur only when the patient's own ventricular rate falls below the rate set for the pacemaker.

If your patient is having PVCs, they'll occur prematurely and won't have pacemaker spikes preceding them. Examples are shown in the shaded areas of the bottom ECG strip.

INTERMITTENT VENTRICULAR PACING

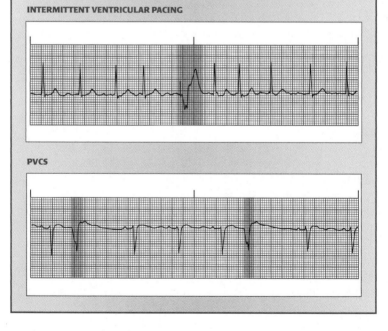

PVCS

pulses only when the heart's intrinsic heart rate falls below the preset rate of the pacemaker. In asynchronous, or fixed, pacing, the pacemaker constantly initiates electrical impulses at a preset rate without regard to the patient's intrinsic electrical activity or heart rate. Asynchronous pacing is rarely used.

Pacemaker description codes

Pacemakers use a uniform code system to describe how they're programmed. This system consists of five letters that indicate the chamber paced, the chamber sensed, the response to sensing, the programmability, and antiarrhythmia function. (See *Pacemaker coding systems*.)

Although the coding system consists of five letters, a three-letter code is typically used to describe pacemaker function. Pacemaker codes include AAI, VVI, DVI, and DDD.

AAI

The AAI, or atrial demand, pacemaker is a single-chambered pacemaker that paces and senses the atria. When the pacemaker senses intrinsic atrial activity, it inhibits pacing and resets itself.

Because AAI pacemakers require a functioning AV node and intact conduction system, they aren't used in AV block. An AAI pacemaker may be used in patients with sinus bradycardia, which may occur after cardiac surgery, or with SSS, as long as the AV node and His-Purkinje system aren't diseased.

VVI

The VVI, or ventricular demand, pacemaker paces and senses the ventricles. When it senses intrinsic ventricular activity, it inhibits pacing.

This single-chambered pacemaker benefits patients with complete heart block and those needing intermittent pacing. Because it doesn't affect atrial activity, it's used for patients who don't need an atrial kick—the extra 15% to 30% of cardiac output that comes from atrial contraction.

If a patient has spontaneous atrial activity, a VVI pacemaker won't synchronize the ventricular activity with it, so tricuspid and mitral insufficiency may develop. Sedentary patients may receive this pacemaker, but it won't adjust its rate for more active patients. (See *AAI and VVI pacemakers*, page 224.)

DVI

The DVI, or AV sequential, pacemaker paces the atria and ventricles. This dual-chambered pacemaker senses only the ventricles' intrinsic activity, inhibiting ventricular pacing.

Two types of DVI pacemakers may be used, a committed DVI and a noncommitted DVI pace-

Pacemaker coding systems

The capabilities of permanent pacemakers can be described by a five-letter coding system. Typically, only the first three letters are used.

First letter

The first letter identifies which heart chambers are paced:
◆ V = Ventricle
◆ A = Atrium
◆ D = Dual—ventricle and atrium
◆ 0 = None.

Second letter

The second letter signifies the heart chamber where the pacemaker senses intrinsic activity:
◆ V = Ventricle
◆ A = Atrium
◆ D = Dual
◆ 0 = None.

Third letter

The third letter indicates the pacemaker's mode of response to the intrinsic electrical activity it senses in the atrium or ventricle:
◆ T = Triggers pacing
◆ I = Inhibits pacing
◆ D = Dual—can trigger or inhibit depending on the mode and where intrinsic activity occurs
◆ 0 = None—doesn't change mode in response to sensed activity.

Fourth letter

The fourth letter describes the degree of programmability and the presence or absence of an adaptive rate response:
◆ P = Basic functions programmable
◆ M = Multiprogrammable parameters
◆ C = Communicating functions such as telemetry
◆ R = Rate responsiveness—rate adjusts to fit the patient's metabolic needs and achieve normal hemodynamic status
◆ 0 = None.

Fifth letter

The fifth letter denotes the pacemaker's response to a tachyarrhythmia:
◆ P = Pacing ability—the pacemaker's rapid burst paces the heart at a rate above its intrinsic rate to override the tachycardia source
◆ S = Shock—an implantable cardioverter-defibrillator identifies ventricular tachycardia and delivers a shock to stop the arrhythmia
◆ D = Dual ability to shock and pace
◆ 0 = None.

maker. The committed DVI pacemaker doesn't sense intrinsic activity during the AV interval—the time between an atrial and ventricular spike. It generates an impulse even with spontaneous ventricular depolarization. The noncommitted DVI pacemaker,

on the other hand, is inhibited if a spontaneous depolarization occurs. (See *DVI pacemaker rhythm strip,* page 225.)

The DVI pacemaker helps patients with AV block or SSS who have a diseased His-Purkinje conduction system. It provides

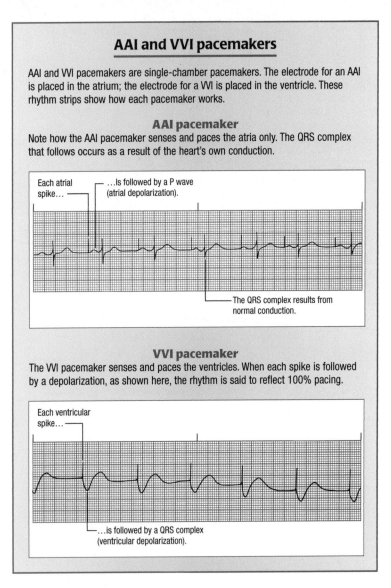

AAI and VVI pacemakers

AAI and VVI pacemakers are single-chamber pacemakers. The electrode for an AAI is placed in the atrium; the electrode for a VVI is placed in the ventricle. These rhythm strips show how each pacemaker works.

AAI pacemaker

Note how the AAI pacemaker senses and paces the atria only. The QRS complex that follows occurs as a result of the heart's own conduction.

Each atrial spike...

...Is followed by a P wave (atrial depolarization).

The QRS complex results from normal conduction.

VVI pacemaker

The VVI pacemaker senses and paces the ventricles. When each spike is followed by a depolarization, as shown here, the rhythm is said to reflect 100% pacing.

Each ventricular spike...

...is followed by a QRS complex (ventricular depolarization).

the benefits of AV synchrony and atrial kick, thus improving cardiac output. However, it can't vary the atrial rate and isn't helpful in atrial fibrillation (AF) because it can't capture the atria. In addition, it may needlessly fire or inhibit its own pacing.

DVI pacemaker rhythm strip

Here's a rhythm strip from a committed DVI pacemaker, which paces both the atria and the ventricles. The pacemaker senses ventricular activity only. In two of the complexes, the pacemaker didn't sense the intrinsic QRS complex because the complex occurred during the AV interval, when the pacemaker was already committed to fire.

With a noncommitted DVI pacemaker, spikes after the QRS complex wouldn't appear because the stimulus to pace the ventricles would be inhibited.

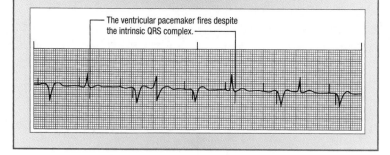

The ventricular pacemaker fires despite the intrinsic QRS complex.

DDD

A DDD, or universal, pacemaker is used with severe AV block. However, because the pacemaker possesses so many capabilities, it may be hard to troubleshoot problems.

Advantages of the DDD pacemaker include its:
◆ versatility
◆ programmability
◆ ability to change modes automatically
◆ ability to mimic the normal physiologic cardiac cycle, maintaining AV synchrony
◆ ability to sense and pace the atria and ventricles at the same time according to the intrinsic atrial rate and maximal rate limit.

Unlike other pacemakers, the DDD pacemaker is set with a rate range, rather than a single critical rate. It senses atrial activity and ensures that the ventricles respond to each atrial stimulation, thereby maintaining normal AV synchrony.

The DDD pacemaker fires when the ventricle doesn't respond on its own, and it paces the atria when the atrial rate falls below the lower set rate. In a patient with a high atrial rate, a safety mechanism allows the pacemaker to follow the intrinsic atrial rate only to a preset upper limit. That limit is usually set at

DDD pacemaker rhythm strip

On this DDD pacemaker rhythm strip, complexes 1, 2, 4, and 7 reveal the atrial-synchronous mode, set at a rate of 70. The patient has an intrinsic P wave; the pacemaker serves only to make sure the ventricles respond.

Complexes 3, 5, 8, 10, and 12 are intrinsic ventricular depolarizations. The pacemaker senses these depolarizations and inhibits firing. In complexes 6, 9, and 11, the pacemaker is pacing both the atria and the ventricles in sequence. In complex 13, only the atria are paced; the ventricles respond on their own.

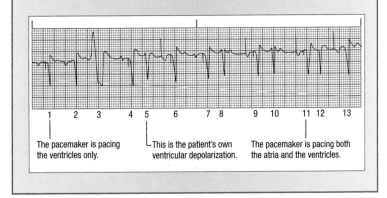

The pacemaker is pacing the ventricles only.

└─This is the patient's own ventricular depolarization.

The pacemaker is pacing both the atria and the ventricles.

about 130 beats/minute and helps to prevent the ventricles from responding to atrial tachycardia or atrial flutter. (See *DDD pacemaker rhythm strip.*)

Assessing pacemaker function

A patient who has a permanent pacemaker should have its function assessed regularly. To assess a pacemaker's function, follow these steps:

◆ Determine the pacemaker's mode and settings. If the patient had a pacemaker implanted previously, ask whether the wallet card from the manufacturer notes the mode and settings. If the pacemaker was recently implanted, check the patient's medical record for information about the pacemaker settings to prevent misinterpretation of the ECG tracing. (For example, if the tracing has ventricular spikes but no atrial pacing spikes, you might assume that it's a VVI pacemaker when it's a DVI pacemaker that has lost its atrial output.)

◆ Review the patient's 12-lead ECG. If it isn't available, examine lead V_1 or MCL_1 instead.

◆ Select a monitoring lead that clearly shows the pacemaker spikes. At the same time, make sure the lead you select doesn't cause the cardiac monitor to misinterpret a spike for a QRS complex and double-count the heart rate. This may cause the alarm to sound, falsely signaling a high heart rate.

◆ When looking at an ECG tracing for a patient with a pacemaker, consider the pacemaker mode, and then interpret the paced rhythm. Does it correlate with what you know about the pacemaker?

◆ Look for information that tells you which chamber is paced. Is there capture? Is there a P wave or QRS complex after each atrial or ventricular spike? Or do the P waves and QRS complexes stem from intrinsic electrical activity?

◆ Look for information about the pacemaker's sensing ability. If intrinsic atrial or ventricular activity is present, what's the pacemaker's response?

◆ Look at the rate. What's the pacing rate per minute? Is it appropriate given the pacemaker settings? Although you can determine the rate quickly by counting the number of complexes in a 6-second ECG strip, a more accurate method is to count the number of small boxes between complexes and divide this into 1,500. (See *A closer look at pacemaker function,* page 228.)

Pacemaker malfunctions

A malfunctioning pacemaker can lead to arrhythmias, hypotension, syncope, and other signs and symptoms of decreased cardiac output. (See *Recognizing a malfunctioning pacemaker,* pages 229 and 230.) Common problems with pacemakers that can lead to low cardiac output and loss of AV synchrony include failure to capture, failure to pace, undersensing, and oversensing.

Failure to capture

Failure to capture appears on an ECG as a pacemaker spike without the appropriate atrial or ventricular response—a spike without a complex. Think of failure to capture as the pacemaker's inability to stimulate the chamber.

Causes of failure to capture include acidosis, electrolyte imbalances, fibrosis, incorrect leadwire position, a low mA or output setting, depletion of the battery, a broken or cracked leadwire, or perforation of the leadwire through the myocardium.

Failure to pace

Failure to pace is indicated by no pacemaker activity on an ECG when pacemaker activity is expected. This problem may be caused by battery or circuit failure, cracked or broken leads, or interference between atrial and ventricular sensing in a dual-

A closer look at pacemaker function

To more thoroughly evaluate pacemaker function, the practitioner may apply a magnet to a pacemaker. When this occurs, the device reverts to a predefined (asynchronous) response mode that allows for assessment of various aspects of pacemaker function. Specifically, applying a magnet allows the practitioner to:

◆ determine which chambers are being paced

◆ assess capture

◆ provide emergency pacing if the device malfunctions

◆ ensure pacing despite electromagnetic interference

◆ assess battery life by checking the magnet rate—a predetermined rate that indicates the need for battery replacement.

Keep in mind, however, that you must know which implanted device the patient has before a magnet is applied. The patient might have an implantable cardioverter-defibrillator (ICD), which only rarely is an appropriate target for magnet application.

It used to be relatively easy to tell a pacemaker from an ICD because of the difference in generator size and implant location. Today it isn't as easy. The generators are similar in size, and both kinds of devices are implanted under the skin of the patient's chest. What's more, a single device may perform multiple functions.

In general, a magnet shouldn't be applied to an ICD or a pacemaker-ICD combination. Applying a magnet to an ICD can cause an unexpected response because various responses can be programmed or determined by the manufacturer. When directed, applying a magnet to an ICD usually suspends therapies for ventricular tachycardia and fibrillation while leaving bradycardia pacing active, which may be helpful in patients who receive multiple, inappropriate shocks. Some models may beep when exposed to a magnetic field.

---

chambered pacemaker. Failure to pace can lead to asystole.

Undersensing

Undersensing is indicated by a pacemaker spike when intrinsic cardiac activity is present. In asynchronous pacemakers that have such codes as VOO or DOO, undersensing is a programming limitation.

When undersensing occurs in synchronous pacemakers, pacing spikes occur on the ECG where they shouldn't. Although they may appear in any part of the cardiac cycle, the spikes are especially dangerous if they fall on the T wave, where they can cause ventricular tachycardia (VT) or ventricular fibrillation (VF).

In synchronous pacemakers, undersensing may be caused by electrolyte imbalances, lead disconnection or dislodgment, improper lead placement, increased sensing threshold from edema or

Recognizing a malfunctioning pacemaker

Occasionally, pacemakers fail to function properly. When this happens, you'll need to take immediate action to correct the problem. The rhythm strips below show examples of problems that can occur with a temporary pacemaker.

Failure to capture

◆ In this situation, the pacemaker can't stimulate the chamber.

◆ The electrocardiogram (ECG) will show a pacemaker spike without the appropriate atrial or ventricular response (spike without a complex), as shown at right.

◆ The patient may be asymptomatic or have signs of decreased cardiac output.

◆ The problem may occur because of increased pacing thresholds related to:
– metabolic or electrolyte imbalance
– antiarrhythmics
– fibrosis or edema at electrode tip.

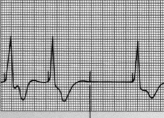

There's a pacemaker spike but no response from the heart.

◆ The problem may also result from lead malfunction because of:
– a dislodged lead
– a broken or damaged lead
– perforation of the myocardium by the lead
– a loose connection between the lead and pulse generator.

◆ Related interventions may solve the problem. For example:
– Treat any metabolic disturbance.
– Replace the damaged lead.
– Change the pulse generator battery.
– Slowly increase the output setting until capture occurs.
– Obtain a chest X-ray to determine electrode placement.

Failure to pace

◆ The ECG shows no pacemaker activity when pacemaker activity should be evident, as shown at the top of the next page.

◆ Magnet application yields no response. (It should cause asynchronous pacing.)

◆ The problem has several common causes, including:
– a depleted battery
– circuit failure
– lead malfunction
– inappropriate programming of sensing function
– electromagnetic interference.

(continued)

Recognizing a malfunctioning pacemaker *(continued)*

Failure to pace *(continued)*

◆ Failure to pace can lead to asystole or a severe decrease in cardiac output in pacemaker-dependent patients.

◆ If you think a pacemaker is failing to pace, a temporary pacemaker (transcutaneous or transvenous) should be used to prevent asystole.

◆ Related interventions may solve the problem. For example:
– Replace the pulse generator battery.
– Replace the pulse generator unit.
– Adjust the sensitivity setting.
– Remove any source of electromagnetic interference.

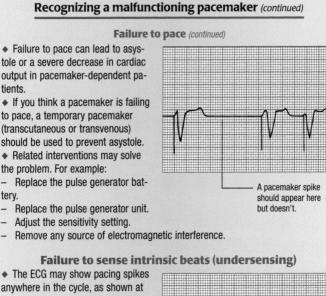

A pacemaker spike should appear here but doesn't.

Failure to sense intrinsic beats (undersensing)

◆ The ECG may show pacing spikes anywhere in the cycle, as shown at right.

◆ A pacemaker spike may appear where intrinsic cardiac activity is present.

◆ The patient may report feeling palpitations or skipped beats.

◆ Spikes are especially dangerous if they fall on the T wave because ventricular tachycardia or fibrillation may result.

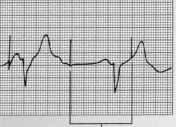

The pacemaker fires anywhere in the cycle.

◆ The problem has several common causes, including:
– battery failure
– fracture of the pacing leadwire
– displacement of the electrode tip
– "cross-talk" between atrial and ventricular channels
– electromagnetic interference mistaken for intrinsic signals.

◆ Related interventions may solve the problem. For example:
– Replace the pulse generator battery.
– Replace the leadwires.
– Adjust the sensitivity setting.

fibrosis at the electrode tip, drug interactions, or a depleted or dead pacemaker battery.

Oversensing

If the pacemaker is too sensitive, it can misinterpret muscle movements or other events in the cardiac cycle as intrinsic cardiac electrical activity. Pacing won't occur when it's needed, and the heart rate and AV synchrony won't be maintained.

Caring for patients with pacemakers

When caring for a patient with a pacemaker, your nursing interventions may vary, depending on the type of pacemaker the patient has. Besides assessing for general function, as discussed previously, also incorporate the following steps into your care plan.

Interventions for permanent pacemakers

◆ Using a systematic approach, obtain the following information about the patient's pacemaker:
– What's the mode?
– What's the base rate and upper rate limit (maximum tracking or sensor rate)?
– Are features, such as mode switching or rate response, activated?
– Is the device a biventricular pacemaker?
– Is the patient pacemaker-dependent?

– Does the patient have signs and symptoms of pacemaker malfunction, such as decreased heart rate, dizziness, or hypotension?
◆ Gather and evaluate information from these sources: the patient, the patient's family, the identification card issued by the pacemaker manufacturer, the patient's history, and the practitioner's notes or printouts from the programmer, if available.
◆ Review the patient's 12-lead ECG to evaluate pacemaker function. If unavailable, examine lead V_1 or MCL_1 instead. Compare at least two leads to verify what you observe. Keep in mind that the visibility of spikes depends on pacing polarity and the type of lead. As part of the ECG evaluation, do the following:
– Measure the rate and interpret the paced rhythm.
– Compare the morphology of paced and intrinsic complexes. (Traditional right ventricular pacing should produce a morphology similar to left bundle-branch block pattern.)
– Differentiate between ventricular ectopy and paced activity.
– Look for information that tells you which chamber is paced and information about the pacemaker's sensing function.
◆ Monitor vital signs.
◆ Observe the patient for complications, such as:

– decreased cardiac output (hypotension, chest pain, dyspnea, syncope)
– infection
– pneumothorax
– abnormal electrical stimulation occurring in synchrony with the pacemaker
– pectoral muscle twitching
– hiccups (stimulation of diaphragm)
– cardiac tamponade.

Interventions for biventricular pacemakers

Follow the same general guidelines for a patient with a permanent pacemaker; in addition, include these specific measures:

◆ Because of the position of the left ventricular lead, watch for stimulation of the diaphragm and left chest wall, which may present as hiccups or visible muscle spasms. Notify the practitioner if this occurs because the left ventricular lead may need repositioning.

◆ Observe the ECG for pacemaker spikes. Although both ventricles are paced, only one pacemaker spike is seen.

◆ Measure the duration of the QRS complex, which should be narrowed. A widened QRS complex may indicate that the left ventricular lead is no longer positioned properly.

Interventions for temporary pacemakers

◆ Check stimulation and sensing thresholds daily because they increase over time.

◆ Assess the patient and pacemaker regularly to check for possible problems, such as failure to capture, undersensing, or oversensing.

◆ Turn or reposition the patient carefully to prevent dislodging the leadwire.

◆ Follow recommended electrical safety precautions.

◆ Make sure the bed and all electrical equipment are grounded properly and that all pacing wires and connections to temporary wires are insulated with moisture-proof material (such as a disposable glove) to avoid microshocks to the patient. *Remember:* Temporary pacing wires have the potential to deliver a shock directly to the heart, resulting in VT or VF.

◆ Obtain a chest X-ray and assist the practitioner with repositioning the leadwire, if required.

◆ Defibrillation and cardioversion (up to 360 joules) don't usually require that the pulse generator be disconnected.

◆ Look for signs of complications, such as:
– decreased cardiac output (hypotension, chest pain, dyspnea, syncope)
– infection

– pneumothorax
– abnormal electrical stimulation occurring in synchrony with the pacemaker
– pectoral muscle twitching
– hiccups (stimulation of diaphragm)
– perforated ventricle and resultant cardiac tamponade. (Signs and symptoms of this complication include persistent hiccups, tachycardia, distant heart sounds, pulsus paradoxus [a drop in the strength of a pulse during inspiration], hypotension with narrowed pulse pressure, cyanosis, distended jugular veins, decreased urine output, restlessness, and complaints of fullness in the chest. If any of these signs or symptoms occur, notify the practitioner immediately.)

◆ If the patient requires pacing but the pacemaker is failing to stimulate the heart (no output), take these steps:
– Verify that the pacemaker is turned on.
– Check the output settings.
– Change the pulse generator battery.
– Change the pulse generator.
– Check for a disconnected or dislodged pacing wire.

Patient education

Explain to the patient undergoing pacemaker insertion why a pacemaker is needed, how it works, and what can be expected from it. Make your teaching specific to the type of pacemaker inserted, being sure to cover the following points with the patient and his family.

Teaching about permanent pacemakers

◆ Teach the patient about the pacemaker's function, including relevant information about anatomy and physiology, and explain why it's necessary. Review postoperative care and routines.

◆ Before discharge, emphasize:
– how to care for the incision
– signs of pocket complications (hematoma, infection, bleeding)
– the need to avoid heavy lifting or vigorous activity for 2 to 4 weeks
– the need to restrict arm movement on the pacemaker side, as prescribed
– the importance of keeping all follow-up appointments
– how to obtain transtelephonic monitoring follow-up, if indicated
– the need to carry the pacemaker identification card at all times
– the procedure for taking his pulse.

◆ Tell the patient to call his practitioner if he experiences light-headedness, syncope, fatigue, palpitations, muscle stimulation, hiccups, or if his heart

Understanding EMI

Electromagnetic interference (EMI) can wreak havoc on patients who have a pacemaker or an implantable cardioverter-defibrillator (ICD). For someone with a pacemaker, EMI may inhibit pacing, cause asynchronous or unnecessary pacing, or mimic intrinsic cardiac activity. For someone with an ICD, EMI may mimic ventricular fibrillation, or it may prevent detection of a problem that needs treatment.

If your patient has a pacemaker or an ICD, review common sources of EMI and urge the patient to avoid them. These may include:

◆ strong electromagnetic fields
◆ large generators and transformers
◆ arc and resistance welders
◆ large magnets
◆ motorized radiofrequency equipment.

EMI may present a risk in medical or hospital settings as well. Make sure your patient knows to notify all health care providers about the implanted device so the provider can evaluate the risk of such therapies as:

◆ magnetic resonance imaging (usually contraindicated)
◆ radiation therapy (excluding diagnostic X-rays, such as mammograms, which typically are safe)
◆ diathermy
◆ electrocautery
◆ transcutaneous electrical nerve stimulation.

---

rate is unusually fast or slower than the base rate.

◆ Because today's pacemakers are well shielded from environmental interactions, explain that the patient can safely use:

– most common household appliances, including microwaves

– cellular phones (on the opposite side of the device)

– spark-ignited combustion engines (leaf blower, lawnmower, automobile)

– office equipment (computer, copier, fax machine)

– light shop equipment.

◆ Caution the patient to avoid close or prolonged exposure to potential sources of electromagnetic interference. (See *Understanding EMI*.)

◆ Remind the patient about these travel-related issues:

– Metal detectors won't disturb device function, but they may detect the device and trigger an alarm.

– Hand-held screening tools shouldn't be used over the device or near it.

– The patient should be prepared to present his pacemaker

identification card to security personnel.

Teaching about biventricular pacemakers

Provide the same basic teaching as for a patient receiving a permanent pacemaker. Additionally, cover these points:

◆ Explain to the patient and his family why a biventricular pacemaker is needed, how it works, and what they can expect.

◆ Before pacemaker insertion, caution the patient and his family that placing the left ventricular lead can be painful and that the procedure may take 3 hours or more.

◆ Stress the importance of calling the practitioner immediately if the patient develops chest pain, shortness of breath, swelling of the hands or feet, or a weight gain of 3 lb (1.4 kg) in 24 hours or 5 lb (2.3 kg) in 48 hours.

Teaching about temporary pacemakers

◆ Provide information to the patient about the pacemaker's function, related anatomy and physiology, the need for the pacemaker, and the potential need for a permanent pacemaker.

◆ Before pacemaker insertion, tell the patient what he can expect postoperatively, especially regarding pain management.

◆ Advise the patient not to get out of bed without assistance.

◆ Instruct the patient not to manipulate the pacemaker wires or the pulse generator.

◆ Instruct the patient to tell the nurse if he experiences lightheadedness, syncope, palpitations, muscle stimulation, or hiccups.

◆ Advise the patient to limit arm movement on the side of the pacemaker.

Implantable cardioverter-defibrillator

An ICD is an electronic device implanted in the body to provide continuous monitoring of the heart for bradycardia, VT, and VF. The device then administers either shocks or paced beats to treat the dangerous arrhythmia. In general, ICDs are indicated for patients for whom drug therapy, surgery, or catheter ablation has failed to prevent the arrhythmia.

Procedure

The procedure for ICD insertion is similar to that of a permanent pacemaker and may take place in a cardiac catheterization laboratory. Occasionally, a patient who requires other surgery, such as coronary artery bypass grafting,

ICD overview

Today's implantable cardioverter-defibrillators (ICDs) are easier to implant and more effective than ever. For most patients, the leads can be threaded through the cephalic vein and positioned in the heart and superior vena cava. The pulse generator is inserted under the skin through a small incision. In some cases, a high-voltage subcutaneous patch electrode is placed inside the superior periaxial area to reduce the amount of energy needed for defibrillation.

Programming features have evolved greatly and now allow tiered therapy, antitachycardia pacing, low-energy cardioversion, antibradycardia pacing, data storage, and diagnostic algorithms. In addition, some devices allow the magnet mode (in which placing a magnet over the generator suppresses ICD programming) to be turned on or off. With the magnet mode turned off, a magnet won't affect ICD function. In some devices, a magnet temporarily suspends detection and tachycardia therapy, while leaving antibradycardia pacing intact.

Originally, the only patients chosen to receive ICDs were those who survived sudden cardiac death and those who sustained ventricular tachycardia and syncope unresponsive to antiarrhythmic drugs. However, reports have revealed a survival rate 40% to 60% higher among at-risk patients with ICDs than among those who received conventional therapies. Consequently, ICDs are now recommended or being investigated for:
◆ ventricular fibrillation without structural heart disease or triggering factors
◆ syncope of an undetermined cause
◆ unsuccessful antiarrhythmic therapy
◆ patients with risk factors for ventricular arrhythmias
◆ patients with extensive anterior wall myocardial infarction (MI) who can't take thrombolytic agents
◆ patients with previous MI and unexplained recurrent syncope
◆ children with congenital long QT-interval syndrome
◆ patients who are waiting for heart transplantations.

may have the device implanted in the operating room. (See *ICD overview*.)

An ICD consists of a programmable pulse generator and one or more leadwires. The pulse generator is a small battery-powered computer that monitors the heart's electrical signals and delivers electrical therapy when it identifies an abnormal rhythm. The leads are insulated wires

that carry the heart signal to the pulse generator and deliver the electrical energy from the pulse generator to the heart.

An ICD also stores information about the heart's activity before, during, and after an arrhythmia, along with tracking which treatment was delivered and the treatment's outcome. Many devices also store electrograms (electrical tracings similar to ECGs). With

Types of ICD therapies

An implantable cardioverter-defibrillator (ICD) can deliver a range of therapies depending on the type of device, how the device is programmed and the arrhythmia it detects. Therapies include antitachycardia pacing, cardioversion, defibrillation, and bradycardia pacing. Some models also provide biventricular pacing.

THERAPY	DESCRIPTION
Antitachycardia pacing	A series of small, rapid electrical pacing pulses used to interrupt atrial fibrillation (AF) or ventricular tachycardia (VT) and return the heart to its normal rhythm. Antitachycardia pacing isn't appropriate for all patients and begins only after appropriate electrophysiology studies.
Cardioversion	A low- or high-energy shock (up to 35 joules) timed to the R wave to terminate VT and return the heart to its normal rhythm.
Defibrillation	A high-energy shock (up to 35 joules) to the heart to terminate ventricular fibrillation or AF and return the heart to its normal rhythm.
Bradycardia pacing	Electrical pacing pulses used when natural electrical signals are too slow. Most ICDs pace one chamber (VVI pacing) of the heart at a preset rate. Some can sense and pace both chambers (DDD pacing).

an interrogation device, a practitioner can retrieve this information to evaluate ICD function and battery status and to adjust ICD system settings.

Today's advanced devices can detect a wide range of arrhythmias and automatically respond with the appropriate therapy, such as bradycardia pacing (both single- and dual-chamber), antitachycardia pacing, cardioversion, and defibrillation. ICDs that provide therapy for atrial arrhythmias, such as AF, are also available. (See *Types of ICD therapies*.)

Interventions

If the patient experiences an arrhythmia or the ICD delivers a therapy, the device's program information helps to evaluate the functioning of the device. This information is available through a status report that can be obtained and printed when the practitioner or specially trained technician interrogates the device. A specialized piece of equipment is placed over the implanted pulse generator to retrieve pacing function.

Program information includes:
◆ type and model of ICD
◆ status of the device (on or off)
◆ detection rates
◆ therapies delivered (pacing, antitachycardia pacing, cardioversion, and defibrillation).

If the patient experiences an arrhythmia:
◆ Assess the patient for signs and symptoms related to decreased cardiac output.
◆ Record the patient's ECG rhythm.
◆ Evaluate the appropriateness of any delivered ICD therapy.

If the patient experiences cardiac arrest:
◆ Initiate cardiopulmonary resuscitation (CPR) and advanced cardiac life support (ACLS).
◆ If the patient needs external defibrillation, position the paddles as far from the device as possible or use the anteroposterior paddle position.

Patient education

◆ Explain to the patient and his family why an ICD is needed, how it works, potential complications, and what they can expect. Make sure they also understand ICD terminology.

◆ Discuss signs and symptoms to report to the practitioner immediately.
◆ Advise the patient to wear a medical identification bracelet indicating ICD placement.
◆ Educate family members in emergency techniques (such as dialing 911 and performing CPR) in case the device fails.
◆ Explain that electrical or electronic devices may disrupt the device.
◆ Warn the patient to avoid placing excessive pressure over the insertion site or moving or jerking the area until the postoperative visit.
◆ Tell the patient to follow normal routines as allowed by the practitioner and to increase exercise as tolerated. After the first 24 hours, show the patient how to perform passive range-of-motion exercises and progress as tolerated.
◆ Remind the patient to carry information regarding his ICD at all times and to inform airline clerks when he travels as well as individuals performing diagnostic functions (such as computed tomography scans and magnetic resonance imaging).
◆ Stress the importance of follow-up care and checkups.

Radiofrequency ablation

Radiofrequency ablation is an invasive procedure that may be used to treat arrhythmias in patients who haven't responded to antiarrhythmic drugs or cardioversion or can't tolerate antiarrhythmic drugs. In this procedure, a burst of radiofrequency energy is delivered through a catheter to the heart tissue to destroy the arrhythmia's focus or block the conduction pathway.

Radiofrequency ablation is effective in treating patients with AF and flutter, VT, AV nodal reentry tachycardia, and Wolff-Parkinson-White (WPW) syndrome.

Procedure

The patient first undergoes electrophysiology studies to identify and map the specific area of the heart that's causing the arrhythmia. The ablation catheters are inserted into a vein, usually the femoral vein, and advanced to the heart where short bursts of radiofrequency waves destroy a small targeted area of heart tissue. The destroyed tissue can no longer conduct electrical impulses. Other types of energy may also be used, such as microwave, sonar, or cryo (freezing). In some patients, the tissue inside the pulmonary vein is responsible for the arrhythmia. Targeted radiofrequency ablation is used to block these abnormal impulses. (See *Destroying the source,* pages 240 and 241.)

If a rapid arrhythmia that originates above the AV node (such as AF) isn't terminated by targeted ablation, AV nodal ablation may be used to block electrical impulses from being conducted to the ventricles. After ablation of the AV node, the patient may need a pacemaker because impulses can no longer be conducted from the atria to the ventricles. If the atria continue to beat irregularly, anticoagulation therapy will also be needed to reduce the risk of stroke.

If the patient has WPW syndrome, electrophysiology studies can locate the accessory pathway and ablation can destroy it. When reentry is the cause of the arrhythmia, such as AV nodal reentry tachycardia, ablation can destroy the pathway without affecting the AV node.

Interventions

When caring for a patient after radiofrequency ablation, follow these guidelines:
◆ Provide continuous cardiac monitoring, assessing for arrhythmias and ischemic changes.

Destroying the source

In radiofrequency ablation, special catheters are inserted in a vein and advanced to the heart. After the arrhythmia's source is identified, radiofrequency energy is used to destroy the source of the abnormal electrical impulses or abnormal conduction pathway.

AV nodal ablation

If a rapid arrhythmia originates above the atrioventricular (AV) node, the AV node may be destroyed to block impulses from reaching the ventricles. The radiofrequency ablation catheter is directed to the AV node (A). Radiofrequency energy is used to destroy the AV node (B).

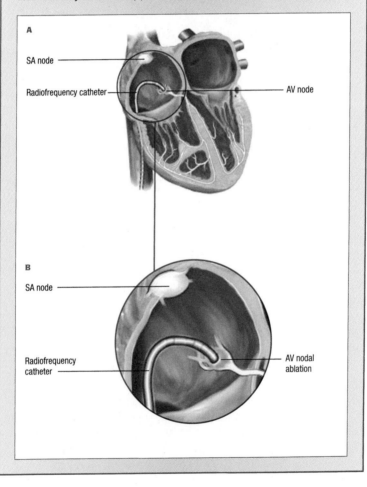

Destroying the source (continued)

Pulmonary vein ablation

If the pulmonary vein is the source of the arrhythmia, radiofrequency energy is used to destroy the tissue at the base of the pulmonary vein. The radiofrequency catheter is directed to the base of the pulmonary vein (A). Radiofrequency energy is used to destroy the tissue at the base of the pulmonary vein (B).

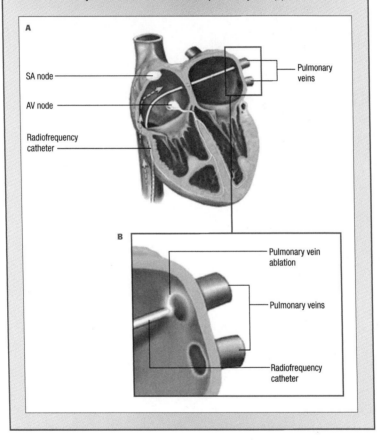

A

SA node

AV node

Radiofrequency catheter

Pulmonary veins

B

Pulmonary vein ablation

Pulmonary veins

Radiofrequency catheter

◆ Place the patient on bed rest for 8 hours, or as ordered, and keep the affected extremity straight. Maintain the head of the bed between 15 and 30 degrees.

◆ Assess the patient's vital signs every 15 minutes for the first hour, then every 30 minutes for 4 hours, unless the patient's condition warrants more frequent checking.

◆ Assess peripheral pulses distal to the catheter insertion site as well as the color, sensation, temperature, and capillary refill of the affected extremity.

◆ Check the catheter insertion site for bleeding and hematoma formation.

◆ **ALERT** Monitor the patient for complications, such as hemorrhage, stroke, perforation of the heart, arrhythmias, phrenic nerve damage, pericarditis, pulmonary vein stenosis or thrombosis, and sudden death.

Patient education

When a patient undergoes radiofrequency ablation, be sure to cover these points:

◆ Discuss with the patient and his family why radiofrequency ablation is needed, how it works, and what they can expect.

◆ Warn the patient and his family that the procedure can be lengthy, up to 6 hours if electrophysiology studies are being done first.

◆ Explain that the patient may be hospitalized for 24 to 48 hours to monitor his heart rhythm.

◆ Provide pacemaker teaching if the patient had a pacemaker inserted.

12-lead ECGs

Basic 12-lead electrocardiography

12

The 12-lead electrocardiogram (ECG) is a diagnostic test that helps identify pathologic conditions, especially ischemia and acute myocardial infarction (MI). It provides a more complete view of the heart's electrical activity than a rhythm strip and can be used to assess left ventricular function more effectively. Patients with conditions that affect the heart's electrical system may also benefit from a 12-lead ECG, including those with:

◆ cardiac arrhythmias
◆ heart chamber enlargement or hypertrophy
◆ digoxin or other drug toxicity
◆ electrolyte imbalances
◆ pulmonary embolism
◆ pericarditis
◆ pacemakers
◆ hypothermia.

Like other diagnostic tests, a 12-lead ECG must be viewed in conjunction with other clinical data. Therefore, always correlate the patient's ECG results with the history, physical assessment findings, and results of laboratory and other diagnostic studies as well as the drug regimen.

Remember, too, that an ECG can be done in various ways, including over a telephone line. (See *Transtelephonic cardiac monitoring*, page 246.) In fact, transtelephonic monitoring has become increasingly important as a tool for assessing patients at home and in other nonclinical settings.

Fundamentals

The 12-lead ECG records the heart's electrical activity using a series of electrodes placed on the patient's extremities and chest wall. The 12 leads include three bipolar limb leads (I, II, III), three unipolar augmented limb leads (aV_R, aV_L, and aV_F), and six unipolar precordial, or chest,

Transstelephonic cardiac monitoring

Using a special recorder-transmitter, patients at home can transmit electrocardiograms (ECGs) by telephone to a central monitoring center for immediate interpretation. This commonly used technique, called *transtelephonic cardiac monitoring* (TTM), reduces health care costs.

Nurses play an important role in TTM. Besides performing extensive patient and family teaching, they may operate the central monitoring center and help interpret ECGs sent by patients.

TTM allows a practitioner to assess transient conditions that cause such symptoms as palpitations, dizziness, syncope, confusion, paroxysmal dyspnea, and chest pain. Such conditions, which aren't commonly apparent while the patient is with a practitioner, can make diagnosis difficult and costly.

With TTM, the patient can transmit an ECG recording from his home when the symptoms appear, avoiding the need to go to the hospital and offering a greater opportunity for early diagnosis. Even if symptoms seldom appear, the patient can keep the equipment for long periods, which further aids in the diagnosis of the patient's condition.

Home care

TTM can also be used by a patient having cardiac rehabilitation at home. He'll be called regularly during this period to assess his progress. Because of this continuous monitoring, TTM can help reduce the anxiety felt by the patient and his family after discharge, especially if the patient suffered a myocardial infarction.

TTM is especially valuable for assessing the effects of drugs and for diagnosing and managing paroxysmal arrhythmias. In both cases, TTM can eliminate the need for admitting the patient for evaluation and a potentially lengthy hospital stay.

Understanding TTM equipment

TTM requires three main pieces of equipment: an ECG recorder-transmitter, a standard telephone line, and a receiver. The ECG recorder-transmitter converts electrical activity from the patient's heart into acoustic waves. Some models contain built-in memory devices that store recordings of cardiac activity for transmission later.

A standard telephone line is used to transmit information. The receiver converts the acoustic waves transmitted over the telephone line into ECG activity, which is then recorded on ECG paper for interpretation and documentation in the patient's chart. The recorder-transmitter uses two types of electrodes applied to the finger and chest. The electrodes produce ECG tracings similar to those of a standard 12-lead ECG.

Credit card-size recorder

This recorder operates on a battery and is about the size of a credit card. When a patient becomes symptomatic, he holds the back of the card firmly to the center of his chest and pushes the start button. Four electrodes located on the back of the card sense electrical activity and record it. The card can store 30 seconds of activity and can later transmit the recording across phone lines for evaluation.

leads (V_1, V_2, V_3, V_4, V_5, and V_6). These leads provide 12 different views of the heart's electrical activity. (See *ECG leads*.)

Scanning up, down, and across, each lead transmits information about a different area of the heart. The waveforms ob-

ECG leads

Each of the leads on a 12-lead electrocardiogram (ECG) views the heart from a different angle. These illustrations show the direction of electrical activity (depolarization) monitored by each lead and the 12 views of the heart.

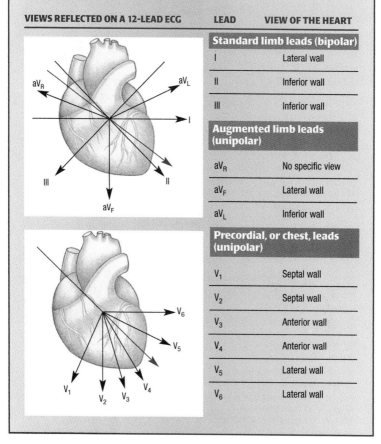

VIEWS REFLECTED ON A 12-LEAD ECG	LEAD	VIEW OF THE HEART
Standard limb leads (bipolar)		
	I	Lateral wall
	II	Inferior wall
	III	Inferior wall
Augmented limb leads (unipolar)		
	aV_R	No specific view
	aV_F	Lateral wall
	aV_L	Inferior wall
Precordial, or chest, leads (unipolar)		
	V_1	Septal wall
	V_2	Septal wall
	V_3	Anterior wall
	V_4	Anterior wall
	V_5	Lateral wall
	V_6	Lateral wall

tained from each lead vary depending on the lead's location in relation to the wave of depolarization passing through the myocardium.

Limb leads

The six limb leads record electrical activity in the heart's frontal plane, a view through the middle of the heart from top to bottom. Electrical activity is recorded from the anterior to the posterior axes.

Precordial leads

The six precordial leads provide information on electrical activity in the heart's horizontal plane, a transverse view through the middle of the heart, dividing it into upper and lower portions. Electrical activity is recorded from either a superior or an inferior approach.

Electrical axis

As well as assessing 12 different leads, a 12-lead ECG records the heart's electrical axis. The term *axis* refers to the direction of depolarization as it spreads through the heart. As impulses travel through the heart, they generate small electrical forces called instantaneous vectors. The mean of these vectors represents the force and direction of the wave of depolarization through the heart— the electrical axis. The electrical axis is also called the *mean instantaneous vector* and the *mean QRS vector.*

In a healthy heart, impulses originate in the sinoatrial node, travel through the atria to the atrioventricular node, and then to the ventricles. Most of the movement of the impulses is down-

ward and to the left, the direction of a normal axis.

In an unhealthy heart, axis direction varies. That's because the direction of electrical activity travels away from areas of damage or necrosis and toward areas of hypertrophy. Knowing the normal deflection of each lead will help you evaluate whether the electrical axis is normal or abnormal.

Obtaining a 12-lead ECG

To perform a 12-lead ECG, you'll need to prepare properly, select the appropriate electrode sites, understand how to perform variations on a standard 12-lead ECG, and make an accurate recording.

Preparation

Gather all necessary supplies, including the ECG machine, recording paper, electrodes, and gauze pads. Tell the patient that the practitioner has ordered an ECG, and explain the procedure. Emphasize that the test takes about 10 minutes and that it's a safe and painless way to evaluate the heart's electrical activity. Answer the patient's questions, and offer reassurance. Preparing the patient properly will help alleviate anxiety and promote cooperation.

Ask the patient to lie in a supine position in the center of the bed with arms at his sides. If he can't tolerate lying flat, raise the head of the bed to semi-Fowler's position. Document the patient's position during the procedure. Ensure privacy, and expose the patient's arms, legs, and chest, draping for comfort.

Site selection

Select the areas where you'll apply the electrodes. Choose areas that are flat and fleshy and not muscular or bony. Clip the area if it's excessively hairy. Remove excess oil and other substances from the skin to enhance electrode contact. Remember, the better the electrode contact, the better the recording.

The 12-lead ECG provides 12 different views of the heart, just as 12 photographers snapping the same picture would produce 12 different photographs. Taking all of those snapshots requires placing four electrodes on the limbs and six across the front of the chest wall.

To help ensure an accurate recording, the electrodes must be applied correctly. Inaccurate placement of an electrode by greater than $5/8''$ (1.5 cm) from its standardized position may lead to inaccurate waveforms and an incorrect ECG interpretation.

Limb lead placement

To record the bipolar limb leads I, II, and III and the unipolar limb leads aV_R, aV_L, and aV_F, place electrodes on both of the patient's arms and on his left leg. The right leg also receives an electrode, but that electrode acts as a ground and doesn't contribute to the waveform. (See *Limb lead placement,* pages 250 and 251.)

Placing the electrodes on the patient is typically easy because each leadwire is labeled or color-coded. For example, a wire (usually white) might be labeled "RA" for right arm. Another (usually red) might be labeled "LL" for left leg.

Precordial lead placement

Precordial leads are also labeled or color-coded according to which wire corresponds to which lead. To record the six precordial leads (V_1 through V_6), position the electrodes on specific areas of the anterior chest wall. (See *Precordial lead placement,* page 252.) If they're placed too low, the ECG tracing will be inaccurate.

◆ Place lead V_1 over the fourth intercostal space at the right ster-

Limb lead placement

Proper lead placement is critical for the accurate recording of cardiac rhythms. The diagrams here show electrode placement for the six limb leads. RA indicates right arm; LA, left arm; RL, right leg; and LL, left leg. The plus sign (+) indicates the positive pole, the minus sign (−) indicates the negative pole, and G indicates the ground. Below each diagram is a sample electrocardiogram recording for that lead.

Lead I
Lead I connects the right arm (negative pole) with the left arm (positive pole).

Lead II
Lead II connects the right arm (negative pole) with the left leg (positive pole).

Lead III
Lead III connects the left arm (negative pole) with the left leg (positive pole).

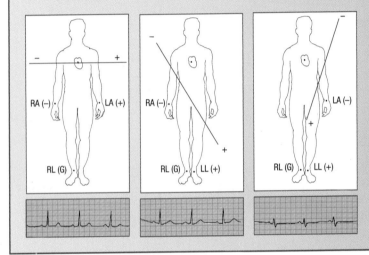

nal border. To find the space, locate the sternal notch at the second rib and feel your way down the sternal border until you reach the fourth intercostal space.

◆ Place lead V_2 just opposite V_1, over the fourth intercostal space at the left sternal border.

◆ Place lead V_4 over the fifth intercostal space at the left midclavicular line. Placing lead V_4 before V_3 makes it easier to see where to place lead V_3.

◆ Place lead V_3 midway between V_2 and V_4.

◆ Place lead V_5 over the fifth intercostal space at the left anterior axillary line.

◆ Place lead V_6 over the fifth intercostal space at the left midaxillary line. If you've placed leads V_4 through V_6 correctly, they should line up horizontally.

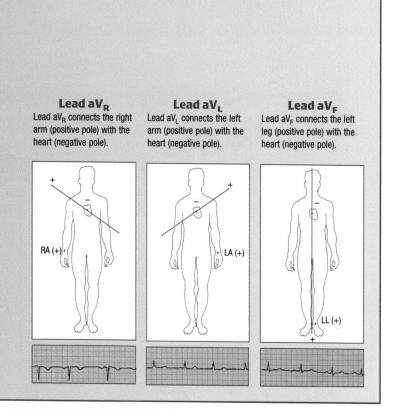

Lead aV_R
Lead aV_R connects the right arm (positive pole) with the heart (negative pole).

Lead aV_L
Lead aV_L connects the left arm (positive pole) with the heart (negative pole).

Lead aV_F
Lead aV_F connects the left leg (positive pole) with the heart (negative pole).

Additional types of ECGs

In addition to the standard 12-lead ECG, two other types of ECGs may be used for diagnostic purposes: the posterior-lead ECG and the right chest lead ECG. These ECGs use chest leads to assess areas that standard 12-lead ECGs can't.

Posterior-lead ECG

Because of lung and muscle barriers, the usual chest leads can't "see" the heart's posterior surface to record myocardial damage there. So, some practitioners add three posterior leads to the 12-lead ECG: leads V_7, V_8, and V_9. These leads are placed opposite anterior leads V_4, V_5, and V_6, on the left side of the patient's back, following the same horizontal

Precordial lead placement

The precordial leads complement the limb leads to provide a complete view of the heart. To record the precordial leads, place the electrodes as shown.

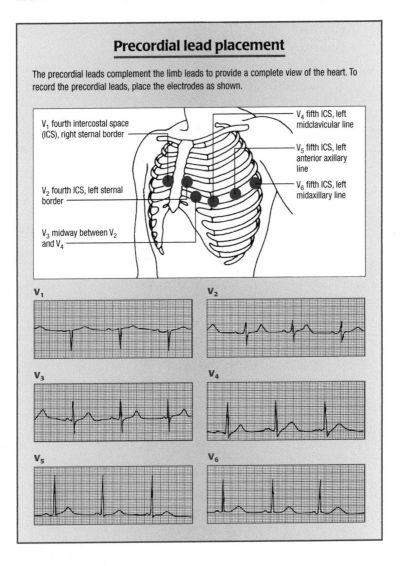

line. (See *Posterior lead placement*.)

Occasionally, a practitioner may request right-sided posterior leads. These leads are labeled V_{7R}, V_{8R}, and V_{9R} and are placed on the right side of the patient's back. Their placement is a mirror image of the electrodes on the left side of the back. This type of ECG provides information on the right posterior area of the heart.

Posterior lead placement

Posterior leads can be used to assess the heart's posterior. To ensure an accurate reading, make sure the posterior electrodes V_7, V_8, and V_9 are placed at the same horizontal level as the V_6 lead at the fifth intercostal space. Place lead V_7 at the posterior axillary line, lead V_9 at the paraspinal line, and lead V_8 halfway between leads V_7 and V_9.

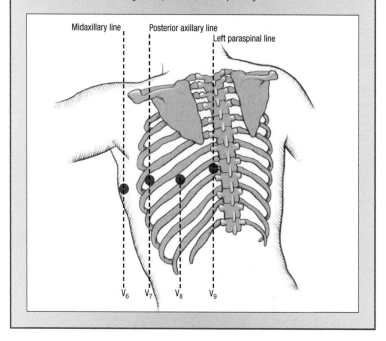

Right chest lead ECG

The standard 12-lead ECG evaluates only the left ventricle. If the right ventricle needs to be assessed for damage or dysfunction, the practitioner may order a right chest lead ECG. For example, a patient with an inferior wall MI might have a right chest lead ECG to rule out right ventricular involvement.

With this type of ECG, the six leads are placed on the right side of the chest in a mirror image of the standard precordial lead placement. Electrodes start at the left sternal border and swing down under the right breast area (See *Right precordial lead placement,* page 254.)

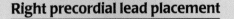

Right precordial lead placement

Right precordial leads can provide specific information about the function of the right ventricle. Place the six leads on the right side of the chest in a mirror image of the standard precordial lead placement, as shown here.

V_{1R}: Fourth intercostal space (ICS), left sternal border
V_{2R}: Fourth ICS, right sternal border
V_{3R}: Halfway between V_{2R} and V_{4R}
V_{4R}: Fifth ICS, right midclavicular line
V_{5R}: Fifth ICS, right anterior axillary line
V_{6R}: Fifth ICS, right midaxillary line

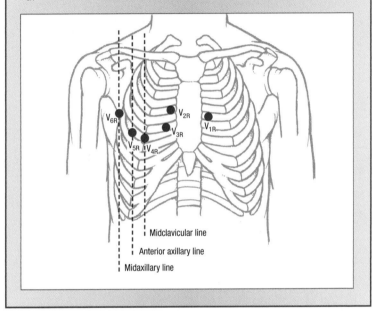

Midclavicular line
Anterior axillary line
Midaxillary line

Recording the ECG

After properly placing the electrodes, record the ECG. ECG machines come in two types: multichannel recorders (most common) and single-channel recorders. With a multichannel recorder, all electrodes are attached to the patient at once and the machine prints a simultaneous view of all leads.

To record a multichannel ECG, follow these steps:

◆ Plug the cord of the ECG machine into a grounded outlet. If the machine operates on a charged battery, it may not need to be plugged in.

◆ Place all of the electrodes on the patient.

◆ Make sure all leads are securely attached, and then turn on the machine.

◆ Instruct the patient to relax, lie still, and breathe normally. Ask him not to talk during the recording, to prevent distortion of the ECG tracing.

◆ Set the ECG paper speed selector to 25 mm per second. If necessary, enter the patient's identification data.

◆ Press the appropriate button on the ECG machine and record the ECG.

◆ Observe the quality of the tracing. When the machine finishes the recording, turn it off.

◆ Remove the electrodes, and clean the patient's skin.

ECG printout

Depending on the information entered, ECG printouts from a multichannel ECG machine will show the patient's name and room number and, possibly, his medical record number. At the top of the printout, you'll see the patient's heart rate and wave durations, measured in seconds. (See *Multichannel ECG recording*, page 256.)

Some machines can record ST-segment elevation and depression. The name of the lead will appear next to each 6-second strip.

If not already included on the printout, write the following information: date, time, practitioner's name, and special circumstances. For example, you might include an episode of chest pain, abnormal electrolyte levels, related drug treatment, abnormal placement of the electrodes, or the presence of an artificial pacemaker and whether a magnet was used while the ECG was obtained.

Remember, ECGs are legal documents. They belong in the patient's medical record and must be saved for future reference and comparison with baseline strips.

Multichannel ECG recording

The top of a 12-lead electrocardiogram (ECG) recording usually shows patient identification information along with an interpretation by the machine. A rhythm strip is commonly included at the bottom of the recording.

Standardization

Look for standardization marks on the recording, normally 10 small squares high. If the patient has high voltage complexes, the marks will be half as high. You'll also notice that lead markers separate the lead recordings on the paper and that each lead is labeled.

Familiarize yourself with the order in which the leads are arranged on an ECG tracing. Getting accustomed to the layout of the tracing will help you interpret the ECG more quickly and accurately.

Patient and ECG information   Lead marker   Lead name   Standardization mark

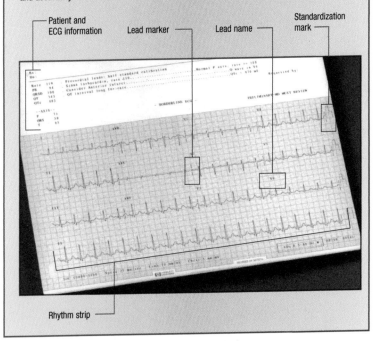

Rhythm strip

Electrocardiogram analysis

13

After obtaining an electrocardiogram (ECG), you'll want to read and interpret the findings. Becoming comfortable with ECG analysis will allow you to detect subtle, and sometimes dangerous, changes in your patient's condition.

Steps in interpretation

When interpreting a patient's 12-lead ECG, first compare the patient's previous ECG with the current one, if available. Doing so helps you identify changes. Then follow a systematic approach, first analyzing the recording for technical accuracy and then evaluating the specific components of the waveform.

Assess for technical accuracy

To ensure that the ECG has been recorded properly, follow these steps:

◆ Make sure the baseline is free from electrical interference and drift.

◆ Scan the limb leads I, II, and III. The R-wave voltage in lead II should equal the sum of the R-wave voltage in leads I and III. Lead aV_R is typically negative. If these rules aren't met, the tracing may be recorded incorrectly.

◆ Locate the lead markers on the waveform. Lead markers are the points where one lead changes to another.

◆ Check the standardization markings (1 millivolt or 10 mm) to make sure all leads were recorded with the ECG machine's amplitude at the same setting. Standardization markings are usually located at the beginning of the strip.

Assess the ECG components

After you've ensured that the recording is accurate, focus your

◆

R-wave progression

R waves should progress normally through the precordial leads. Note that the R wave in this example is the first positive deflection in the QRS complex. Also note that the S wave gets smaller, or regresses, from lead V_1 to V_6 until it finally disappears.

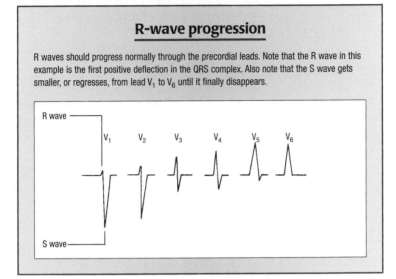

analysis on the various components of the ECG.

◆ Assess the heart's rate and rhythm.

◆ Determine the heart's electrical axis. Use either the quadrant method or the degree method, which are described later in this chapter.

◆ Examine limb leads I, II, and III. The R wave in lead II should be taller than in lead I. The R wave in lead III should be a smaller version of the R wave in lead I. The P wave or QRS complex may be inverted. Each lead should have flat ST segments and upright T waves. Pathologic Q waves should be absent.

◆ Examine limb leads aV_L, aV_F, and aV_R. The tracings from leads aV_L and aV_F should be similar, but lead aV_F should have taller P and R waves. Lead aV_R has little diagnostic value. Its P wave, QRS complex, and T wave should be deflected downward.

◆ Examine the R wave in the precordial leads. Normally, the R wave—the first positive deflection of the QRS complex—gets progressively taller from lead V_1 to V_5. It gets slightly smaller in lead V_6. (See *R-wave progression*.)

◆ Examine the S wave (the negative deflection after an R wave) in the precordial leads. It should appear extremely deep in lead V_1 and become progressively more shallow, usually disappearing by lead V_5.

Analyzing the waveform

On the ECG tracing, each wave represents a component of the cardiac cycle. Therefore, as you examine each lead, note where changes occur so you can identify the area of the heart affected.

P waves

P waves should be upright; however, they may be inverted in lead aV_R or biphasic or inverted in leads III, aV_L, and V_1. Peaked, notched, or enlarged P waves may signify atrial hypertrophy or enlargement. Inverted P waves may signify retrograde conduction. Absent P waves may signify conduction by a route other than the sinoatrial (SA) node.

PR intervals

PR intervals should always be constant, just like QRS-complex durations. Short PR intervals (less than 0.12 second) signify impulses originating somewhere other than the SA node, as in junctional arrhythmias or preexcitation syndromes. Prolonged PR intervals (greater than 0.20 second) signify a conduction delay, such as in heart block or digoxin toxicity.

QRS complex

QRS-complex deflections vary in different leads. A duration greater than 0.12 second may signify ventricular conduction. One or more missing QRS complexes may signify atrioventricular (AV) block or ventricular standstill. Observe for pathologic Q waves. A normal Q wave generally has a duration of under 0.04 second. An abnormal Q wave has either a duration of 0.04 second or more, a depth greater than 4 mm, or a height one-fourth of the R wave.

Abnormal Q waves indicate myocardial necrosis. These waves develop when depolarization can't follow its normal path due to damaged tissue in the area. Lead aV_R normally has a large Q wave, so disregard this lead when searching for abnormal Q waves.

ST segment

ST segments should be isoelectric or have minimal deviation. ST-segment elevation greater than 1 mm above the baseline and ST-segment depression greater than 0.5 mm below the baseline are considered abnormal. Leads facing an injured area have ST-segment elevations, and leads facing away show ST-segment depressions.

T wave

The T wave normally deflects upward in leads I, II, and V_3 through V_6. It's inverted in lead aV_R and variable in the other leads. Tall, peaked or tented T waves may signify myocardial injury or hyperkalemia. Inverted T waves may signify myocardial ischemia.

QT interval

A prolonged QT interval (greater than 0.44 second) indicates prolonged ventricular repolarization or congenital prolonged QT syndrome. A short QT interval (less than 0.36 second) may result from digoxin toxicity or hypercalcemia.

Analyzing the electrical axis

The electrical axis is the average direction of the heart's electrical activity during ventricular depolarization. Leads placed on the body sense the sum of the heart's electrical activity and record it as waveforms.

Electrical axis determination

You can determine your patient's electrical axis by examining the waveforms recorded from the six frontal plane leads: I, II, III, aV_R, aV_L, and aV_F. Imaginary lines drawn from each of the leads intersect at the center of the heart and form a diagram known as the hexaxial reference system. (See *Hexaxial reference system.*)

An axis that falls between 0 and 90 degrees is considered normal (some sources consider –30 to 90 degrees to be normal). An axis between 90 and 180 degrees indicates right axis deviation, and one between 0 and –90 degrees indicates left axis deviation (some sources consider –30 to –90 degrees to be left axis deviation). An axis between –180 and –90 degrees indicates extreme right axis deviation and is called an indeterminate axis.

Left axis deviation commonly occurs in elderly patients. This axis shift may result from fibrosis of the anterior fascicle of the left bundle branch and because the thickness of the left ventricular wall increases by 25% between ages 30 and 80.
To determine your patient's electrical axis, use the quadrant method or the degree method.

Quadrant method
The quadrant method, a fast, easy way to plot the heart's axis, involves observing the main deflection of the QRS complex in leads I and aV_F. Lead I indicates whether impulses are moving to the right or left, and lead aV_F in-

Hexaxial reference system

The hexaxial reference system consists of six bisecting lines, each representing one of the six limb leads, and a circle, representing the heart. The intersection of all lines divides the circle into equal, 30-degree segments.

Shifting degrees

Note that 0 degrees appears at the 3 o'clock position (positive pole lead I). Moving counterclockwise, the degrees become increasingly negative, until reaching ±180 degrees, at the 9 o'clock position (negative pole lead I).

The bottom one-half of the circle contains the corresponding positive degrees. However, a positive-degree designation doesn't necessarily mean that the pole is positive.

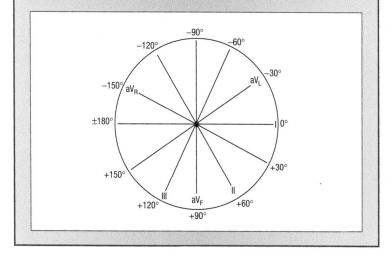

dicates whether they're moving up or down.

If the QRS-complex deflection is positive or upright in both leads, the electrical axis is normal. If lead I is upright and lead aV_F points down, left axis deviation exists. When lead I points down and lead aV_F is upright, right axis deviation exists. Both waves pointing down signal extreme right axis deviation. (See *Quadrant method,* page 262.)

Degree method

A more precise axis calculation, the degree method provides an exact measurement of the electrical axis. It also allows you to determine the axis even if the QRS complex isn't clearly positive or negative in leads I and aV_F. To

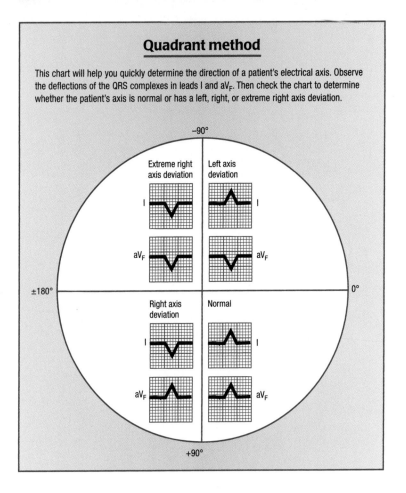

Quadrant method

This chart will help you quickly determine the direction of a patient's electrical axis. Observe the deflections of the QRS complexes in leads I and aV$_F$. Then check the chart to determine whether the patient's axis is normal or has a left, right, or extreme right axis deviation.

use the degree method, follow these steps.

1. Review all six leads, and identify the one that contains either the smallest QRS complex or the complex with an equal deflection above and below the baseline.

2. Use the hexaxial diagram to identify the lead perpendicular to this lead. For example, if lead I has the smallest QRS complex, then the lead perpendicular to the line representing lead I would be lead aV$_F$.

3. After you've identified the perpendicular lead, examine its QRS complex. If the electrical activity is moving toward the positive pole of a lead, the

Degree method

The degree method of determining axis deviation allows you to identify a patient's electrical axis by degrees on the hexaxial system, not just by quadrant. To use this method, take the following steps.

Step 1

Identify the limb lead with the smallest QRS complex or the equiphasic QRS complex. In this example, it's lead III.

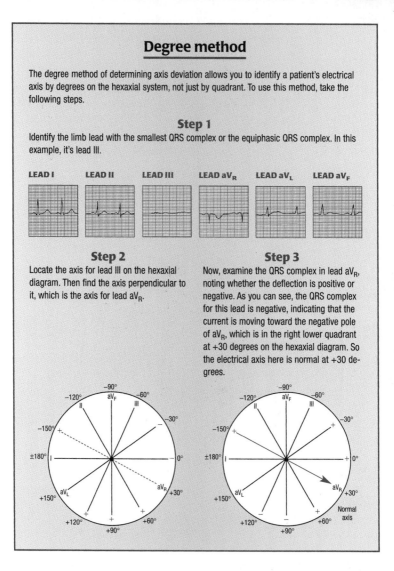

Step 2

Locate the axis for lead III on the hexaxial diagram. Then find the axis perpendicular to it, which is the axis for lead aV_R.

Step 3

Now, examine the QRS complex in lead aV_R, noting whether the deflection is positive or negative. As you can see, the QRS complex for this lead is negative, indicating that the current is moving toward the negative pole of aV_R, which is in the right lower quadrant at +30 degrees on the hexaxial diagram. So the electrical axis here is normal at +30 degrees.

QRS complex deflects upward. If it's moving away from the positive pole of a lead, the QRS complex deflects downward.

4. Plot this information on the hexaxial diagram to determine the direction of the electrical axis. (See *Degree method*.)

Axis deviation

Finding a patient's electrical axis can help confirm a diagnosis or narrow the range of possible diagnoses. Factors that influence the location of the axis include the heart's position in the chest, the heart's size, the patient's body size or type, the conduction pathways, and the force of the electrical impulses being generated. Causes of left axis deviation include:

◆ normal variation
◆ inferior-wall myocardial infarction (MI)
◆ left anterior hemiblock
◆ Wolff-Parkinson-White syndrome
◆ mechanical shifts (ascites, pregnancy, tumors)
◆ left bundle-branch block
◆ left ventricular hypertrophy
◆ aortic stenosis
◆ aging.

Causes of right axis deviation include:

◆ normal variation
◆ lateral-wall MI
◆ left posterior hemiblock
◆ right bundle-branch block (RBBB)
◆ emphysema
◆ right ventricular hypertrophy
◆ pulmonary hypertension
◆ pulmonic stenosis.

Remember that electrical activity in the heart swings away from areas of damage or necrosis, so the heart's damaged part is the last area depolarized. For example, in RBBB, the impulse travels quickly down the normal left side and then moves slowly down the right side. This impulse activity shifts the electrical forces to the right, causing right axis deviation.

Axis deviation isn't always clinically significant, and it isn't always cardiac in origin. For example, infants and children normally have right axis deviation. Pregnant women normally have left axis deviation.

Disorders affecting 12-lead ECGs

14

A 12-lead electrocardiogram (ECG) is a key tool in diagnosing and evaluating certain disorders, such as angina, Prinzmetal's angina, myocardial infarction (MI), pericarditis, left ventricular hypertrophy (LVH), and bundle-branch block (BBB). In some disorders, such as angina, ECG changes are fleeting, making a quick response crucial to diagnosis. In other disorders, such as MI, subtle ECG changes could signal a life-threatening complication. Take time to become familiar with these disorders and the ECG changes they produce. Doing so allows you to respond promptly to changes in the patient's condition.

Angina

During an episode of angina, the myocardium demands more oxygen than the coronary arteries can deliver. An episode of angina usually lasts between 2 and 10 minutes. If the patient's pain persists as long as 30 minutes, he's more likely suffering from an MI than angina.

Angina is classified as an acute coronary syndrome. Types of angina include stable angina—which occurs in a predictable, repetitive pattern—and unstable angina—which commonly signals an impending MI.

Causes

Narrowing of the arteries from coronary artery disease (CAD) restricts the amount of blood flowing to the myocardium. Platelet clumping, thrombus formation, and vasospasm may further restrict blood flow. When conditions arise in which the myocardium demands more oxygen than the narrowed arteries can supply—such as exertion, stress, or even a large meal—myocardial ischemia and pain result.

◆

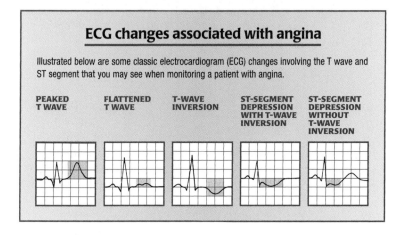

ECG changes associated with angina

Illustrated below are some classic electrocardiogram (ECG) changes involving the T wave and ST segment that you may see when monitoring a patient with angina.

PEAKED T WAVE	FLATTENED T WAVE	T-WAVE INVERSION	ST-SEGMENT DEPRESSION WITH T-WAVE INVERSION	ST-SEGMENT DEPRESSION WITHOUT T-WAVE INVERSION

Clinical significance

Stable angina suggests a narrowing of the coronary arteries, usually resulting from atherosclerosis. If ignored, the arteries may continue to narrow, eventually leading to unstable angina.

◆ **ALERT** Unstable angina is considered a medical emergency because its onset usually indicates an MI.

ECG characteristics

Most patients with either form of angina show ischemic changes on an ECG only during an attack. Because these changes may be fleeting, obtain an order for, and perform, a 12-lead ECG as soon as the patient reports chest pain. Once obtained, the ECG can reveal the area of the heart being affected. By recognizing danger early, you may possibly prevent an MI or even death. (See *ECG changes associated with angina*.)

Signs and symptoms

In stable angina, patients describe the pain as substernal or precordial burning, squeezing, or tightness. The pain may radiate to the left arm, neck, or jaw. Triggered by exertion or stress, the pain is typically relieved by rest. Each episode of stable angina follows the same pattern.

Unstable angina, on the other hand, is more easily provoked, commonly waking the patient. Compared with stable angina, the pain is more intense, lasts longer, and may not radiate. The episodes of pain are also unpredictable and worsen over time. During an attack, the patient's skin may be become pale and clammy, and he may complain of feeling nauseous and anxious.

Interventions

Drug therapy is a key component of angina treatment. Nitrates help reduce myocardial oxygen consumption, while beta-adrenergic blockers reduce the heart's workload and oxygen demands. Patients with angina caused by coronary vasospasm typically receive calcium channel blockers. Antiplatelet drugs may be given to minimize platelet aggregation and reduce the risk of coronary occlusion. Antilipemic drugs may also be given to help lower elevated serum cholesterol or triglycerides levels.

If the patient has continued unstable angina or acute chest pain, glycoprotein IIb/IIIa inhibitors may be given to reduce platelet aggregation. Coronary artery bypass surgery or percutaneous transluminal coronary angioplasty may be performed to remove obstructive lesions.

Prinzmetal's angina

Prinzmetal's angina is a relatively uncommon form of unstable angina. Ischemic pain usually occurs at rest or awakens the patient from sleep. Pain doesn't follow physical activity or emotional stress.

Causes

Prinzmetal's angina results from a focal episodic spasm of a coronary artery, with or without an obstructing coronary artery lesion. Cocaine use has been implicated as one possible cause of Prinzmetal's angina.

Clinical significance

Besides causing episodes of disabling pain, Prinzmetal's angina may lead to ventricular arrhythmias, atrioventricular block, MI and, rarely, sudden death.

ECG characteristics

◆ *Rhythm:* Atrial and ventricular rhythms are normal.
◆ *Rate:* Atrial and ventricular rates are within normal limits.
◆ *P wave:* Normal size and configuration.
◆ *PR interval:* Normal.
◆ *QRS complex:* Normal.
◆ *ST segment:* Marked elevation in leads monitoring the area of coronary spasm. This elevation occurs during chest pain and resolves when pain subsides.
◆ *T wave:* Usually of normal size and configuration.
◆ *QT interval:* Normal.
◆ *Other:* None.

ECG changes associated with Prinzmetal's angina

This 12-lead electrocardiogram (ECG) illustrates the changes resulting from Prinzmetal's angina.

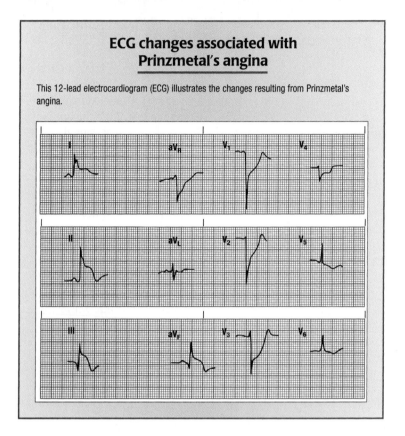

(See *ECG changes associated with Prinzmetal's angina.*)

Signs and symptoms

A patient with Prinzmetal's angina typically experiences substernal chest pain ranging from a feeling of heaviness to a crushing discomfort, usually while at rest. He may also experience dyspnea, nausea, vomiting, diaphoresis, and arrhythmias.

Interventions

Acute management includes the administration of nitroglycerin (Nitro-Bid), which should provide prompt relief from pain by dilating the coronary arteries. For chronic management, long-acting nitrates and calcium channel blockers may be used to help prevent coronary artery spasm. Patients with obstructing coronary artery lesions may benefit from revascularization.

Myocardial infarction

Categorized as an acute coronary syndrome, MI occurs when reduced blood flow through one or more coronary arteries causes myocardial ischemia, injury, and necrosis. Damage usually occurs in the left ventricle, although the location varies depending on the coronary artery affected. For as long as the myocardium is deprived of an oxygen-rich blood supply, an ECG will reflect the three pathologic changes of an MI: ischemia, injury, and infarction.

Causes

Causes of MI include atherosclerosis and embolus. In atherosclerosis, plaque (an unstable and lipid-rich substance) forms and subsequently ruptures or erodes, resulting in platelet adhesions, fibrin clot formation, and activation of thrombin.

Risk factors for MI include:
◆ diabetes
◆ family history of heart disease
◆ high-fat, high-carbohydrate diet
◆ hyperlipoproteinemia
◆ hypertension
◆ menopause
◆ obesity
◆ sedentary lifestyle
◆ smoking
◆ stress.

Clinical significance

The location of the MI is a key factor in determining the most appropriate treatment and in predicting probable complications. Locations include the anterior wall, septal wall, lateral wall, inferior wall, posterior wall, and right ventricle.

Anterior wall

The left anterior descending artery supplies blood to the anterior portion of the left ventricle, ventricular septum, and portions of the right and left bundle-branch systems. When the left anterior descending artery becomes occluded, an anterior-wall MI occurs. Complications include second-degree AV blocks, BBBs, ventricular irritability, and left-sided heart failure.

Septal wall

The patient with a septal-wall MI is at increased risk for developing a ventricular septal defect. Because the left anterior descending artery also supplies blood to the ventricular septum, a septal-wall MI typically accompanies an anterior-wall MI.

Lateral wall

A lateral-wall MI usually results from a blockage in the left circumflex artery. It typically accompanies an anterior- or inferior-wall MI and causes premature ventricular contractions (PVCs) and varying degrees of heart block.

Inferior wall

An inferior-wall MI commonly results from occlusion of the right coronary artery. This type of MI may occur alone or with a lateral-wall or right-ventricular MI. Patients with inferior-wall MI risk developing sinus bradycardia, sinus arrest, heart block, and PVCs.

Posterior wall

A posterior-wall MI results from occlusion of the right coronary artery or the left circumflex arteries. Posterior infarctions may accompany inferior infarctions.

Right ventricle

A right-ventricular MI usually follows occlusion of the right coronary artery. This type of MI rarely occurs alone. In 40% of patients, a right-ventricular MI accompanies an inferior-wall MI. A right-ventricular MI can lead to right ventricular failure.

ECG characteristics

As myocardial cells undergo ischemia and necrosis, they become unable to depolarize normally. In turn, this produces several ECG abnormalities, including the appearance of a Q wave as well as changes in the ST segment and the T wave.

◆ *Q wave:* The cardinal ECG change associated with an area of myocardial necrosis (called the *zone of infarction*) is a pathologic Q wave. The pathologic Q wave results from a lack of depolarization in the necrotic area. Eventually, scar tissue replaces the dead tissue, making the damage, and the resultant Q waves, permanent. Some MIs, however, don't produce Q waves; they're called non–Q-wave MIs.

◆ *ST segment:* ST-segment elevation results from a prolonged lack of blood supply to the zone of injury, which surrounds the zone of infarction. (In a non–Q-wave MI, abnormalities may include non–ST-segment elevation or ST-segment depression.) The ST-segment typically elevates at the onset of an MI—indicating that myocardial injury is occurring—and then returns to baseline within 2 weeks.

◆ *T wave:* T-wave inversion results from ischemia to the outermost area of the zone of infarction, which is called the *zone of ischemia.* When ischemia persists and injury begins, T waves generally flatten and eventually invert. Inverted T waves may persist for several months, but they eventually return to their upright position.

Reciprocal changes in MI

Ischemia, injury, and infarction—the three "Is" of myocardial infarction (MI)—disrupt normal depolarization and produce characteristic electrocardiogram changes. These changes arise in the leads reflecting electrical activity in the damaged areas (shown on the right side of the illustration below).

Reciprocal changes occur in leads opposite the damaged areas. These changes are shown on the left side of the illustration.

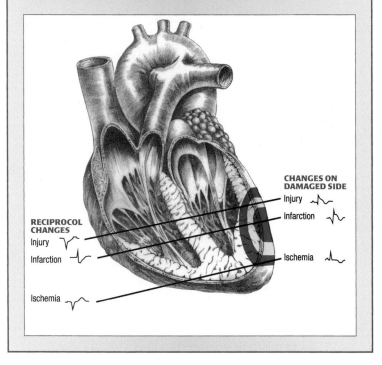

CHANGES ON DAMAGED SIDE

Injury

Infarction

Ischemia

RECIPROCOL CHANGES

Injury

Infarction

Ischemia

Leads showing ECG changes

The leads showing the changes characteristic of an MI will vary, depending on the area of infarction. (See *Reciprocal changes in MI* and *Locating myocardial damage,* page 272.)

Anterior-wall MI

An anterior-wall MI causes characteristic ECG changes in leads V_2 to V_4. Because the left ventricle can't depolarize normally, the precordial leads show poor R-wave progression, ST-segment elevation, and T-wave inversion. The reciprocal leads for the ante-

Locating myocardial damage

After you've noted characteristic lead changes in an acute myocardial infarction, use this table to identify the areas of damage. Match the lead changes (ST elevation, abnormal Q waves) in the second column with the affected wall in the first column and the artery involved in the third column. The fourth column shows reciprocal lead changes.

WALL AFFECTED	LEADS	ARTERY INVOLVED	RECIPROCAL CHANGES
Anterior	V_2, V_3, V_4	Left coronary artery, left anterior descending (LAD)	II, III, aV_F
Anterolateral	I, aV_L, V_3, V_4, V_5, V_6	LAD and diagonal branches, circumflex and marginal branches	II, III, aV_F
Anteroseptal	V_1, V_2, V_3, V_4	LAD	None
Inferior	II, III, aV_F	Right coronary artery (RCA)	I, aV_L
Lateral	I, aV_L, V_5, V_6	Circumflex branch of left coronary artery	II, III, aV_F
Posterior	V_8, V_9	RCA or circumflex	V_1, V_2, V_3, V_4 (R greater than S in V_1 and V_2, ST-segment depression, elevated T wave)
Right ventricular	V_{4R}, V_{5R}, V_{6R}	RCA	None

rior wall are the inferior leads II, III, and aV_F. They initially show tall R waves and depressed ST segments. (See *Recognizing an anterior-wall MI.*)

Septal-wall MI

In a septal-wall MI, the R wave disappears, the ST segment rises, and the T wave inverts in leads V_1 and V_2.

Lateral-wall MI

In a lateral-wall MI, the ECG shows changes in the left lateral leads I, aV_L, V_5, and V_6. The reciprocal leads for a lateral wall infarction are leads V_1 and V_2. (See *Recognizing a lateral-wall MI,* page 274.)

Inferior-wall MI

In an inferior-wall MI, ECG changes appear in the inferior leads II, III, and aV_F. Reciprocal

Recognizing an anterior-wall MI

This 12-lead electrocardiogram shows typical characteristics of an anterior-wall myocardial infarction (MI). Note that the R waves don't progress through the precordial leads. Also note the ST-segment elevation in leads V_2 and V_3. As expected, the reciprocal leads II, III, and aV_F show slight ST-segment depression. Axis deviation is normal at +60 degrees.

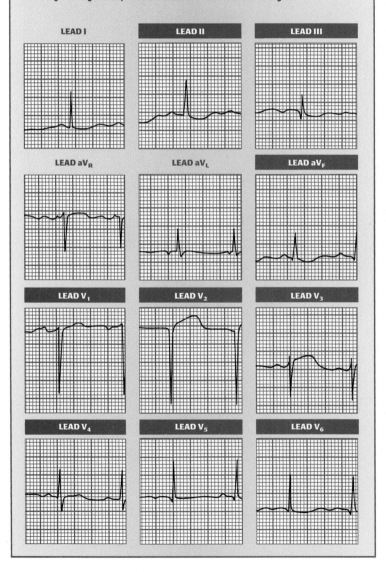

Recognizing a lateral-wall MI

This 12-lead electrocardiogram shows changes characteristic of a lateral-wall myocardial infarction (MI). In leads I and aV$_L$, note the pathologic Q waves, the slight ST-segment elevation, and the T-wave inversion. Reciprocal changes are noted in leads V$_1$ and V$_2$.

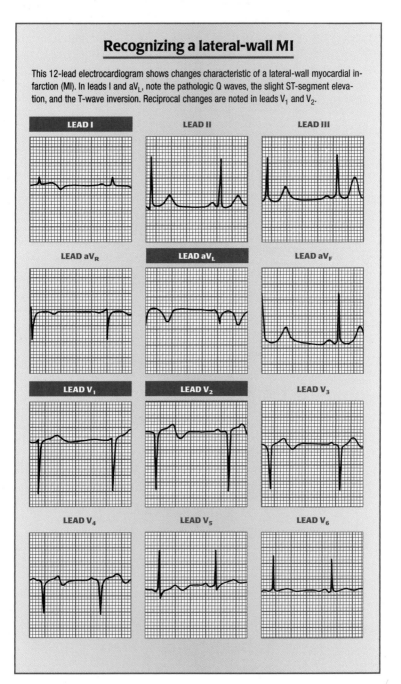

changes occur in the lateral leads I and aV_L. (See *Recognizing an inferior-wall MI,* page 276.)

Posterior-wall MI

In a posterior-wall MI, changes include tall R waves, ST-segment depression, and upright T waves. Obtaining information about the posterior wall requires the use of a posterior ECG; leads V_8 and V_9 may show pathologic Q waves. Reciprocal changes occur in leads V_1 to V_4. (See *Recognizing a posterior-wall MI,* page 277.)

Right-ventricular MI

The classic changes that occur with a right-ventricular MI include ST-segment elevation, pathologic Q waves, and inverted T waves in the right precordial leads V_{2R} to V_{6R}. Identifying a right ventricular MI is difficult without information from the right precordial leads. If these leads aren't available, observe leads II, III, and aV_F or watch leads V_1, V_2, and V_3 for ST-segment elevation. If a right ventricular MI has occurred, use lead II to monitor for further damage. (See *Recognizing a right-ventricular MI,* page 278.)

Signs and symptoms

Patients experiencing an MI typically complain of chest pain, which they may describe as severe, persistent, burning, squeezing, or crushing. Usually substernal or precordial, the pain may radiate to the left arm, neck, jaw, or shoulder blade. The pain is unrelieved by rest and lasts at least 20 minutes, although it may persist for several hours. Other signs and symptoms include anxiety, cool extremities, fatigue, a feeling of impending doom, hypertension, hypotension, nausea, shortness of breath, and vomiting.

Women, elderly patients, and patients with diabetes are more likely to have atypical symptoms. In these patients, chest pain may be vague or even absent. Other complaints include jaw, back, or shoulder pain; shortness of breath; fatigue; or abdominal discomfort.

Interventions

Patients with an MI require vigilant monitoring to detect changes in their ECG and in their general condition. (See *Monitoring MI patients,* page 279.)

To prevent myocardial necrosis, patients must receive treatment within 6 hours of the onset of symptoms. If treatment is sought within 3 hours of the onset of symptoms, prepare the patient for thrombolytic therapy to restore vessel patency and mini-

(Text continues on page 279.)

Recognizing an inferior-wall MI

This 12-lead electrocardiogram (ECG) shows the characteristic changes of an inferior-wall myocardial infarction (MI). In leads II, III, and aV_F, note the T-wave inversion, ST-segment elevation, and pathologic Q waves. In leads I and aV_L, note the slight ST-segment depression—a reciprocal change. This ECG shows left axis deviation at –60 degrees.

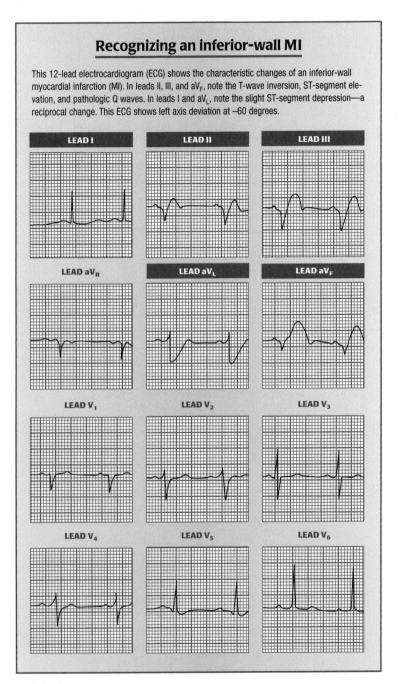

Recognizing a posterior-wall MI

This 12-lead electrocardiogram (ECG) shows typical characteristics of a posterior-wall myocardial infarction (MI). Note the tall R waves, the depressed ST segments, and the upright T waves in leads V_1, V_2, and V_3. These are reciprocal changes because the leads that best monitor a posterior-wall MI (V_7, V_8, and V_9) aren't on a standard 12-lead ECG.

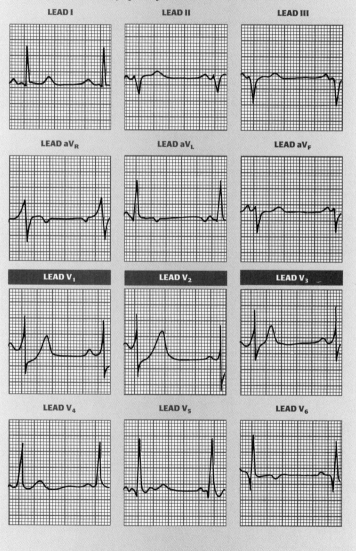

Recognizing a right-ventricular MI

This 12-lead electrocardiogram shows typical characteristics of a right-ventricular myocardial infarction (MI). Note the T wave inversion in leads V_{3R}, V_{4R}, V_{5R}, and V_{6R}. Pathologic Q waves and ST-segment elevation are also present.

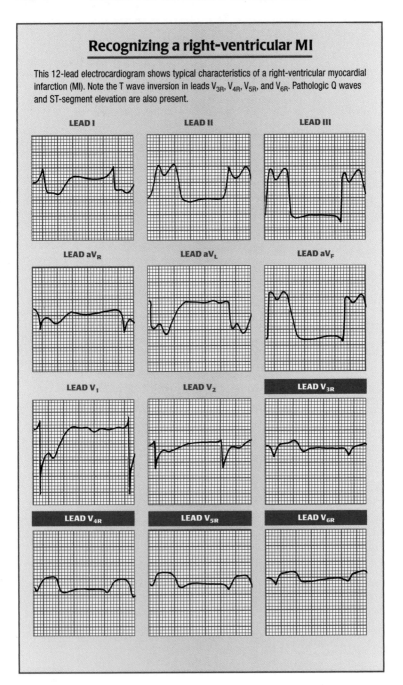

mize necrosis, unless contraindicated.

Treatment measures aim to decrease cardiac workload and increase the supply of oxygen to the myocardium. Specific measures include oxygen administration, sublingual nitroglycerin to relieve chest pain (unless systolic blood pressure is less than 90 mm Hg or heart rate is less than 50 or more than 100 beats/minute), and morphine.

Additional drug therapy includes beta-adrenergic blockers, ACE inhibitors, and aspirin and clopidogrel (Plavix) to inhibit platelet aggregation. Statin therapy may be given to help lower serum lipid levels. If the patient received tissue plasminogen activator, I.V. heparin may be given to promote patency in the affected coronary artery. Patients without hypotension, bradycardia, or excessive tachycardia may receive I.V. nitroglycerin for 24 to 48 hours to reduce afterload and preload and to relieve chest pain.

If the patient has an arrhythmia, he'll require an antiarrhythmic or epinephrine; he may also require transcutaneous pacing patches, a transvenous pacemaker, or defibrillation, as indicated. If the patient has unstable angina or acute chest pain, or if he's had an invasive cardiac procedure, glycoprotein IIb/IIIa in-

hibitors may be given to reduce platelet aggregation.

The patient may also require percutaneous transluminal angioplasty, stent placement, coronary artery atherectomy; or a surgical procedure (such as coronary artery bypass graft) to open blocked or narrowed arteries.

> ## Monitoring MI patients
>
> Remember that specific leads monitor specific walls of the heart. Here's a quick overview of those leads.
> ◆ For an anterior-wall myocardial infarction (MI), monitor lead V_1 or MCL_1.
> ◆ For a septal-wall MI, monitor lead V_1 or MCL_1 to pick up hallmark changes.
> ◆ For a lateral-wall MI, monitor lead V_6 or MCL_6.
> ◆ For an inferior-wall MI, monitor lead II.

Pericarditis

Pericarditis is an inflammation of the pericardium, the fibroserous sac that envelops the heart. Pericarditis can be either acute or chronic. The acute form may be fibrinous or effusive, with purulent, serous, or hemorrhagic exudate. Chronic constrictive pericarditis causes dense fibrous thickening of the pericardium.

Causes

Possible causes of pericarditis include:

◆ viral, bacterial, or fungal disorders
◆ rheumatic fever
◆ autoimmune disorders
◆ complications of cardiac injury, such as following an MI or cardiotomy.

Clinical significance

Pericarditis may cause cardiac tamponade if fluid accumulates too quickly. If constriction occurs, heart failure may result.

ECG characteristics

In pericarditis, ECG changes occur secondary to myocardial inflammation and excessive pericardial fluid or a thickened pericardium. In the earliest stage, elevation of ST segments accompanies upright T waves. Typically, resolution of the ST-segment elevation marks the beginning of the second stage of acute pericarditis, with widespread T-wave inversion.

The primary ECG abnormality in acute pericarditis is ST-segment elevation. In contrast to the convex ST-segment elevation in acute MI, the ST segments appear somewhat concave in pericarditis. Because pericarditis usually affects the entire myocardial surface, ST segments are usually elevated in most—if not all—leads, except lead aV_R. (See *Comparing MI with acute pericarditis*.)

◆ *Rhythm:* Atrial and ventricular rhythms are usually regular.
◆ *Rate:* Atrial and ventricular rates usually remain within normal limits.
◆ *P wave:* Normal size and configuration.
◆ *PR interval:* Usually normal.
◆ *QRS complex:* Normal, but a possible decrease in amplitude may occur.
◆ *ST segment:* In stage 1, the ST segment is elevated 1 to 2 mm in leads II, III, and aV_F as well as in the precordial leads.
◆ *T wave:* Remains elevated during the acute phase of pericarditis. As the pericarditis resolves, the T waves become inverted in the leads that had the ST-segment elevation.
◆ *QT interval:* Normal.
◆ *Other:* Atrial fibrillation, atrial flutter, or tachycardia may occur as a result of sinoatrial node irritation.

Signs and symptoms

A patient with acute pericarditis may complain of chest pain, dyspnea, and chills. The chest pain typically worsens with deep inspiration and improves when the patient sits up and leans forward.

Comparing MI with acute pericarditis

Myocardial infarction (MI) and acute pericarditis cause ST-segment elevation on an electro-cardiogram (ECG). However, the ST segment and T wave (shaded areas) on an MI waveform are quite different from those on the pericarditis waveform.

In addition, because pericarditis involves the surrounding pericardium, several leads will show ST-segment and T-wave changes (typically leads I, II, aV_F, and V_4 through V_6). In MI, however, only those leads reflecting the area of infarction will show the characteristic changes.

These rhythm strips demonstrate the ECG variations between MI and acute pericarditis.

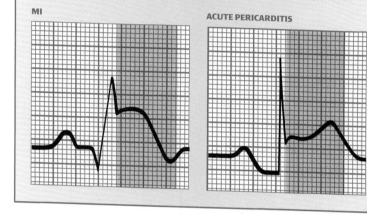

MI   **ACUTE PERICARDITIS**

The patient may also experience fever, diaphoresis, and arrhythmias. Patients with chronic pericarditis usually experience symptoms similar to chronic right-sided heart failure, including edema, ascites, and hepatomegaly.

A pericardial friction rub is commonly audible upon auscultation. However, the most distinctive clinical feature is a palpable, and sometimes audible, sharp knock or rub in early diastole, which occurs as the rapidly filling ventricle touches the unexpansive pericardium.

Interventions

Acute pericarditis is treated with bed rest and corticosteroids or nonsteroidal anti-inflammatory drugs (NSAIDs) to relieve pain and inflammation. Infectious pericarditis is treated with antibiotics. Pericardiocentesis is performed for cardiac tamponade, and a complete pericardectomy may be performed for constrictive pericarditis. Keep in mind that the underlying cause of the pericarditis needs to be identified and treated.

Left ventricular hypertrophy

In LVH, the left ventricular wall thickens. LVH usually results from conditions that cause chronic increases in pressures within the ventricle.

Causes

LVH may result from mitral insufficiency, cardiomyopathy, aortic stenosis or insufficiency, or systemic hypertension (the most common cause). LVH may lead to left-sided heart failure, which subsequently leads to increased left atrial pressure, pulmonary vascular congestion, and pulmonary arterial hypertension.

Clinical significance

LVH can decrease coronary artery perfusion, causing MI. It can also alter the papillary muscle, causing mitral insufficiency.

ECG characteristics

◆ *Rhythm:* Atrial and ventricular rhythms are normal.
◆ *Rate:* Atrial and ventricular rates are normal.
◆ *P wave:* May be normal in size and configuration, or may reflect left atrial enlargement.
◆ *PR interval:* Normal.

◆ *QRS complex:* May be prolonged or widened with increased amplitude. In lead I, the R wave's amplitude exceeds 1.4 mV. In leads V_1 and V_2, deeper S waves appear. The sum of the S wave in lead V_1 or V_2 and the R wave in lead V_5 or V_6 exceeds 3.5 mV. The R wave is taller in lead V_6 than in V_5. The R wave's amplitude in lead V_5 or V_6 exceeds 2.6 mV. (See *Recognizing LVH.*)
◆ *ST segment:* Possibly depressed in the precordial leads when associated with T-wave inversion. This pattern is known as LVH with strain.
◆ *T wave:* May be inverted in leads V_5 and V_6, depending on the degree of hypertrophy.
◆ *QT interval:* Usually normal.
◆ *Other:* The axis is usually normal, but left axis deviation may be present.

Signs and symptoms

Signs and symptoms are related to the underlying disorder.

Interventions

Interventions are focused on managing the underlying disorder (such as hypertension).

Recognizing LVH

Left ventricular hypertrophy (LVH) can lead to heart failure or myocardial infarction. This rhythm strip illustrates key electrocardiogram changes of LVH as they occur in selected leads: a large S wave (shaded area below left) in V_1 and a large R wave (shaded area below right) in V_5. If the depth (in mm) of the S wave in V_1 added to the height (in mm) of the R wave in V_5 is greater than 35 mm, then LVH is present.

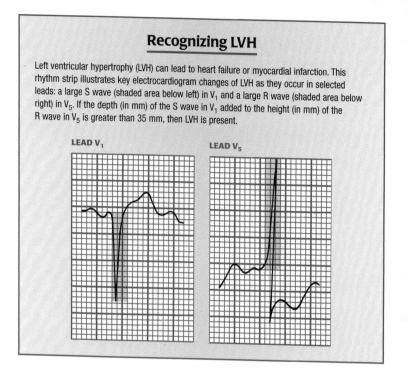

LEAD V_1 LEAD V_5

Bundle-branch block

One potential complication of an MI is BBB. In this disorder, either the left or the right bundle branch fails to conduct impulses normally. A BBB that occurs toward the distal end of the left bundle, in the posterior or anterior fasciculus, is called a *hemiblock*.

In a BBB, the impulse travels down the unaffected bundle branch and then from one myocardial cell to the next to depolarize the ventricle. Because this cell-to-cell conduction progresses much more slowly than along the specialized cells of the conduction system, ventricular depolarization is prolonged.

Causes

Right bundle-branch block (RBBB) occurs with such conditions as anterior wall MI, coronary artery disease (CAD), and pulmonary embolism. It may also occur without cardiac disease. If it develops as the heart rate increases, it's called rate-related RBBB. (See *Understanding RBBB*, page 284.)

Understanding RBBB

In right bundle-branch block (RBBB), the initial impulse activates the interventricular septum from left to right, just as in normal activation (arrow 1). Next, the left bundle branch activates the left ventricle (arrow 2). The impulse then crosses the interventricular septum to activate the right ventricle (arrow 3).

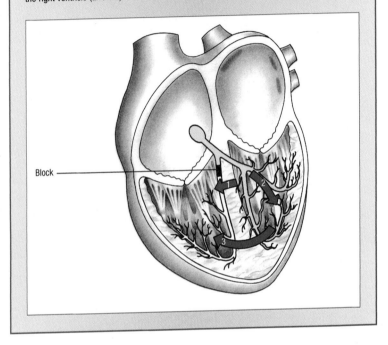

Block

Left bundle-branch block (LBBB) never occurs normally. This block usually results from hypertensive heart disease, aortic stenosis, degenerative changes of the conduction system, or CAD. (See *Understanding LBBB*.)

Clinical significance

Because BBB typically occurs secondary to underlying cardiac disease, patients should undergo testing to identify the cause of the arrhythmia.

ECG characteristics

Prolonged ventricular depolarization means that the QRS complex widens. The normal width is 0.06 to 0.10 second. If it increases to more than 0.12 second, BBB is present. After identifying

Understanding LBBB

In left bundle-branch block (LBBB), the impulse first travels down the right bundle branch (arrow 1). Then the impulse activates the interventricular septum from right to left (arrow 2), the opposite of normal activation. Finally, the impulse activates the left ventricle (arrow 3).

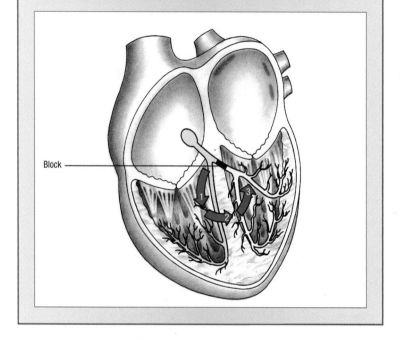

Block

BBB, examine lead V_1 and lead V_6. You'll use these leads to determine whether the block is in the right or the left bundle branch.

Right bundle-branch block
◆ *Rhythm:* Atrial and ventricular rhythms are regular.
◆ *Rate:* Atrial and ventricular rates are within normal limits.
◆ *P wave:* Usually less than 0.12 second.

◆ *QRS complex:* Duration is greater than 0.12 second and the configuration sometimes resembles rabbit ears or the letter "M." Septal depolarization isn't affected in lead V_1, so the initial small R wave remains. The R wave is followed by an S wave, which represents left ventricular depolarization, and a tall R wave (called *R prime,* or *R′*), which represents late right ventricular depolarization. The opposite occurs in lead V_6. A small Q wave is followed by depolarization of the left ventricle, which produces a tall R wave. Depolarization of the right ventricle then causes a broad S wave.

◆ *T wave:* Negative in lead V_1; however, the negative deflection is called a secondary T-wave change and isn't clinically significant. Again, the opposite occurs in lead V_6, with the T wave being positive.

◆ *QT interval:* Normal. (See *Recognizing RBBB.*)

Left bundle-branch block

◆ *Rhythm:* Atrial and ventricular rhythms are regular.

◆ *Rate:* Atrial and ventricular rates are within normal limits.

◆ *P wave:* Usually less than 0.12 second.

◆ *QRS complex:* Duration is greater than 0.12 second because the ventricles are activated sequentially, not simultaneously. As the wave of depolarization spreads from the right ventricle to the left, a wide S wave is produced in lead V_1. The S wave may be preceded by a Q wave or a small R wave. In lead V_6, no initial Q wave occurs. A tall, notched R wave, or a slurred one, is produced as the impulse spreads from right to left. This initial positive deflection is a sign of LBBB.

◆ *T wave:* Positive in lead V_1; negative in lead V_6.

◆ *QT interval:* Normal. (See *Recognizing LBBB,* page 288.)

It may be difficult to differentiate between BBB and Wolff-Parkinson-White (WPW) syndrome. Whenever you spot BBB, check for WPW syndrome. (See *Distinguishing BBB from WPW syndrome,* page 289.)

Signs and symptoms

Patients are usually asymptomatic unless the arrhythmia leads to a more complete block. In rare instances, patients may develop symptoms of low cardiac output, such as dizziness and diaphoresis.

Interventions

Many times, BBB is monitored only to detect whether it progresses to a more complete block. However, some blocks require treatment with a temporary pacemaker. For example, when a LBBB occurs along with an anterior-wall MI, and if complete heart block occurs, the patient may require the insertion of a pacemaker.

Recognizing RBBB

This 12-lead electrocardiogram shows the characteristic changes of right bundle-branch block (RBBB). In lead V_1, note the rsR′ pattern and T-wave inversion. In lead V_6, see the widened S wave and the upright T wave. Also note the prolonged QRS complexes.

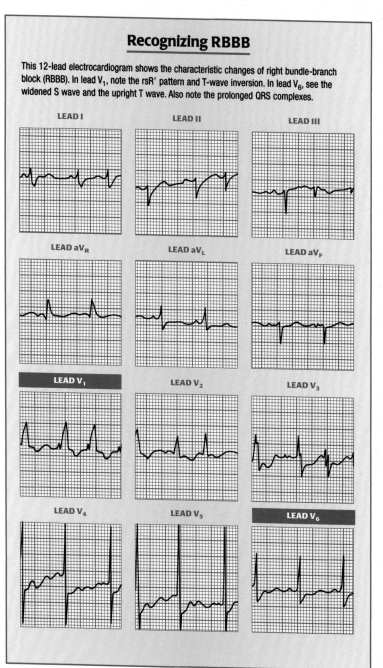

Recognizing LBBB

This 12-lead electrocardiogram shows characteristic changes of a left bundle-branch block (LBBB). All leads have prolonged QRS complexes. In lead V_1, note the QS wave pattern. In lead V_6, you'll see the slurred R wave and T-wave inversion. The elevated ST segments and upright T waves in leads V_1 to V_4 are also common in LBBB.

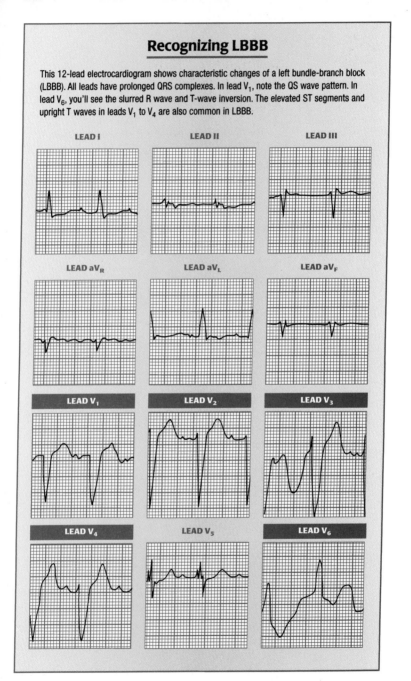

LOOK-ALIKES

Distinguishing BBB from WPW syndrome

Wolff-Parkinson-White (WPW) syndrome is a common type of preexcitation syndrome, an abnormal condition in which electrical impulses enter the ventricles from the atria by using an accessory pathway that bypasses the atrioventricular (AV) junction. This activity results in a short PR interval and a wide QRS complex with an initial slurring of the upward slope of the QRS complex, called a *delta wave*. Because the delta wave prolongs the QRS complex, its presence may be confused with a bundle-branch block (BBB).

Bundle-branch block

◆ Carefully examine the QRS complex, noting which part of the complex is widened. A BBB involves a defective conduction of electrical impulses through the right or left bundle branch from the bundle of His to the Purkinje network causing a right or left BBB.

◆ This conduction disturbance results in an overall increase in QRS duration, or widening of the last part of the QRS complex, whereas the initial part of the QRS complex commonly appears normal.

◆ Carefully examine the 12-lead electrocardiogram (ECG). With BBB, the prolonged duration of the QRS complexes is generally consistent in all leads.

◆ Measure the PR interval. BBB has no effect on the PR interval, so the PR intervals are generally normal. However, if the patient has a preexisting AV conduction defect, such as first-degree AV block, the PR interval is prolonged.

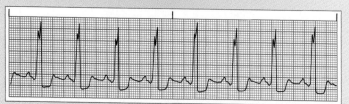

Wolff-Parkinson-White syndrome

◆ A delta wave occurs at the beginning of the QRS complex, usually causing a distinctive slurring or hump in its initial slope. A delta wave isn't present in BBB.

◆ On the 12-lead ECG, the delta wave is most pronounced in the leads "looking at" the part of the heart where the accessory pathway is located.

◆ The delta wave shortens the PR interval in WPW syndrome.

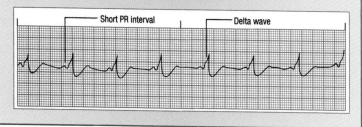

Short PR interval   Delta wave

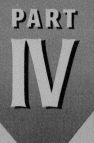

PART
IV

Practice strips

1.

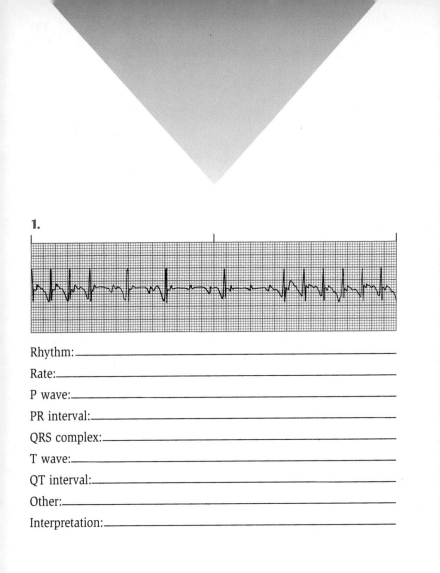

Rhythm:_____

Rate:_____

P wave:_____

PR interval:_____

QRS complex:_____

T wave:_____

QT interval:_____

Other:_____

Interpretation:_____

2.

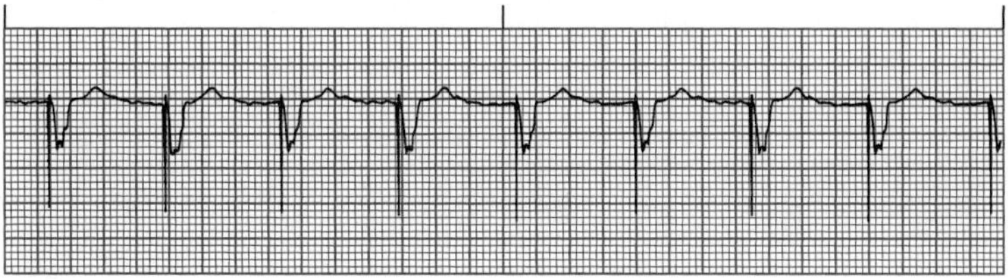

Rhythm: _____

Rate: _____

P wave: _____

PR interval: _____

QRS complex: _____

T wave: _____

QT interval: _____

Other: _____

Interpretation: _____

3.

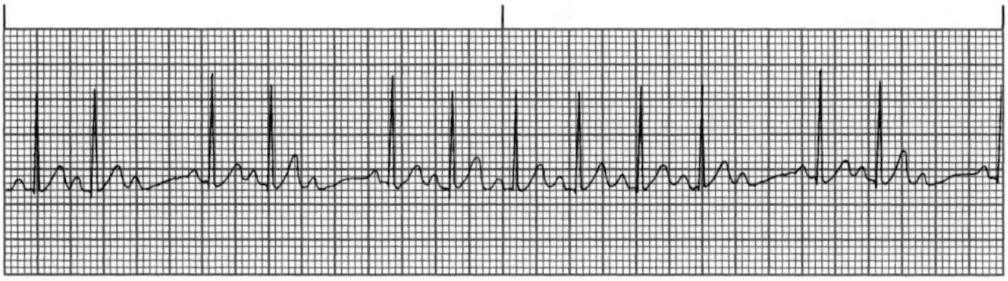

Rhythm: _____

Rate: _____

P wave: _____

PR interval: _____

QRS complex: _____

T wave: _____

QT interval: _____

Other: _____

Interpretation: _____

4.

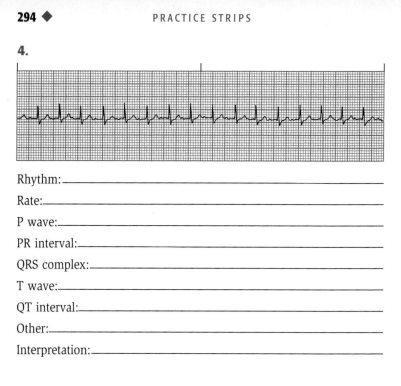

Rhythm:_____

Rate:_____

P wave:_____

PR interval:_____

QRS complex:_____

T wave:_____

QT interval:_____

Other:_____

Interpretation:_____

5.

Rhythm:_____

Rate:_____

P wave:_____

PR interval:_____

QRS complex:_____

T wave:_____

QT interval:_____

Other:_____

Interpretation:_____

6.

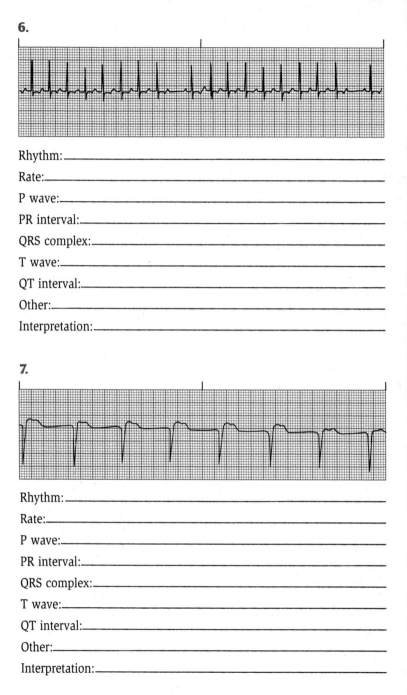

Rhythm: _____

Rate: _____

P wave: _____

PR interval: _____

QRS complex: _____

T wave: _____

QT interval: _____

Other: _____

Interpretation: _____

7.

Rhythm: _____

Rate: _____

P wave: _____

PR interval: _____

QRS complex: _____

T wave: _____

QT interval: _____

Other: _____

Interpretation: _____

8.

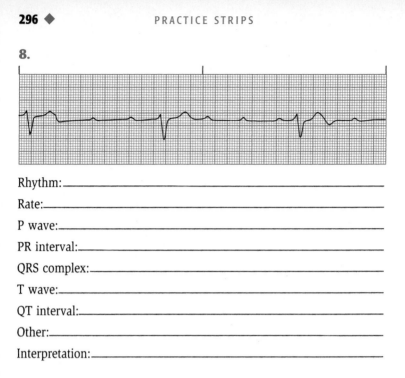

Rhythm: _____

Rate: _____

P wave: _____

PR interval: _____

QRS complex: _____

T wave: _____

QT interval: _____

Other: _____

Interpretation: _____

9.

Rhythm: _____

Rate: _____

P wave: _____

PR interval: _____

QRS complex: _____

T wave: _____

QT interval: _____

Other: _____

Interpretation: _____

10.

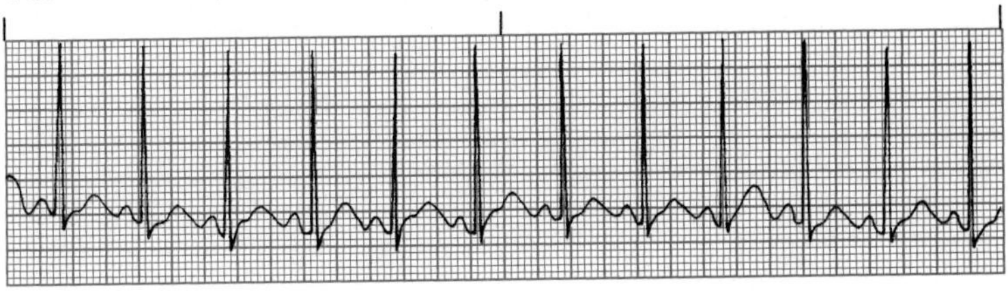

Rhythm:_____

Rate:_____

P wave:_____

PR interval:_____

QRS complex:_____

T wave:_____

QT interval:_____

Other:_____

Interpretation:_____

11.

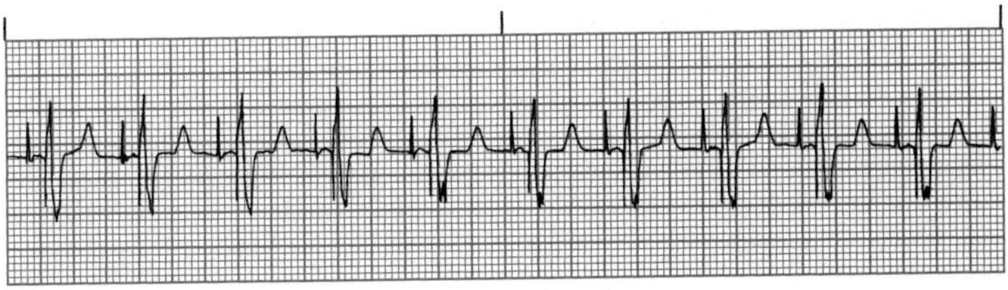

Rhythm:_____

Rate:_____

P wave:_____

PR interval:_____

QRS complex:_____

T wave:_____

QT interval:_____

Other:_____

Interpretation:_____

12.

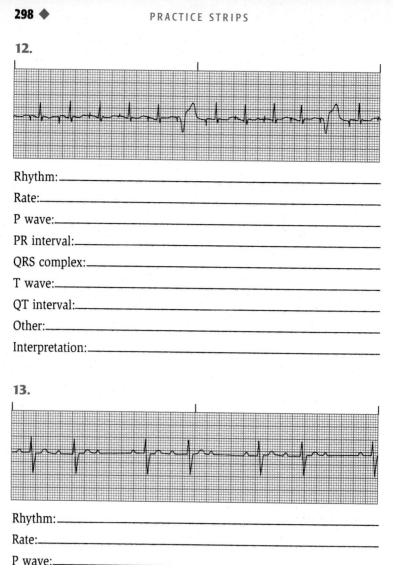

Rhythm: _____

Rate: _____

P wave: _____

PR interval: _____

QRS complex: _____

T wave: _____

QT interval: _____

Other: _____

Interpretation: _____

13.

Rhythm: _____

Rate: _____

P wave: _____

PR interval: _____

QRS complex: _____

T wave: _____

QT interval: _____

Other: _____

Interpretation: _____

14.

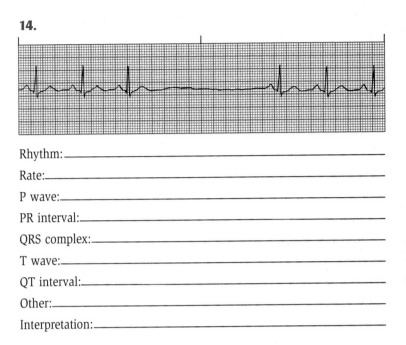

Rhythm:_____

Rate:_____

P wave:_____

PR interval:_____

QRS complex:_____

T wave:_____

QT interval:_____

Other:_____

Interpretation:_____

15.

Rhythm:_____

Rate:_____

P wave:_____

PR interval:_____

QRS complex:_____

T wave:_____

QT interval:_____

Other:_____

Interpretation:_____

16.

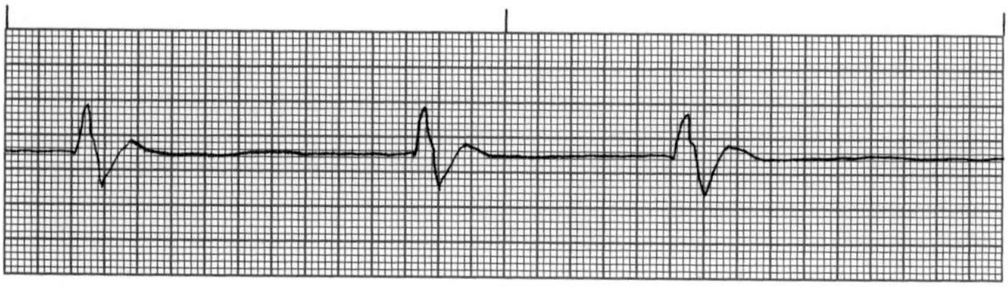

Rhythm:_____

Rate:_____

P wave:_____

PR interval:_____

QRS complex:_____

T wave:_____

QT interval:_____

Other:_____

Interpretation:_____

17.

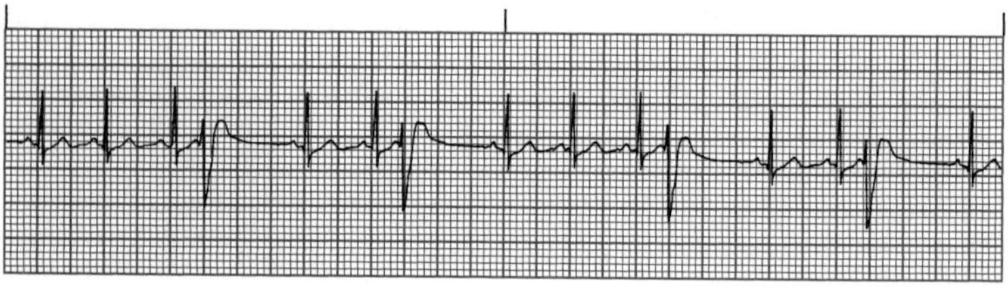

Rhythm:_____

Rate:_____

P wave:_____

PR interval:_____

QRS complex:_____

T wave:_____

QT interval:_____

Other:_____

Interpretation:_____

18.

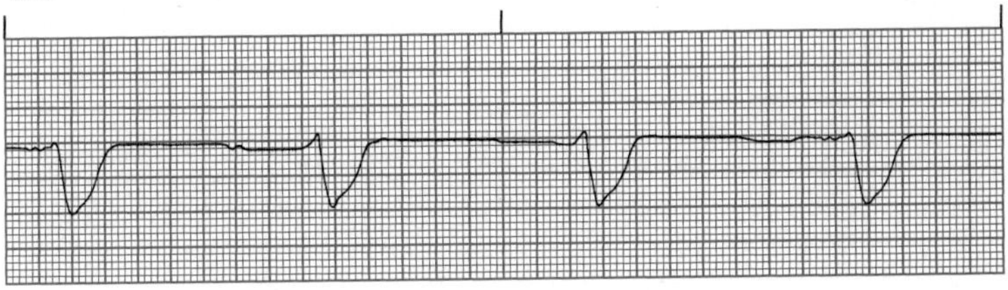

Rhythm: _____

Rate: _____

P wave: _____

PR interval: _____

QRS complex: _____

T wave: _____

QT interval: _____

Other: _____

Interpretation: _____

19.

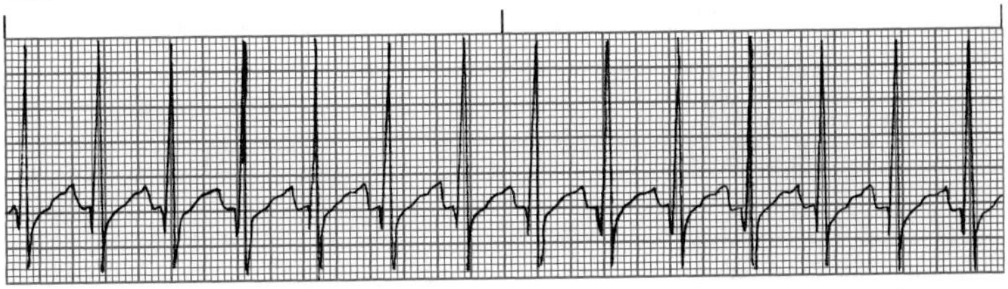

Rhythm: _____

Rate: _____

P wave: _____

PR interval: _____

QRS complex: _____

T wave: _____

QT interval: _____

Other: _____

Interpretation: _____

20.

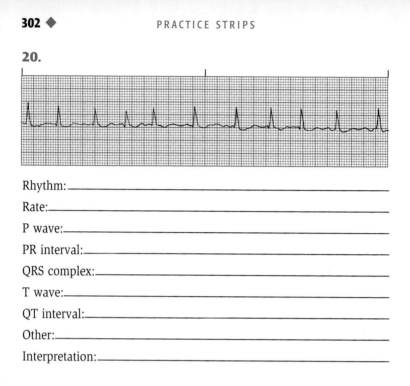

Rhythm:_____

Rate:_____

P wave:_____

PR interval:_____

QRS complex:_____

T wave:_____

QT interval:_____

Other:_____

Interpretation:_____

21.

Rhythm:_____

Rate:_____

P wave:_____

PR interval:_____

QRS complex:_____

T wave:_____

QT interval:_____

Other:_____

Interpretation:_____

22.

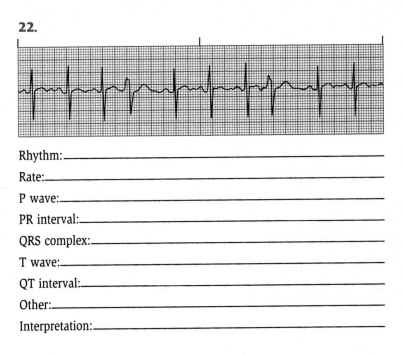

Rhythm:_____

Rate:_____

P wave:_____

PR interval:_____

QRS complex:_____

T wave:_____

QT interval:_____

Other:_____

Interpretation:_____

23.

Rhythm:_____

Rate:_____

P wave:_____

PR interval:_____

QRS complex:_____

T wave:_____

QT interval:_____

Other:_____

Interpretation:_____

24.

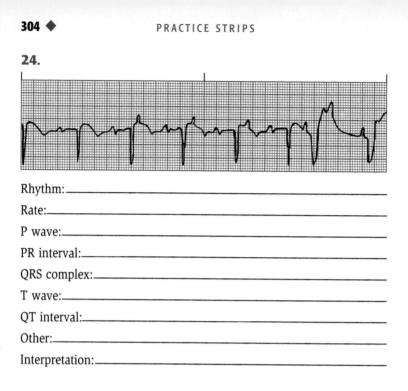

Rhythm:_____

Rate:_____

P wave:_____

PR interval:_____

QRS complex:_____

T wave:_____

QT interval:_____

Other:_____

Interpretation:_____

25.

Rhythm:_____

Rate:_____

P wave:_____

PR interval:_____

QRS complex:_____

T wave:_____

QT interval:_____

Other:_____

Interpretation:_____

26.

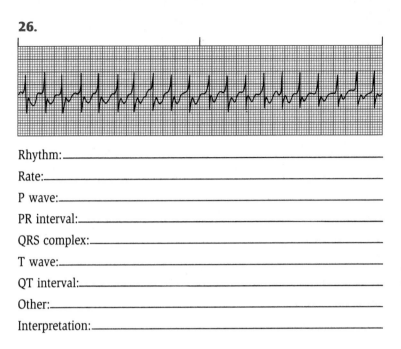

Rhythm: _____

Rate: _____

P wave: _____

PR interval: _____

QRS complex: _____

T wave: _____

QT interval: _____

Other: _____

Interpretation: _____

27.

Rhythm: _____

Rate: _____

P wave: _____

PR interval: _____

QRS complex: _____

T wave: _____

QT interval: _____

Other: _____

Interpretation: _____

28.

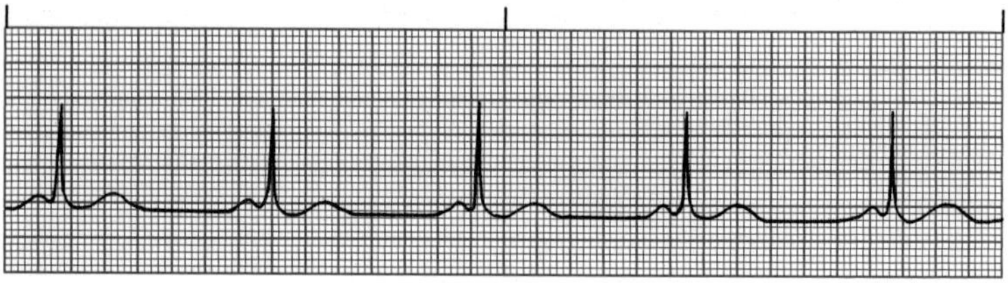

Rhythm: _____

Rate: _____

P wave: _____

PR interval: _____

QRS complex: _____

T wave: _____

QT interval: _____

Other: _____

Interpretation: _____

29.

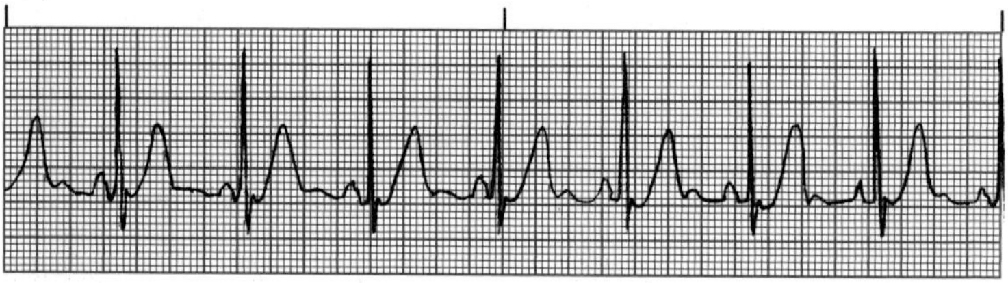

Rhythm: _____

Rate: _____

P wave: _____

PR interval: _____

QRS complex: _____

T wave: _____

QT interval: _____

Other: _____

Interpretation: _____

30.

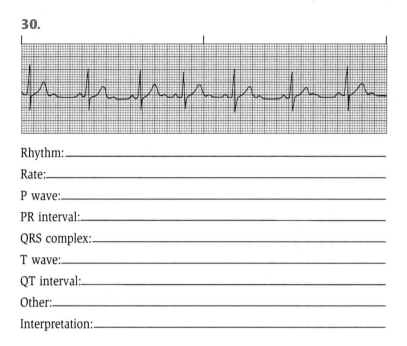

Rhythm: _____

Rate: _____

P wave: _____

PR interval: _____

QRS complex: _____

T wave: _____

QT interval: _____

Other: _____

Interpretation: _____

31.

Rhythm: _____

Rate: _____

P wave: _____

PR interval: _____

QRS complex: _____

T wave: _____

QT interval: _____

Other: _____

Interpretation: _____

32.

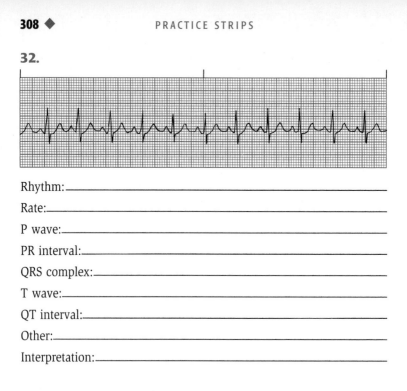

Rhythm:_____

Rate:_____

P wave:_____

PR interval:_____

QRS complex:_____

T wave:_____

QT interval:_____

Other:_____

Interpretation:_____

33.

Rhythm:_____

Rate:_____

P wave:_____

PR interval:_____

QRS complex:_____

T wave:_____

QT interval:_____

Other:_____

Interpretation:_____

34.

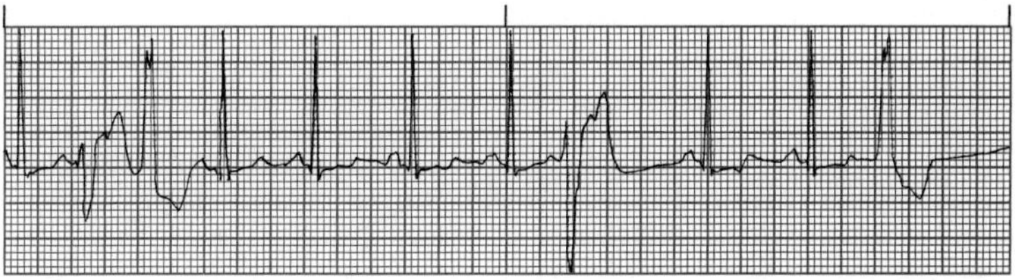

Rhythm: _____

Rate: _____

P wave: _____

PR interval: _____

QRS complex: _____

T wave: _____

QT interval: _____

Other: _____

Interpretation: _____

35.

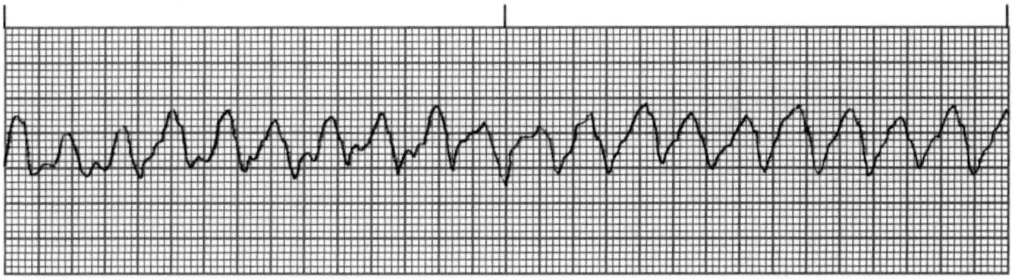

Rhythm: _____

Rate: _____

P wave: _____

PR interval: _____

QRS complex: _____

T wave: _____

QT interval: _____

Other: _____

Interpretation: _____

36.

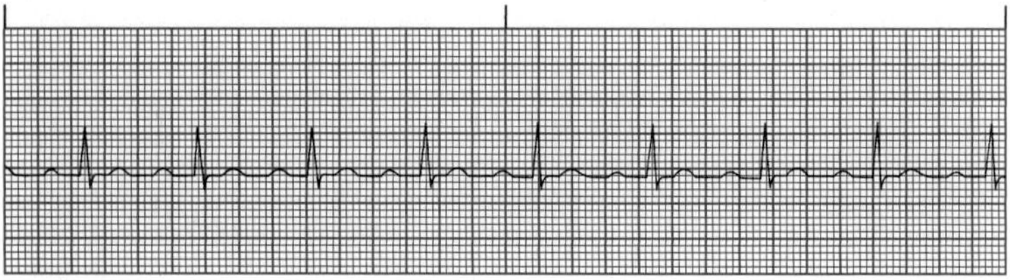

Rhythm:_____

Rate:_____

P wave:_____

PR interval:_____

QRS complex:_____

T wave:_____

QT interval:_____

Other:_____

Interpretation:_____

37.

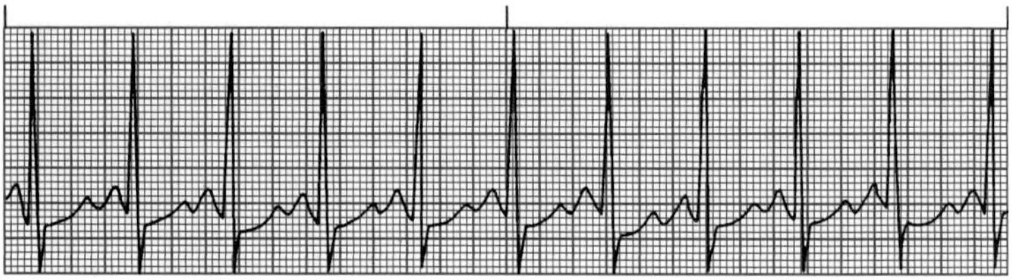

Rhythm:_____

Rate:_____

P wave:_____

PR interval:_____

QRS complex:_____

T wave:_____

QT interval:_____

Other:_____

Interpretation:_____

38.

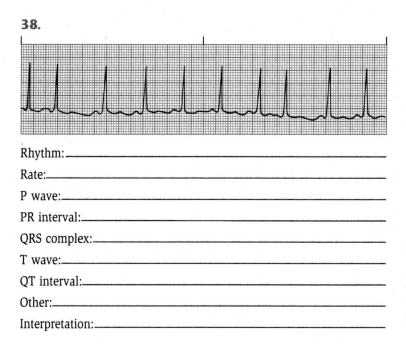

Rhythm: _____

Rate: _____

P wave: _____

PR interval: _____

QRS complex: _____

T wave: _____

QT interval: _____

Other: _____

Interpretation: _____

39.

Rhythm: _____

Rate: _____

P wave: _____

PR interval: _____

QRS complex: _____

T wave: _____

QT interval: _____

Other: _____

Interpretation: _____

40.

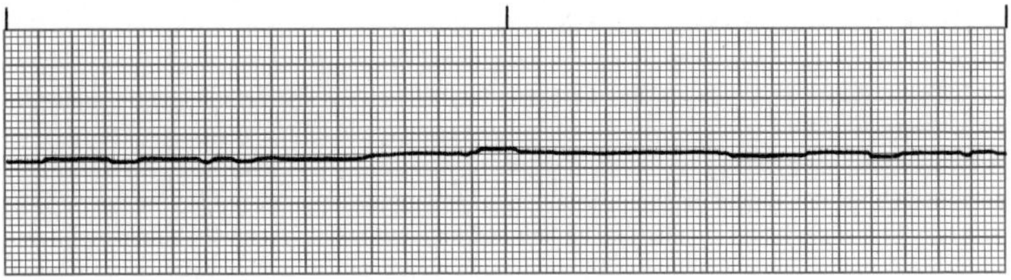

Rhythm:_____

Rate:_____

P wave:_____

PR interval:_____

QRS complex:_____

T wave:_____

QT interval:_____

Other:_____

Interpretation:_____

41.

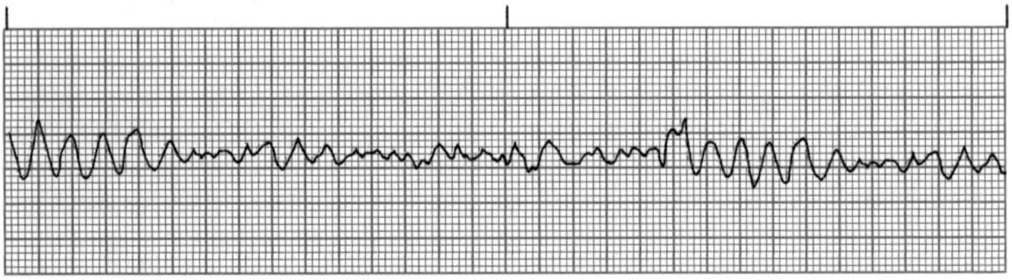

Rhythm:_____

Rate:_____

P wave:_____

PR interval:_____

QRS complex:_____

T wave:_____

QT interval:_____

Other:_____

Interpretation:_____

42.

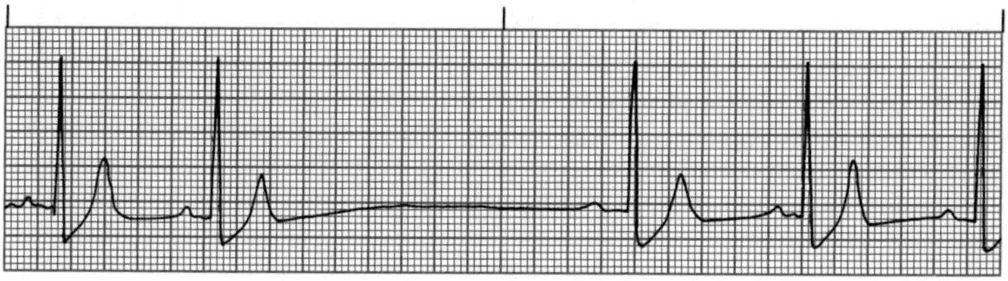

Rhythm: _____

Rate: _____

P wave: _____

PR interval: _____

QRS complex: _____

T wave: _____

QT interval: _____

Other: _____

Interpretation: _____

43.

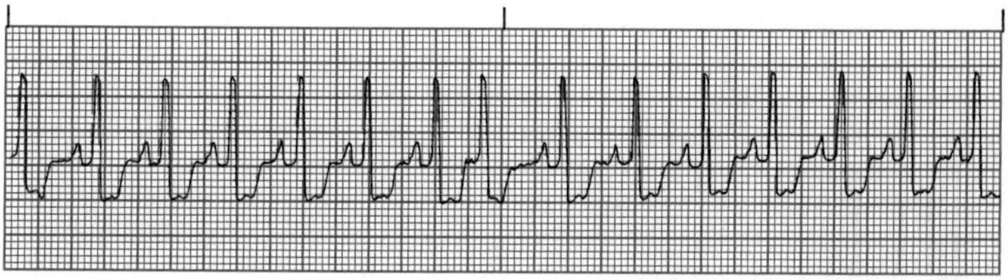

Rhythm: _____

Rate: _____

P wave: _____

PR interval: _____

QRS complex: _____

T wave: _____

QT interval: _____

Other: _____

Interpretation: _____

44.

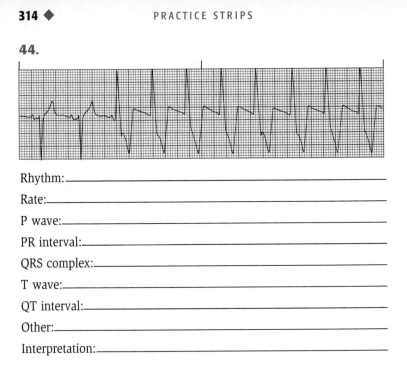

Rhythm:_____

Rate:_____

P wave:_____

PR interval:_____

QRS complex:_____

T wave:_____

QT interval:_____

Other:_____

Interpretation:_____

45.

Rhythm:_____

Rate:_____

P wave:_____

PR interval:_____

QRS complex:_____

T wave:_____

QT interval:_____

Other:_____

Interpretation:_____

46.

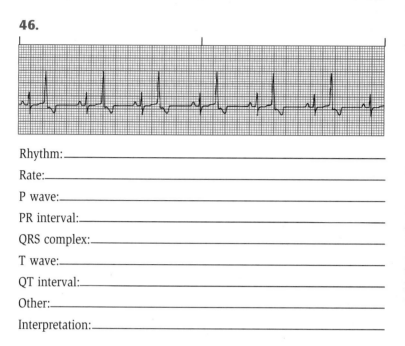

Rhythm:_____

Rate:_____

P wave:_____

PR interval:_____

QRS complex:_____

T wave:_____

QT interval:_____

Other:_____

Interpretation:_____

47.

Rhythm:_____

Rate:_____

P wave:_____

PR interval:_____

QRS complex:_____

T wave:_____

QT interval:_____

Other:_____

Interpretation:_____

48.

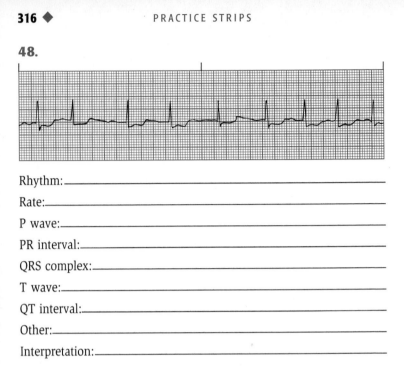

Rhythm: _____

Rate: _____

P wave: _____

PR interval: _____

QRS complex: _____

T wave: _____

QT interval: _____

Other: _____

Interpretation: _____

49.

Rhythm: _____

Rate: _____

P wave: _____

PR interval: _____

QRS complex: _____

T wave: _____

QT interval: _____

Other: _____

Interpretation: _____

50.

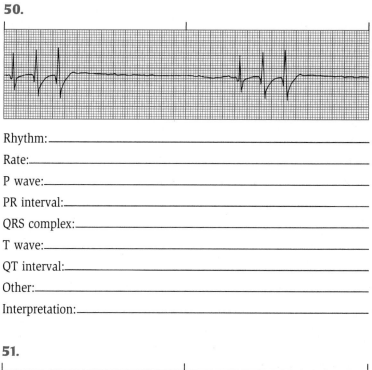

Rhythm: _____

Rate: _____

P wave: _____

PR interval: _____

QRS complex: _____

T wave: _____

QT interval: _____

Other: _____

Interpretation: _____

51.

Rhythm: _____

Rate: _____

P wave: _____

PR interval: _____

QRS complex: _____

T wave: _____

QT interval: _____

Other: _____

Interpretation: _____

52.

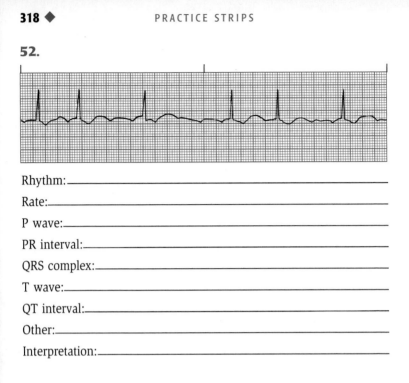

Rhythm: _____

Rate: _____

P wave: _____

PR interval: _____

QRS complex: _____

T wave: _____

QT interval: _____

Other: _____

Interpretation: _____

53.

Rhythm: _____

Rate: _____

P wave: _____

PR interval: _____

QRS complex: _____

T wave: _____

QT interval: _____

Other: _____

Interpretation: _____

54.

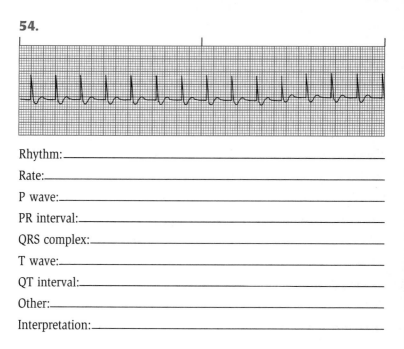

Rhythm: _____

Rate: _____

P wave: _____

PR interval: _____

QRS complex: _____

T wave: _____

QT interval: _____

Other: _____

Interpretation: _____

55.

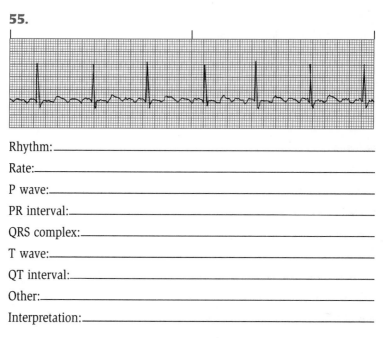

Rhythm: _____

Rate: _____

P wave: _____

PR interval: _____

QRS complex: _____

T wave: _____

QT interval: _____

Other: _____

Interpretation: _____

56.

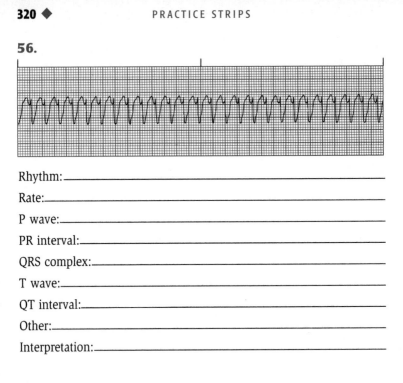

Rhythm: _____

Rate: _____

P wave: _____

PR interval: _____

QRS complex: _____

T wave: _____

QT interval: _____

Other: _____

Interpretation: _____

57.

Rhythm: _____

Rate: _____

P wave: _____

PR interval: _____

QRS complex: _____

T wave: _____

QT interval: _____

Other: _____

Interpretation: _____

58.

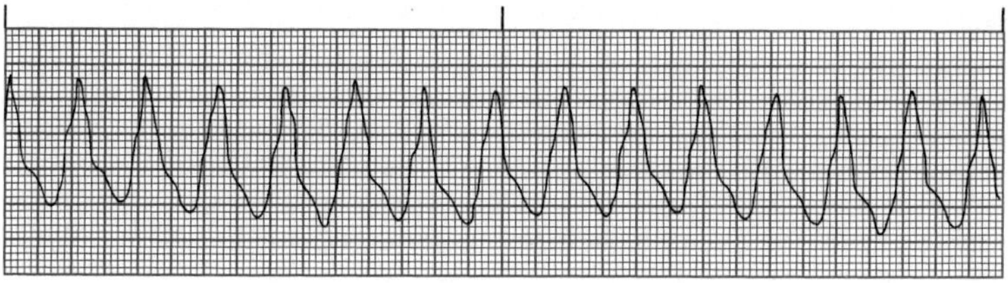

Rhythm:_____

Rate:_____

P wave:_____

PR interval:_____

QRS complex:_____

T wave:_____

QT interval:_____

Other:_____

Interpretation:_____

59.

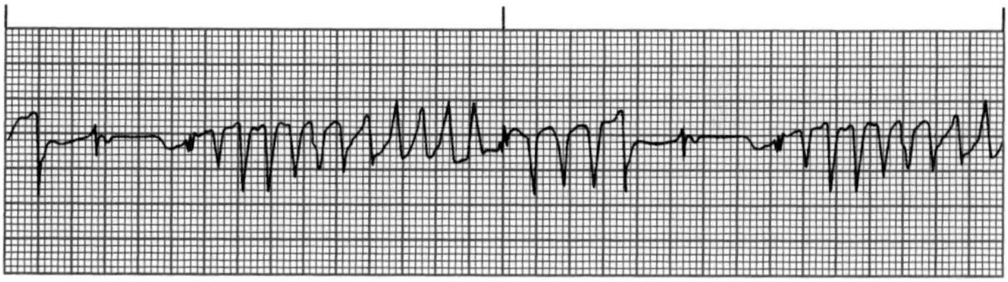

Rhythm:_____

Rate:_____

P wave:_____

PR interval:_____

QRS complex:_____

T wave:_____

QT interval:_____

Other:_____

Interpretation:_____

60.

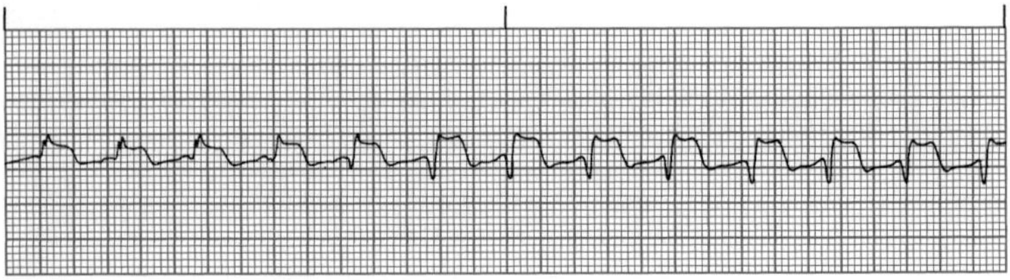

Rhythm: _____

Rate: _____

P wave: _____

PR interval: _____

QRS complex: _____

T wave: _____

QT interval: _____

Other: _____

Interpretation: _____

61.

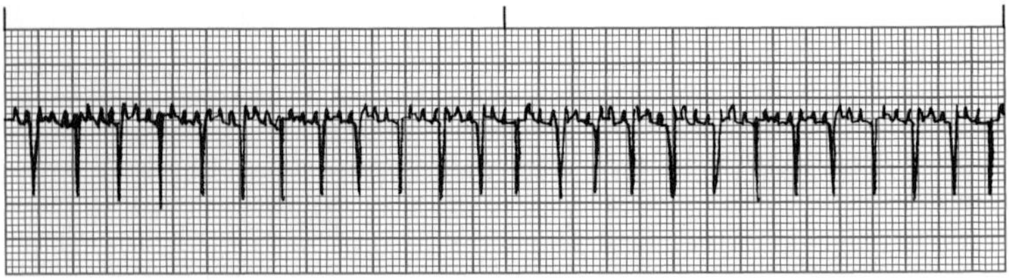

Rhythm: _____

Rate: _____

P wave: _____

PR interval: _____

QRS complex: _____

T wave: _____

QT interval: _____

Other: _____

Interpretation: _____

62.

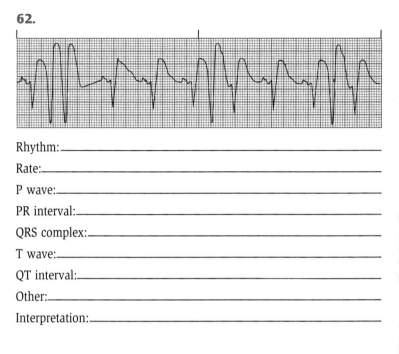

Rhythm: _____

Rate: _____

P wave: _____

PR interval: _____

QRS complex: _____

T wave: _____

QT interval: _____

Other: _____

Interpretation: _____

63.

Rhythm: _____

Rate: _____

P wave: _____

PR interval: _____

QRS complex: _____

T wave: _____

QT interval: _____

Other: _____

Interpretation: _____

64.

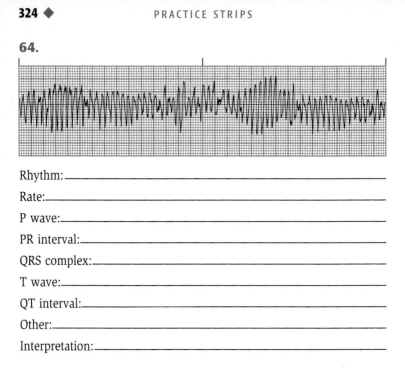

Rhythm:_____

Rate:_____

P wave:_____

PR interval:_____

QRS complex:_____

T wave:_____

QT interval:_____

Other:_____

Interpretation:_____

65.

Rhythm:_____

Rate:_____

P wave:_____

PR interval:_____

QRS complex:_____

T wave:_____

QT interval:_____

Other:_____

Interpretation:_____

66.

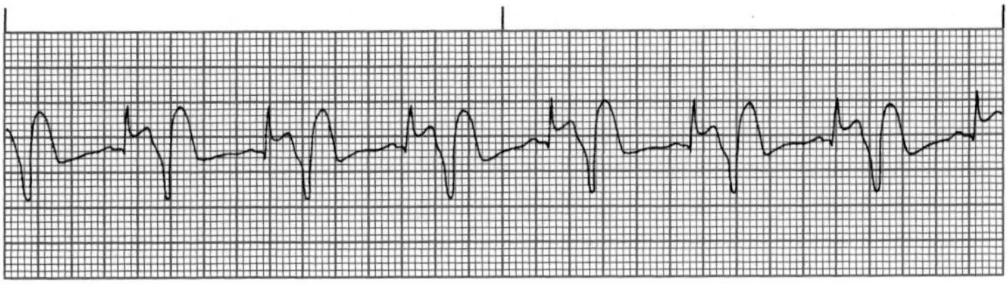

Rhythm:_____

Rate:_____

P wave:_____

PR interval:_____

QRS complex:_____

T wave:_____

QT interval:_____

Other:_____

Interpretation:_____

67.

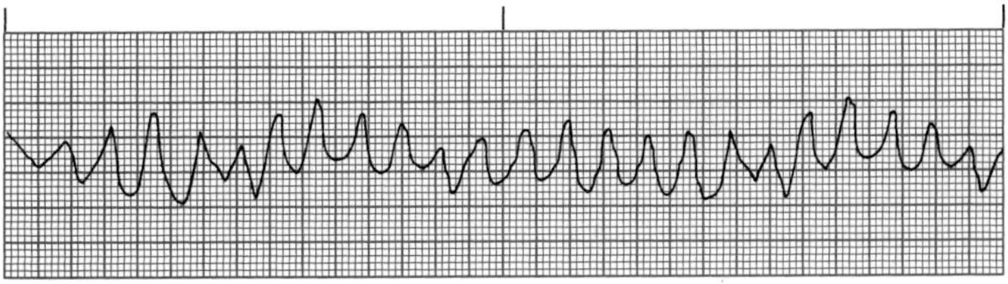

Rhythm:_____

Rate:_____

P wave:_____

PR interval:_____

QRS complex:_____

T wave:_____

QT interval:_____

Other:_____

Interpretation:_____

68.

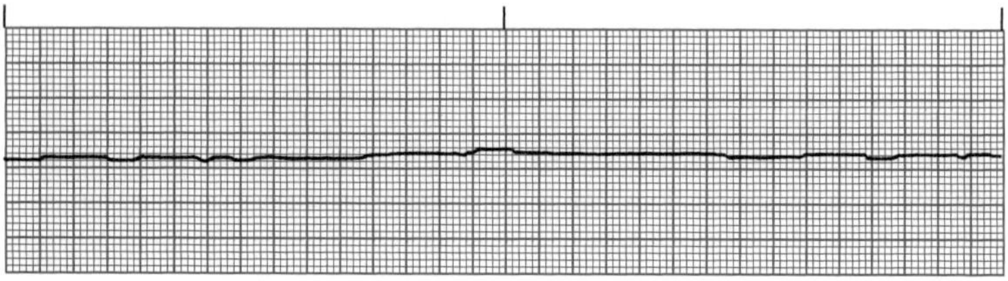

Rhythm:_____

Rate:_____

P wave:_____

PR interval:_____

QRS complex:_____

T wave:_____

QT interval:_____

Other:_____

Interpretation:_____

69.

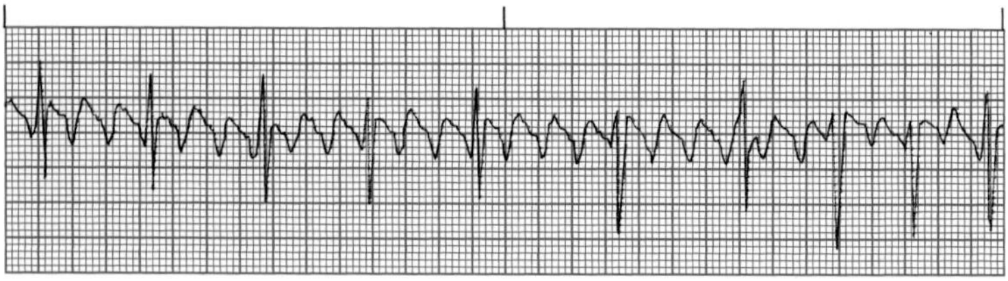

Rhythm:_____

Rate:_____

P wave:_____

PR interval:_____

QRS complex:_____

T wave:_____

QT interval:_____

Other:_____

Interpretation:_____

70.

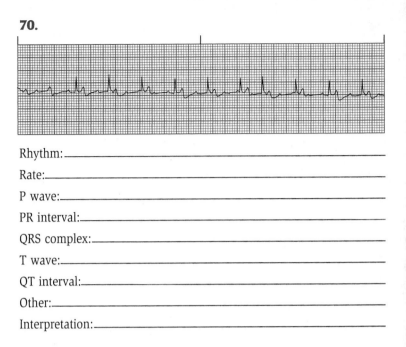

Rhythm: _____

Rate: _____

P wave: _____

PR interval: _____

QRS complex: _____

T wave: _____

QT interval: _____

Other: _____

Interpretation: _____

71.

Rhythm: _____

Rate: _____

P wave: _____

PR interval: _____

QRS complex: _____

T wave: _____

QT interval: _____

Other: _____

Interpretation: _____

72.

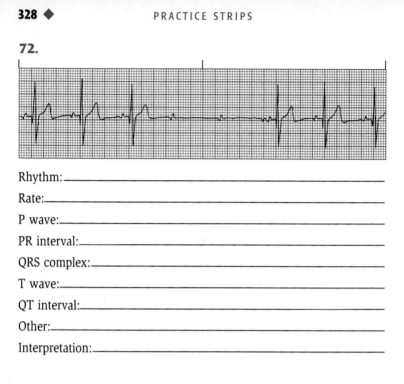

Rhythm:_____

Rate:_____

P wave:_____

PR interval:_____

QRS complex:_____

T wave:_____

QT interval:_____

Other:_____

Interpretation:_____

73.

Rhythm:_____

Rate:_____

P wave:_____

PR interval:_____

QRS complex:_____

T wave:_____

QT interval:_____

Other:_____

Interpretation:_____

74.

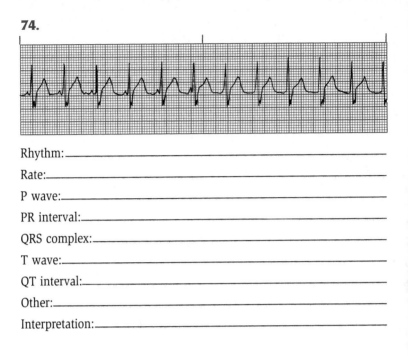

Rhythm:_____

Rate:_____

P wave:_____

PR interval:_____

QRS complex:_____

T wave:_____

QT interval:_____

Other:_____

Interpretation:_____

75.

Rhythm:_____

Rate:_____

P wave:_____

PR interval:_____

QRS complex:_____

T wave:_____

QT interval:_____

Other:_____

Interpretation:_____

76.

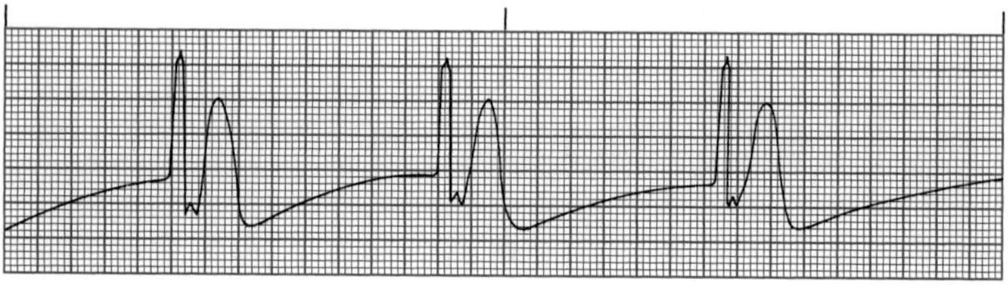

Rhythm: _____

Rate: _____

P wave: _____

PR interval: _____

QRS complex: _____

T wave: _____

QT interval: _____

Other: _____

Interpretation: _____

77.

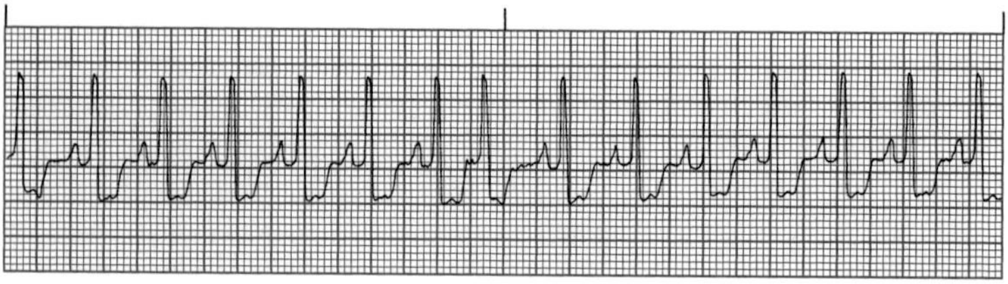

Rhythm: _____

Rate: _____

P wave: _____

PR interval: _____

QRS complex: _____

T wave: _____

QT interval: _____

Other: _____

Interpretation: _____

78.

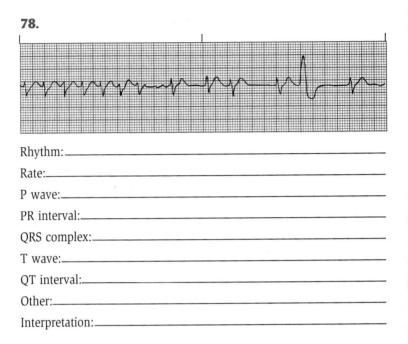

Rhythm:_____

Rate:_____

P wave:_____

PR interval:_____

QRS complex:_____

T wave:_____

QT interval:_____

Other:_____

Interpretation:_____

79.

Rhythm:_____

Rate:_____

P wave:_____

PR interval:_____

QRS complex:_____

T wave:_____

QT interval:_____

Other:_____

Interpretation:_____

80.

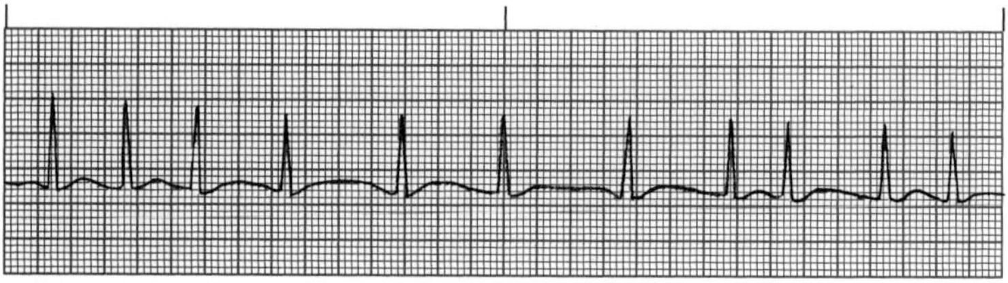

Rhythm:

Rate:

P wave:

PR interval:

QRS complex:

T wave:

QT interval:

Other:

Interpretation:

81.

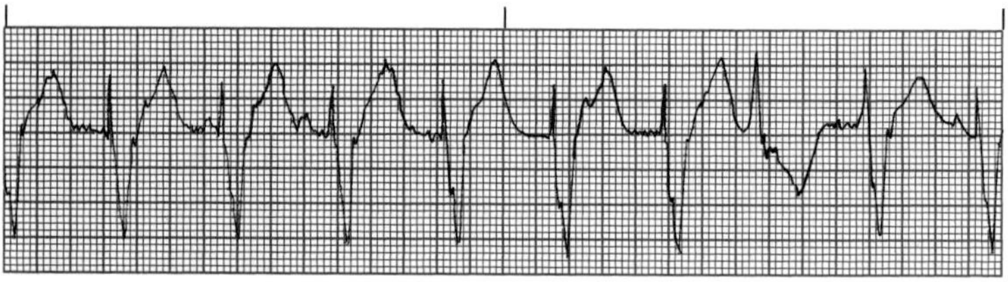

Rhythm:

Rate:

P wave:

PR interval:

QRS complex:

T wave:

QT interval:

Other:

Interpretation:

82.

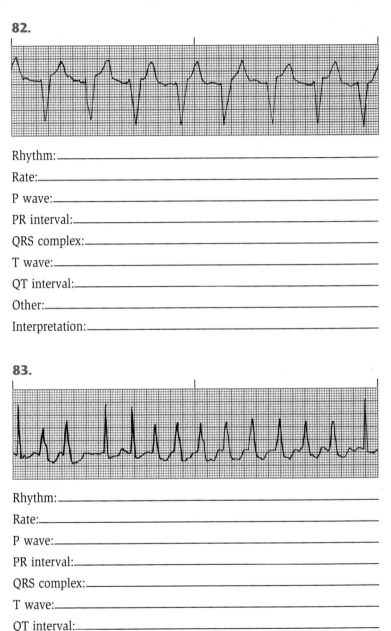

Rhythm: _____

Rate: _____

P wave: _____

PR interval: _____

QRS complex: _____

T wave: _____

QT interval: _____

Other: _____

Interpretation: _____

83.

Rhythm: _____

Rate: _____

P wave: _____

PR interval: _____

QRS complex: _____

T wave: _____

QT interval: _____

Other: _____

Interpretation: _____

84.

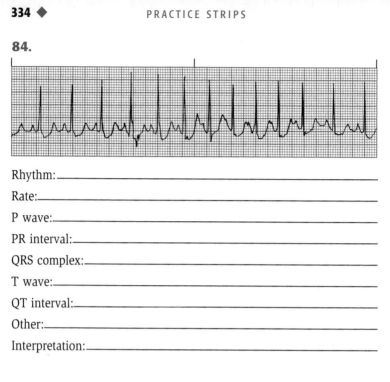

Rhythm:————————————————————————————

Rate:——————————————————————————————

P wave:————————————————————————————

PR interval:————————————————————————

QRS complex:————————————————————————

T wave:—————————————————————————————

QT interval:————————————————————————

Other:——————————————————————————————

Interpretation:————————————————————————

85.

Rhythm:————————————————————————————

Rate:——————————————————————————————

P wave:————————————————————————————

PR interval:————————————————————————

QRS complex:————————————————————————

T wave:—————————————————————————————

QT interval:————————————————————————

Other:——————————————————————————————

Interpretation:————————————————————————

86.

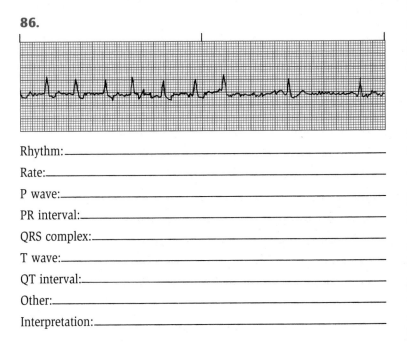

Rhythm:_____

Rate:_____

P wave:_____

PR interval:_____

QRS complex:_____

T wave:_____

QT interval:_____

Other:_____

Interpretation:_____

87.

Rhythm:_____

Rate:_____

P wave:_____

PR interval:_____

QRS complex:_____

T wave:_____

QT interval:_____

Other:_____

Interpretation:_____

88.

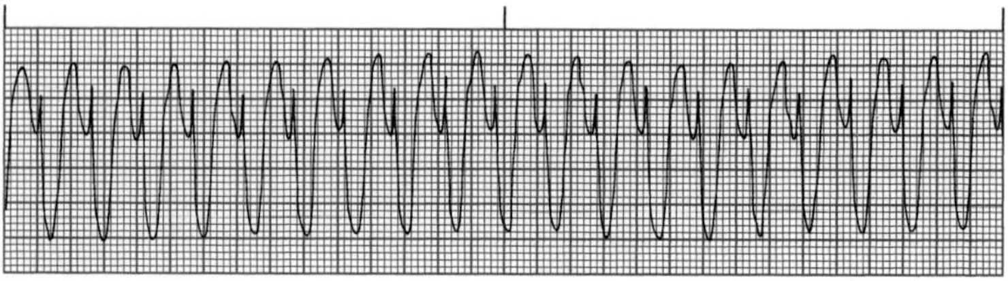

Rhythm:_____

Rate:_____

P wave:_____

PR interval:_____

QRS complex:_____

T wave:_____

QT interval:_____

Other:_____

Interpretation:_____

89.

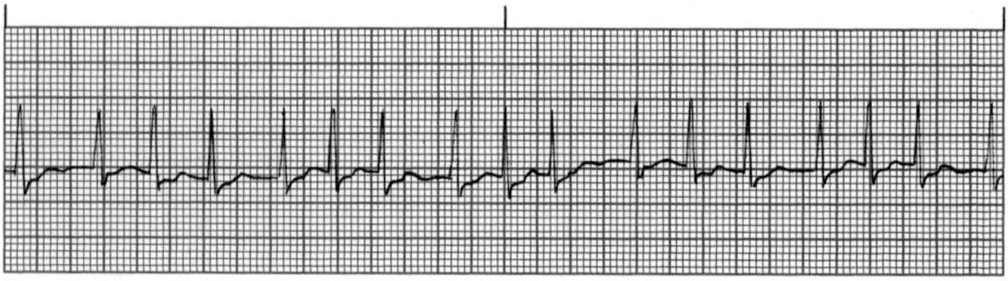

Rhythm:_____

Rate:_____

P wave:_____

PR interval:_____

QRS complex:_____

T wave:_____

QT interval:_____

Other:_____

Interpretation:_____

90.

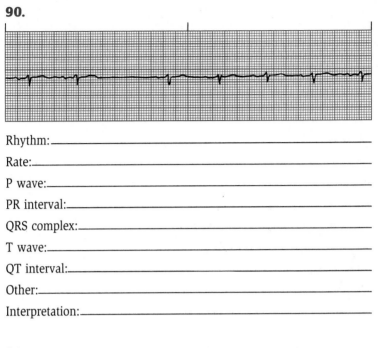

Rhythm:_____

Rate:_____

P wave:_____

PR interval:_____

QRS complex:_____

T wave:_____

QT interval:_____

Other:_____

Interpretation:_____

91.

Rhythm:_____

Rate:_____

P wave:_____

PR interval:_____

QRS complex:_____

T wave:_____

QT interval:_____

Other:_____

Interpretation:_____

92.

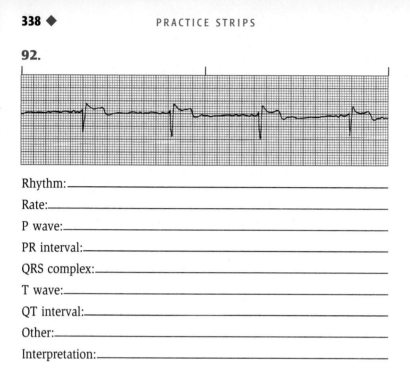

Rhythm:_____

Rate:_____

P wave:_____

PR interval:_____

QRS complex:_____

T wave:_____

QT interval:_____

Other:_____

Interpretation:_____

93.

Rhythm:_____

Rate:_____

P wave:_____

PR interval:_____

QRS complex:_____

T wave:_____

QT interval:_____

Other:_____

Interpretation:_____

94.

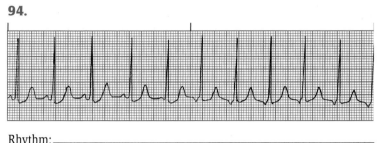

Rhythm: _____

Rate: _____

P wave: _____

PR interval: _____

QRS complex: _____

T wave: _____

QT interval: _____

Other: _____

Interpretation: _____

95.

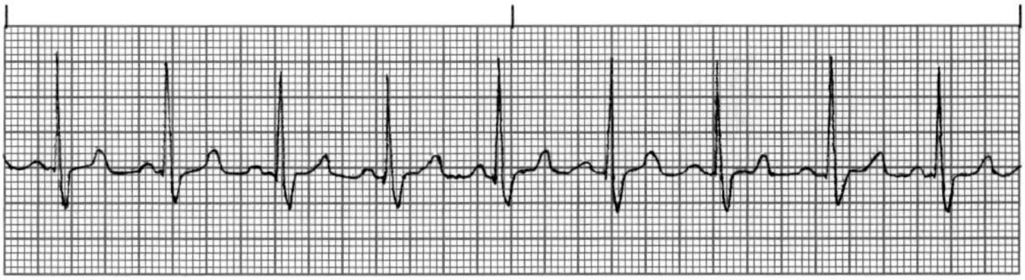

Rhythm: _____

Rate: _____

P wave: _____

PR interval: _____

QRS complex: _____

T wave: _____

QT interval: _____

Other: _____

Interpretation: _____

96.

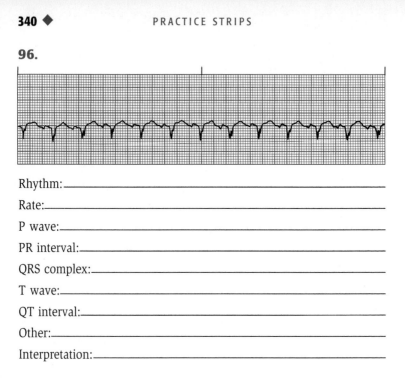

Rhythm:_____

Rate:_____

P wave:_____

PR interval:_____

QRS complex:_____

T wave:_____

QT interval:_____

Other:_____

Interpretation:_____

97.

Rhythm:_____

Rate:_____

P wave:_____

PR interval:_____

QRS complex:_____

T wave:_____

QT interval:_____

Other:_____

Interpretation:_____

98.

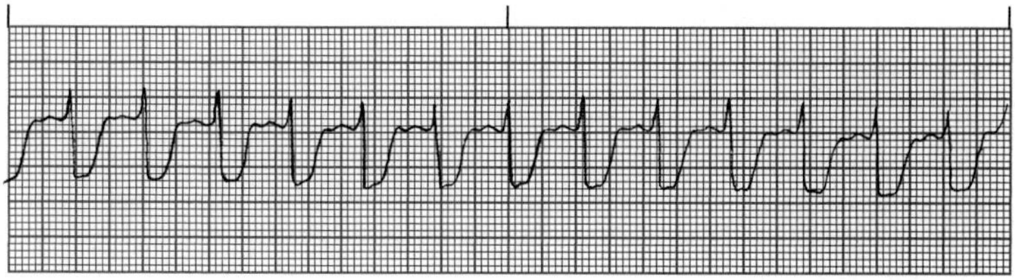

Rhythm:_____

Rate:_____

P wave:_____

PR interval:_____

QRS complex:_____

T wave:_____

QT interval:_____

Other:_____

Interpretation:_____

99.

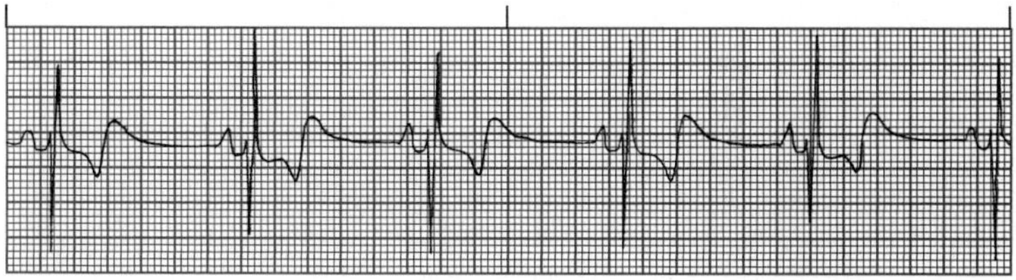

Rhythm:_____

Rate:_____

P wave:_____

PR interval:_____

QRS complex:_____

T wave:_____

QT interval:_____

Other:_____

Interpretation:_____

100.

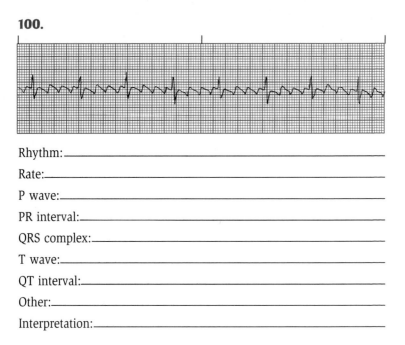

Rhythm: _____

Rate: _____

P wave: _____

PR interval: _____

QRS complex: _____

T wave: _____

QT interval: _____

Other: _____

Interpretation: _____

101.

Rhythm: _____

Rate: _____

P wave: _____

PR interval: _____

QRS complex: _____

T wave: _____

QT interval: _____

Other: _____

Interpretation: _____

102.

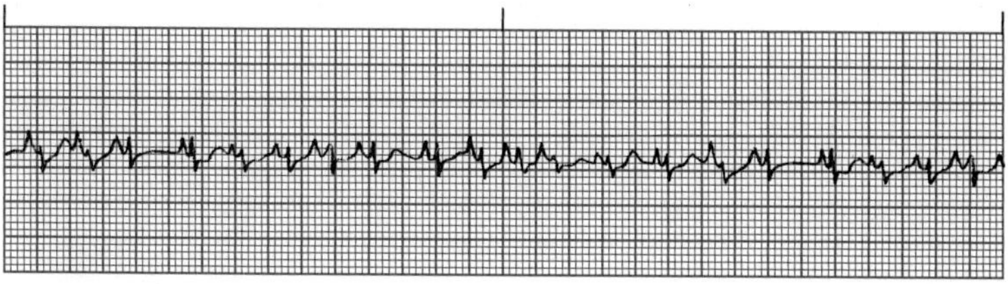

Rhythm:

Rate:

P wave:

PR interval:

QRS complex:

T wave:

QT interval:

Other:

Interpretation:

103.

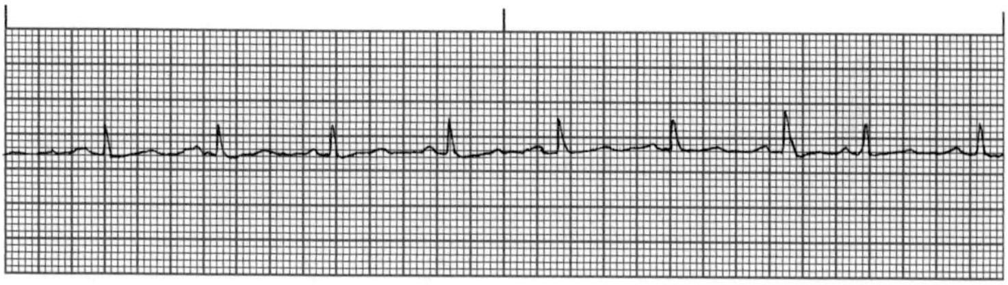

Rhythm:

Rate:

P wave:

PR interval:

QRS complex:

T wave:

QT interval:

Other:

Interpretation:

104.

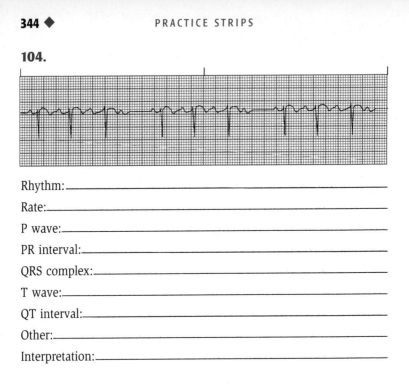

Rhythm:

Rate:

P wave:

PR interval:

QRS complex:

T wave:

QT interval:

Other:

Interpretation:

105.

Rhythm:

Rate:

P wave:

PR interval:

QRS complex:

T wave:

QT interval:

Other:

Interpretation:

106.

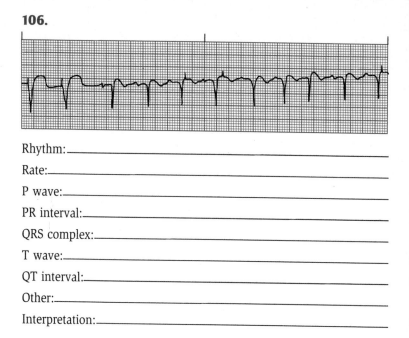

Rhythm:_____

Rate:_____

P wave:_____

PR interval:_____

QRS complex:_____

T wave:_____

QT interval:_____

Other:_____

Interpretation:_____

107.

Rhythm:_____

Rate:_____

P wave:_____

PR interval:_____

QRS complex:_____

T wave:_____

QT interval:_____

Other:_____

Interpretation:_____

108.

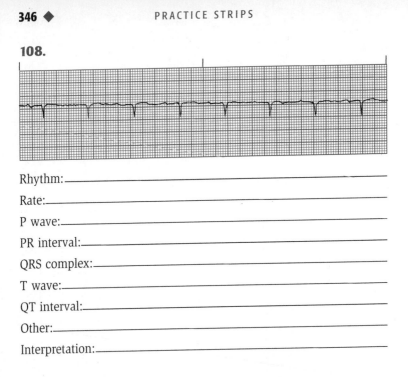

Rhythm:—————————————————————————————

Rate:———————————————————————————————

P wave:——————————————————————————————

PR interval:————————————————————————————

QRS complex:————————————————————————————

T wave:—————————————————————————————

QT interval:—————————————————————————————

Other:——————————————————————————————

Interpretation:————————————————————————————

109.

Rhythm:—————————————————————————————

Rate:———————————————————————————————

P wave:——————————————————————————————

PR interval:————————————————————————————

QRS complex:————————————————————————————

T wave:—————————————————————————————

QT interval:—————————————————————————————

Other:——————————————————————————————

Interpretation:————————————————————————————

110.

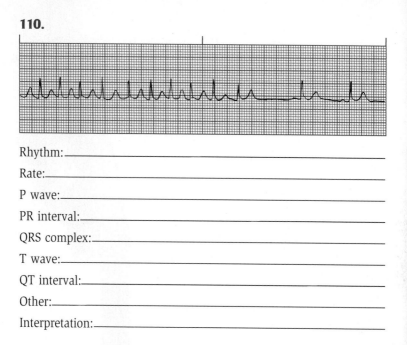

Rhythm:_____

Rate:_____

P wave:_____

PR interval:_____

QRS complex:_____

T wave:_____

QT interval:_____

Other:_____

Interpretation:_____

111.

Rhythm:_____

Rate:_____

P wave:_____

PR interval:_____

QRS complex:_____

T wave:_____

QT interval:_____

Other:_____

Interpretation:_____

112.

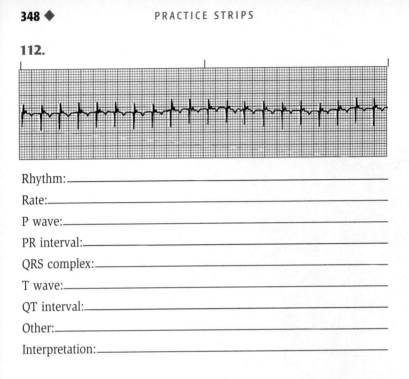

Rhythm:_____

Rate:_____

P wave:_____

PR interval:_____

QRS complex:_____

T wave:_____

QT interval:_____

Other:_____

Interpretation:_____

113.

Rhythm:_____

Rate:_____

P wave:_____

PR interval:_____

QRS complex:_____

T wave:_____

QT interval:_____

Other:_____

Interpretation:_____

114.

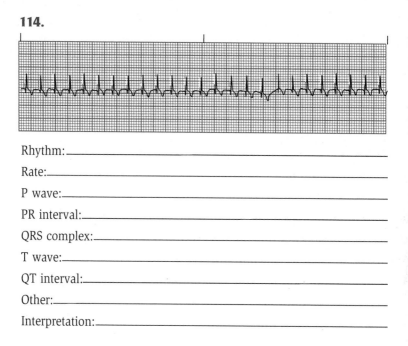

Rhythm:_____

Rate:_____

P wave:_____

PR interval:_____

QRS complex:_____

T wave:_____

QT interval:_____

Other:_____

Interpretation:_____

115.

Rhythm:_____

Rate:_____

P wave:_____

PR interval:_____

QRS complex:_____

T wave:_____

QT interval:_____

Other:_____

Interpretation:_____

116.

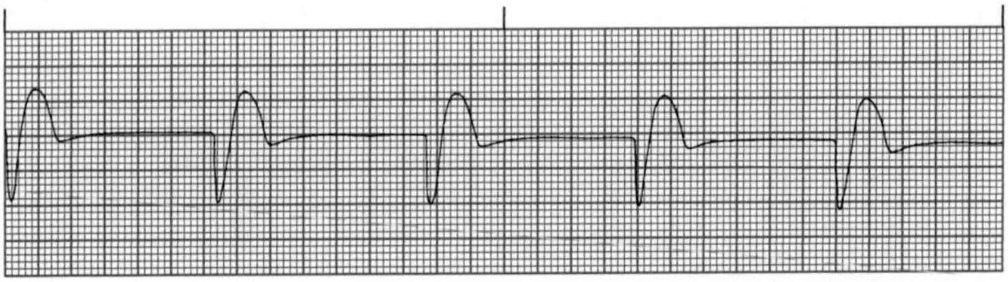

Rhythm:_____

Rate:_____

P wave:_____

PR interval:_____

QRS complex:_____

T wave:_____

QT interval:_____

Other:_____

Interpretation:_____

117.

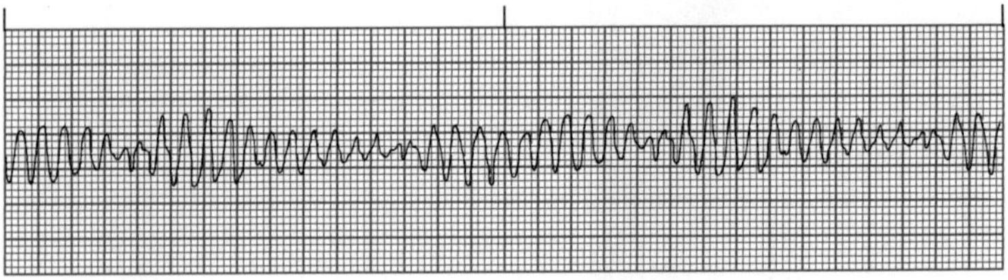

Rhythm:_____

Rate:_____

P wave:_____

PR interval:_____

QRS complex:_____

T wave:_____ _____

QT interval:_____

Other:_____

Interpretation:_____

118.

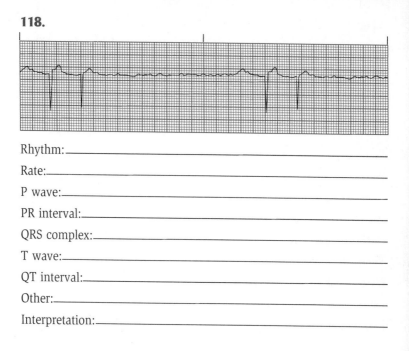

Rhythm:_____

Rate:_____

P wave:_____

PR interval:_____

QRS complex:_____

T wave:_____

QT interval:_____

Other:_____

Interpretation:_____

119.

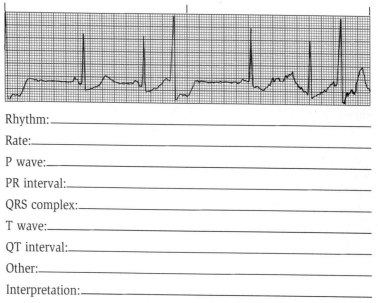

Rhythm:_____

Rate:_____

P wave:_____

PR interval:_____

QRS complex:_____

T wave:_____

QT interval:_____

Other:_____

Interpretation:_____

120.

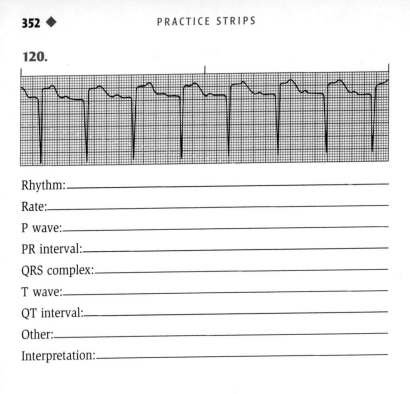

Rhythm:————————————————————————

Rate:——————————————————————————

P wave:—————————————————————————

PR interval:————————————————————————

QRS complex:———————————————————————

T wave:—————————————————————————

QT interval:————————————————————————

Other:——————————————————————————

Interpretation:———————————————————————

Answers

1.
Rhythm: Irregular
Rate: 130 beats/minute
P wave: Normal
PR interval: Unmeasurable
QRS complex: 0.08 second
T wave: Variable
QT interval: Unmeasurable
Other: None
Interpretation: Atrial tachycardia with block

2.
Rhythm: Regular
Rate: 88 beats/minute
P wave: None
PR interval: Unmeasurable
QRS complex: 0.12 second; pacemaker generated
T wave: Normal
QT interval: 0.32 second
Other: None
Interpretation: Ventricular pacing

3.
Rhythm: Irregular
Rate: 120 beats/minute
P wave: Normal
PR interval: 0.12 second
QRS complex: 0.06 second
T wave: Normal
QT interval: 0.20 second
Other: None
Interpretation: Second-degree AV block, type II

4.
Rhythm: Irregular
Rate: 80 beats/minute
P wave: Normal in sinus beats; inverted in PACs
PR interval: 0.28 second in sinus beats
QRS complex: 0.10 second
T wave: Normal
QT interval: 0.40 second
Other: None
Interpretation: First-degree AV block with PACs

5.
Rhythm: Regular
Rate: 100 beats/minute
P wave: Flattened
PR interval: 0.22 second
QRS complex: 0.06 second
T wave: Inverted
QT interval: 0.30 second
Other: None
Interpretation: Sinus tachycardia with first-degree AV block

6.
Rhythm: Irregular
Rate: 180 beats/minute
P wave: Normal
PR interval: Variable
QRS complex: 0.06 second
T wave: Inverted
QT interval: 0.12 second
Other: None
Interpretation: Second-degree AV block, type II

7.
Rhythm: Regular
Rate: 75 beats/minute
P wave: Abnormal within T wave
PR interval: Unmeasurable
QRS complex: 0.08 second
T wave: Distorted by P wave
QT interval: Unmeasurable
Other: None
Interpretation: Accelerated junctional rhythm

8.
Rhythm: Regular
Rate: 28 beats/minute
P wave: Normal
PR interval: Unmeasurable
QRS complex: 0.16 second
T wave: Distorted by P wave
QT interval: Unmeasurable
Other: P wave not related to QRS complex
Interpretation: Third-degree AV block

9.
Rhythm: Regular
Rate: 65 beats/minute
P wave: Normal
PR interval: 0.40 second
QRS complex: 0.08 second
T wave: Normal
QT interval: 0.28 second
Other: None
Interpretation: NSR with first-degree AV block

10.
Rhythm: Regular
Rate: 115 beats/minute
P wave: Normal
PR interval: 0.16 second
QRS complex: 0.08 second
T wave: Normal
QT interval: 0.36 second
Other: None
Interpretation: Sinus tachycardia

11.
Rhythm: Regular
Rate: 107 beats/minute
P wave: None
PR interval: Variable; pacemaker generated
QRS complex: 0.12 second; pacemaker generated
T wave: Normal
QT interval: 0.32 second
Other: None
Interpretation: AV pacing

12.
Rhythm: Irregular
Rate: 120 beats/minute
P wave: None
PR interval: Unmeasurable
QRS complex: 0.08 second
T wave: Flattened
QT interval: 0.32 second
Other: None
Interpretation: Atrial pacing with PVCs

13.
Rhythm: Irregular
Rate: 70 beats/minute
P wave: Normal
PR interval: Variable
QRS complex: 0.12 second
T wave: Normal
QT interval: 0.30 second
Other: PR interval increases until dropped beat
Interpretation: Second-degree AV block, type I

14.
Rhythm: Regular except for pause
Rate: Underlying, 79 beats/minute
P wave: Normal
PR interval: 0.18 second
QRS complex: 0.08 second
T wave: Normal
QT interval: 0.38 second
Other: None
Interpretation: Sinus arrest

15.
Rhythm: Regular
Rate: 44 beats/minute
P wave: Normal
PR interval: Unmeasurable
QRS complex: 0.12 second
T wave: Normal
QT interval: 0.44 second
Other: P wave not related to QRS complex
Interpretation: Third-degree AV block

16.
Rhythm: Slightly irregular
Rate: 30 beats/minute
P wave: Absent
PR interval: Unmeasurable
QRS complex: 0.24 second
T wave: Abnormal
QT interval: 0.44 second
Other: None
Interpretation: Idioventricular rhythm

17.
Rhythm: Irregular
Rate: 150 beats/minute
P wave: Normal with sinus beats
PR interval: 0.12 second
QRS complex: 0.04 second
T wave: Normal
QT interval: 0.22 second
Other: None
Interpretation: Sinus tachycardia with PVCs

18.
Rhythm: Regular
Rate: 38 beats/minute
P wave: Indiscernible
PR interval: Unmeasurable
QRS complex: 0.36 second
T wave: Indiscernible
QT interval: Unmeasurable
Other: None
Interpretation: Idioventricular rhythm

19.
Rhythm: Regular
Rate: 150 beats/minute
P wave: Indiscernible
PR interval: Unmeasurable
QRS complex: 0.08 second
T wave: Indiscernible
QT interval: Unmeasurable
Other: None
Interpretation: Atrial tachycardia

20.
Rhythm: Irregular
Rate: 110 beats/minute
P wave: Fine fibrillation waves
PR interval: Indiscernible
QRS complex: 0.08 second
T wave: Indiscernible
QT interval: Unmeasurable
Other: None
Interpretation: Atrial fibrillation

21.
Rhythm: Irregular
Rate: 90 beats/minute
P wave: Normal with sinus beats
PR interval: 0.16 second
QRS complex: 0.06 second
T wave: Normal
QT interval: 0.28 second
Other: None
Interpretation: NSR with PVCs (trigeminy)

22.
Rhythm: Irregular
Rate: 100 beats/minute
P wave: Normal with sinus beats
PR interval: 0.16 second
QRS complex: 0.08 second
T wave: Normal
QT interval: 0.28 second
Other: None
Interpretation: Sinus tachycardia with PVCs

23.
Rhythm: Regular
Rate: 100 beats/minute
P wave: None present
PR interval: Unmeasurable
QRS complex: 0.10 second
T wave: Normal
QT interval: 0.44 second
Other: ST-segment depression
Interpretation: Accelerated junctional rhythm

24.
Rhythm: Irregular
Rate: 80 beats/minute
P wave: Normal when present
PR interval: 0.32 second
QRS complex: 0.08 second
T wave: Normal; occasionally distorted by spike
QT interval: 0.36 second
Other: ST-segment elevation; erratic pacer spikes present
Interpretation: Failure to sense

25.
Rhythm: Absent
Rate: Absent
P wave: Absent
PR interval: Unmeasurable
QRS complex: Absent
T wave: Absent
QT interval: Unmeasurable
Other: None
Interpretation: Asystole

26.
Rhythm: Regular
Rate: 188 beats/minute
P wave: Indiscernible
PR interval: Unmeasurable
QRS complex: 0.12 second
T wave: Distorted by P wave
QT interval: Unmeasurable
Other: None
Interpretation: Atrial tachycardia

27.
Rhythm: Regular
Rate: 65 beats/minute
P wave: Absent
PR interval: Absent
QRS complex: 0.20 second; pacemaker generated
T wave: Distorted by pacer beat
QT interval: Unmeasurable
Other: None
Interpretation: Ventricular pacing

28.
Rhythm: Regular
Rate: 47 beats/minute
P wave: Normal
PR interval: 0.20 second
QRS complex: 0.08 second
T wave: Normal
QT interval: 0.52 second
Other: None
Interpretation: Sinus bradycardia

29.
Rhythm: Regular
Rate: 79 beats/minute
P wave: Normal
PR interval: 0.16 second
QRS complex: 0.08 second
T wave: Normal
QT interval: 0.40 second
Other: None
Interpretation: NSR

30.
Rhythm: Irregular
Rate: 70 beats/minute
P wave: Normal
PR interval: 0.16 second
QRS complex: 0.10 second
T wave: Biphasic
QT interval: 0.38 second
Other: None
Interpretation: Sinus arrhythmia

31.
Rhythm: Regular
Rate: 50 beats/minute
P wave: Normal
PR interval: 0.16 second
QRS complex: 0.08 second
T wave: Flattened
QT interval: 0.44 second
Other: None
Interpretation: Sinus bradycardia

32.
Rhythm: Regular
Rate: 115 beats/minute
P wave: Normal
PR interval: 0.16 second
QRS complex: 0.08 second
T wave: Normal
QT interval: 0.30 second
Other: None
Interpretation: Sinus tachycardia

33.
Rhythm: Regular
Rate: 88 beats/minute
P wave: Absent
PR interval: Absent
QRS complex: Abnormal
T wave: Indiscernible
QT interval: Unmeasurable
Other: None
Interpretation: Monomorphic VT

34.
Rhythm: Irregular
Rate: 107 beats/minute for underlying rhythm
P wave: Normal; absent with premature beats
PR interval: 0.12 second
QRS complex: 0.08 second for underlying rhythm
T wave: Variable
QT interval: Unmeasurable
Other: None
Interpretation: Sinus tachycardia with multifocal PVCs (one couplet)

35.
Rhythm: Regular
Rate: 188 beats/minute
P wave: Absent
PR interval: Unmeasurable
QRS complex: Abnormal
T wave: Indiscernible
QT interval: Unmeasurable
Other: None
Interpretation: VT

36.
Rhythm: Regular
Rate: 88 beats/minute
P wave: Normal
PR interval: 0.24 second
QRS complex: 0.08 second
T wave: Normal
QT interval: 0.32 second
Other: None
Interpretation: NSR with first-degree AV block

37.
Rhythm: Regular
Rate: 107 beats/minute
P wave: Normal
PR interval: 0.16 second
QRS complex: 0.12 second
T wave: Normal
QT interval: 0.36 second
Other: None
Interpretation: Sinus tachycardia

38.
Rhythm: Irregular
Rate: 100 beats/minute
P wave: Normal
PR interval: 0.16 second
QRS complex: 0.08 second
T wave: Normal
QT interval: 0.40 second
Other: None
Interpretation: NSR with PACs

39.

Rhythm: Regular
Rate: 43 beats/minute
P wave: Normal
PR interval: Unmeasurable
QRS complex: 0.12 second
T wave: Normal
QT interval: Unmeasurable
Other: P wave not related to QRS complex
Interpretation: Third-degree AV block

40.

Rhythm: Absent
Rate: Absent
P wave: Absent
PR interval: Unmeasurable
QRS complex: Absent
T wave: Absent
QT interval: Unmeasurable
Other: None
Interpretation: Asystole

41.

Rhythm: Chaotic
Rate: Greater than 300 beats/ minute
P wave: None
PR interval: Unmeasurable
QRS complex: Abnormal
T wave: Indiscernible
QT interval: Unmeasurable
Other: None
Interpretation: VF

42.

Rhythm: Irregular
Rate: 50 beats/minute
P wave: Normal
PR interval: 0.20 second
QRS complex: 0.08 second
T wave: Normal
QT interval: 0.40 second
Other: Pause present
Interpretation: Sinus bradycardia with PAC

43.

Rhythm: Irregular
Rate: 150 beats/minute
P wave: Normal except during premature beats
PR interval: 0.12 second
QRS complex: 0.08 second
T wave: Inverted
QT interval: 0.24 second
Other: None
Interpretation: Sinus tachycardia with PJC

44.

Rhythm: Irregular
Rate: 110 beats/minute
P wave: Normal with sinus beats
PR interval: 0.12 second
QRS complex: 0.08 second
T wave: Peaked
QT interval: 0.28 second
Other: None
Interpretation: Sinus tachycardia leading to AIVR

45.
Rhythm: Irregular
Rate: 80 beats/minute
P wave: Indiscernible
PR interval: Unmeasurable
QRS complex: 0.08 second
T wave: Normal
QT interval: 0.32 second
Other: None
Interpretation: Controlled atrial fibrillation

46.
Rhythm: Irregular
Rate: 130 beats/minute
P wave: Normal with sinus beats
PR interval: 0.12 second
QRS complex: 0.06 second
T wave: Flattened
QT interval: 0.18 second
Other: None
Interpretation: NSR with PVCs (bigeminy)

47.
Rhythm: Regular
Rate: 58 beats/minute
P wave: Flutter waves
PR interval: Unmeasurable
QRS complex: 0.08 second
T wave: Not discernible
QT interval: Unmeasurable
Other: None
Interpretation: 4:1 atrial flutter

48.
Rhythm: Irregular
Rate: 90 beats/minute
P wave: Indiscernible
PR interval: Unmeasurable
QRS complex: 0.08 second
T wave: Inverted
QT interval: 0.32 second
Other: None
Interpretation: Controlled atrial fibrillation

49.
Rhythm: Irregular
Rate: 90 beats/minute
P wave: Variable
PR interval: Variable
QRS complex: 0.08 second
T wave: Inverted
QT interval: 0.36 second
Other: None
Interpretation: PAT leading back to NSR

50.
Rhythm: Irregular
Rate: 60 beats/minute
P wave: Indiscernible
PR interval: Unmeasurable
QRS complex: 0.10 second
T wave: Indiscernible
QT interval: Unmeasurable
Other: None
Interpretation: AIVR with periods of asystole

51.
Rhythm: Irregular
Rate: 50 beats/minute
P wave: Indiscernible
PR interval: Unmeasurable
QRS complex: 0.14 second
T wave: Abnormal
QT interval: 0.36 second
Other: None
Interpretation: AIVR

52.
Rhythm: Irregular
Rate: 60 beats/minute
P wave: Indiscernible
PR interval: Unmeasurable
QRS complex: 0.08 second
T wave: Indiscernible
QT interval: Unmeasurable
Other: None
Interpretation: Controlled atrial fibrillation

53.
Rhythm: Irregular
Rate: 40 beats/minute
P wave: Variable; not always present
PR interval: 0.20 second
QRS complex: 0.08 second
T wave: Normal
QT interval: 0.38 second
Other: None
Interpretation: Sinus bradycardia with junctional beat

54.
Rhythm: Regular
Rate: 150 beats/minute
P wave: Indiscernible
PR interval: Unmeasurable
QRS complex: 0.12 second
T wave: Normal
QT interval: 0.24 second
Other: None
Interpretation: Junctional tachycardia

55.
Rhythm: Slightly irregular
Rate: 70 beats/minute
P wave: Flutter waves
PR interval: Unmeasurable
QRS complex: 0.08 second
T wave: Indiscernible
QT interval: Unmeasurable
Other: None
Interpretation: Atrial flutter (4:1 block)

56.
Rhythm: Regular
Rate: 250 beats/minute
P wave: Indiscernible
PR interval: Unmeasurable
QRS complex: 0.12 second
T wave: Indiscernible
QT interval: Unmeasurable
Other: None
Interpretation: VT

57.
Rhythm: Irregular
Rate: 200 beats/minute
P wave: Normal with sinus beats
PR interval: 0.12 second
QRS complex: 0.06 second
T wave: Inverted
QT interval: 0.16 second
Other: Artifact present
Interpretation: Sinus tachycardia with PVCs

58.
Rhythm: Regular
Rate: 150 beats/minute
P wave: Indiscernible
PR interval: Unmeasurable
QRS complex: Abnormal
T wave: Indiscernible
QT interval: Unmeasurable
Other: None
Interpretation: VT

59.
Rhythm: Chaotic
Rate: Unmeasurable
P wave: Indiscernible
PR interval: Unmeasurable
QRS complex: Abnormal
T wave: Indiscernible
QT interval: Unmeasurable
Other: Complex size increases and decreases
Interpretation: Torsades de pointes

60.
Rhythm: Regular
Rate: 125 beats/minute
P wave: Indiscernible
PR interval: Unmeasurable
QRS complex: 0.08 second
T wave: Indiscernible
QT interval: Unmeasurable
Other: None
Interpretation: AIVR

61.
Rhythm: Regular
Rate: 250 beats/minute
P wave: Indiscernible
PR interval: Unmeasurable
QRS complex: 0.06 second
T wave: Indiscernible
QT interval: Unmeasurable
Other: None
Interpretation: Atrial tachycardia

62.
Rhythm: Irregular
Rate: 120 beats/minute
P wave: Biphasic when present
PR interval: 0.16 second
QRS complex: 0.10 second
T wave: Elevated
QT interval: 0.40 second when measurable
Other: None
Interpretation: NSR with PVCs

63.
Rhythm: Irregular
Rate: 140 beats/minute
P wave: Normal with sinus beats
PR interval: 0.12 second
QRS complex: 0.08 second
T wave: Flattened
QT interval: 0.20 second
Other: None
Interpretation: Sinus tachycardia with PVCs (quadrigeminy)

64.
Rhythm: Chaotic
Rate: Greater than 300 beats/ minute
P wave: Indiscernible
PR interval: Unmeasurable
QRS complex: Abnormal
T wave: Indiscernible
QT interval: Unmeasurable
Other: Complex size increases and decreases
Interpretation: Torsades de pointes

65.
Rhythm: Irregular
Rate: 170 beats/minute
P wave: Normal with sinus beats
PR interval: 0.08 second
QRS complex: 0.04 second
T wave: Normal
QT interval: 0.16 second
Other: None
Interpretation: Sinus tachycardia with PVCs

66.
Rhythm: Irregular
Rate: 140 beats/minute
P wave: Normal with sinus beats
PR interval: 0.14 second
QRS complex: 0.08 second
T wave: Distorted
QT interval: Unmeasurable
Other: None
Interpretation: NSR with PVCs (bigeminy)

67.
Rhythm: Irregular
Rate: 230 beats/minute
P wave: None
PR interval: Unmeasurable
QRS complex: Abnormal
T wave: None
QT interval: Unmeasurable
Other: None
Interpretation: VF

68.
Rhythm: Absent
Rate: None
P wave: None
PR interval: Unmeasurable
QRS complex: None
T wave: None
QT interval: Unmeasurable
Other: None
Interpretation: Asystole

69.
Rhythm: Irregular
Rate: Approximately 160 beats/minute
P wave: Flutter waves
PR interval: Unmeasurable
QRS complex: 0.08 second
T wave: Indiscernible
QT interval: Unmeasurable
Other: None
Interpretation: Atrial flutter with varying conduction ratios

70.
Rhythm: Slightly irregular
Rate: 110 beats/minute
P wave: Normal
PR interval: Unmeasurable
QRS complex: 0.06 second
T wave: Occasionally distorted by P waves
QT interval: 0.16 second
Other: P wave not related to QRS complex
Interpretation: Third-degree AV block

71.
Rhythm: Regular
Rate: 30 beats/minute
P wave: Normal
PR interval: Unmeasurable
QRS complex: 0.20 second
T wave: Distorted by P wave
QT interval: 0.50 second
Other: None
Interpretation: Third-degree AV block

72.
Rhythm: Irregular
Rate: 60 beats/minute
P wave: Biphasic
PR interval: 0.12 second
QRS complex: 0.12 second
T wave: Normal
QT interval: 0.34 second
Other: None
Interpretation: Second-degree AV block, type II

73.
Rhythm: Regular
Rate: 63 beats/minute
P wave: Flattened
PR interval: 0.20 second
QRS complex: 0.06 second
T wave: Inverted
QT interval: 0.32 second
Other: None
Interpretation: NSR

74.
Rhythm: Regular
Rate: 115 beats/minute
P wave: Abnormal or absent
PR interval: Unmeasurable
QRS complex: 0.10 second
T wave: Normal
QT interval: 0.32 second
Other: Phasic slowing and quickening
Interpretation: Junctional tachycardia

75.

Rhythm: Regular
Rate: 52 beats/minute
PR interval: 0.20 second
QRS complex: 0.10 second
T wave: Normal
QT interval: 0.48 second
Other: None
Interpretation: Sinus bradycardia

76.

Rhythm: Irregular
Rate: 30 beats/minute
P wave: None
PR interval: Absent
QRS complex: 0.20 second
T wave: Abnormal
QT interval: Unmeasurable
Other: None
Interpretation: Idioventricular rhythm

77.

Rhythm: Irregular
Rate: 150 beats/minute
P wave: Normal except during premature beats
PR interval: 0.12 second
QRS complex: 0.08 second
T wave: Inverted
QT interval: 0.24 second
Other: None
Interpretation: Sinus tachycardia with PJCs

78.

Rhythm: Irregular
Rate: 214 down to 50 beats/minute
P wave: Indiscernible
PR interval: Unmeasurable
QRS complex: 0.12 second
T wave: Normal
QT interval: 0.28 second
Other: None
Interpretation: Atrial tachycardia changing to atrial fibrillation with PVCs

79.

Rhythm: Regular
Rate: 214 beats/minute
P wave: Indiscernible
PR interval: Unmeasurable
QRS complex: 0.08 second
T wave: Indiscernible
QT interval: Unmeasurable
Other: None
Interpretation: Atrial tachycardia

80.

Rhythm: Irregular
Rate: 110 beats/minute
P wave: Absent
PR interval: Unmeasurable
QRS complex: 0.06 second
T wave: Indiscernible
QT interval: Unmeasurable
Other: None
Interpretation: Uncontrolled atrial fibrillation

81.

Rhythm: Irregular
Rate: 88 beats/minute
P wave: Absent
PR interval: Unmeasurable
QRS complex: 0.24 second;
pacemaker generated
T wave: Normal
QT interval: 0.44 second
Other: None
Interpretation: VVI pacing

82.

Rhythm: Irregular
Rate: 80 beats/minute
P wave: Absent
PR interval: Unmeasurable
QRS complex: 0.16 second for
underlying rhythm
T wave: Normal
QT interval: 0.44 second
Other: None
Interpretation: Accelerated
idioventricular rhythm

83.

Rhythm: Irregular
Rate: 140 beats/minute
P wave: Fine fibrillatory waves
present for underlying rhythm;
absent for pair and run
PR interval: Absent
QRS complex: 0.04 second for
underlying rhythm
T wave: Indiscernible
QT interval: Indiscernible
Other: None
Interpretation: Atrial fibrillation
with a pair of PVCs and a run of
VT

84.

Rhythm: Irregular
Rate: 125 beats/minute for
underlying rhythm; 150 to
167 beats/minute for run
P wave: Normal with sinus beats
PR interval: 0.12 second
QRS complex: 0.04 second
T wave: Normal
QT interval: 0.32 second
Other: None
Interpretation: Sinus tachycardia
with PAT

85.

Rhythm: Irregular
Rate: 94 beats/minute for under-
lying rhythm; 167 beats/minute
for run
P wave: Normal with sinus beats
PR interval: 0.20 second
QRS complex: 0.08 second
T wave: Normal with sinus beats
QT interval: 0.40 second
Other: None
Interpretation: PAT leading to
NSR

86.

Rhythm: Irregular
Rate: 90 beats/minute
P wave: Fibrillatory waves
PR interval: Unmeasurable
QRS complex: 0.08 second
T wave: Indiscernible
QT interval: Unmeasurable
Other: None
Interpretation: Controlled atrial
fibrillation

87.

Rhythm: Irregular
Rate: 45 beats/minute
P wave: Normal
PR interval: Unmeasurable
QRS complex: 0.10 second
T wave: Normal
QT interval: 0.32 second
Other: P wave not related to QRS complex
Interpretation: Idioventricular rhythm

88.

Rhythm: Regular
Rate: 215 beats/minute
P wave: Indiscernible
PR interval: Unmeasurable
QRS complex: 0.16 second
T wave: Indiscernible
QT interval: Unmeasurable
Other: None
Interpretation: VT

89.

Rhythm: Irregular
Rate: 170 beats/minute
P wave: Indiscernible
PR interval: Unmeasurable
QRS complex: 0.08 second
T wave: Indiscernible
QT interval: Unmeasurable
Other: None
Interpretation: Uncontrolled atrial fibrillation

90.

Rhythm: Irregular
Rate: 70 beats/minute
P wave: Normal
PR interval: 0.20 second
QRS complex: 0.08 second
T wave: Normal
QT interval: 0.32 second
Other: None
Interpretation: NSR with blocked PAC

91.

Rhythm: Irregular
Rate: 60 beats/minute
P wave: Flutter waves
PR interval: Unmeasurable
QRS complex: 0.12 second
T wave: Indiscernible
QT interval: 0.36 second
Other: None
Interpretation: Atrial flutter with variable block

92.

Rhythm: Regular
Rate: 42 beats/minute
P wave: Normal
PR interval: 0.16 second
QRS complex: 0.08 second
T wave: Normal
QT interval: 0.42 second
Other: ST-segment elevation
Interpretation: Sinus bradycardia

93.
Rhythm: Chaotic
Rate: Unmeasurable
P wave: Indiscernible
PR interval: Unmeasurable
QRS complex: Indiscernible
QT interval: Unmeasurable
Other: Complex size increases and decreases
Interpretation: Torsades de pointes

94.
Rhythm: Regular
Rate: 100 beats/minute
P wave: Normal initially, then becomes inverted with shortened PR interval
PR interval: 0.14 second initially then unmeasurable
QRS complex: 0.08 second
T wave: Normal
QT interval: 0.36 second
Other: None
Interpretation: Sinus tachycardia leading to junctional tachycardia

95.
Rhythm: Regular
Rate: 94 beats/minute
P wave: Normal
PR interval: 0.16 second
QRS complex: 0.12 second
T wave: Normal
QT interval: 0.34 second
Other: None
Interpretation: NSR

96.
Rhythm: Regular
Rate: 125 beats/minute
P wave: Slightly peaked
PR interval: 0.12 second
QRS complex: 0.10 second
T wave: Normal
QT interval: 0.28 second
Other: None
Interpretation: Sinus tachycardia

97.
Rhythm: Regular
Rate: 54 beats/minute
P wave: Peaked
PR interval: 0.20 second
QRS complex: 0.08 second
T wave: Inverted
QT interval: 0.44 second
Other: None
Interpretation: Sinus bradycardia

98.
Rhythm: Regular
Rate: 136 beats/minute
P wave: Normal
PR interval: 0.12 second
QRS complex: 0.04 second
T wave: Inverted
QT interval: 0.26 second
Other: None
Interpretation: Sinus tachycardia

99.

Rhythm: Regular
Rate: 54 beats/minute
P wave: Normal
PR interval: 0.20 second
QRS complex: 0.12 second
T wave: Inverted
QT interval: 0.36 second
Other: None
Interpretation: Sinus bradycardia

100.

Rhythm: Regular
Rate: 79 beats/minute
P wave: Flutter waves
PR interval: Unmeasurable
QRS complex: 0.12 second
T wave: Indiscernible
QT interval: Unmeasurable
Other: None
Interpretation: Atrial flutter (4:1 block)

101.

Rhythm: Irregular
Rate: 240 beats/minute
P wave: Indiscernible
PR interval: Unmeasurable
QRS complex: Abnormal
T wave: Indiscernible
QT interval: Unmeasurable
Other: Complex size increases and decreases
Interpretation: Torsades de pointes

102.

Rhythm: Irregular
Rate: 200 beats/minute
P wave: Normal
PR interval: 0.12 second
QRS complex: 0.06 second
T wave: Inverted
QT interval: 0.16 second
Other: None
Interpretation: Atrial tachycardia with PACs

103.

Rhythm: Regular
Rate: 88 beats/minute
P wave: Normal
PR interval: 0.18 second
QRS complex: 0.08 second
T wave: Normal
QT interval: 0.36 second
Other: None
Interpretation: NSR

104.

Rhythm: Irregular
Rate: 90 beats/minute
P wave: Peaked
PR interval: Variable
QRS complex: 0.08 second
T wave: Elevated
QT interval: 0.20 second
Other: PR interval increases until dropped beat
Interpretation: Second-degree AV block, type I

105.
Rhythm: Regular
Rate: 75 beats/minute
P wave: Pacemaker generated
PR interval: 0.24 second
QRS complex: 0.08 second
T wave: Normal
QT interval: 0.28 second
Other: None
Interpretation: Atrial pacing

106.
Rhythm: Regular
Rate: 110 beats/minute
P wave: Indiscernible
PR interval: Unmeasurable
QRS complex: Variable
T wave: Indiscernible
QT interval: Unmeasurable
Other: None
Interpretation: Ventricular pacing leading to atrial fibrillation with failure to sense

107.
Rhythm: Irregular
Rate: 125 beats/minute
P wave: None
PR interval: Unmeasurable
QRS complex: 0.16 second; pacemaker generated
T wave: Normal
QT interval: 0.32 second
Other: None
Interpretation: Ventricular pacing

108.
Rhythm: Regular
Rate: 80 beats/minute
P wave: Flattened
PR interval: 0.24 second
QRS complex: 0.08 second
T wave: Flattened
QT interval: 0.32 second
Other: None
Interpretation: NSR with first-degree AV block

109.
Rhythm: Regular
Rate: 60 beats/minute
P wave: Normal
PR interval: Unmeasurable
QRS complex: 0.08 second
T wave: Distorted by P waves
QT interval: Unmeasurable
Other: None
Interpretation: Second-degree AV block, type II

110.
Rhythm: Irregular
Rate: 120 beats/minute
P wave: Normal with sinus beats
PR interval: 0.16 second
QRS complex: 0.06 second
T wave: Normal
QT interval: 0.32 second
Other: None
Interpretation: Atrial tachycardia converting to NSR

111.

Rhythm: Irregular
Rate: 120 beats/minute
P wave: Normal
PR interval: 0.16 second
QRS complex: 0.08 second
T wave: Inverted
QT interval: 0.24 second
Other: Bundle-branch block
Interpretation: Sinus tachycardia with period of junctional tachycardia

112.

Rhythm: Regular
Rate: 188 beats/minute
P wave: Retrograde
PR interval: Unmeasurable
QRS complex: 0.04 second
T wave: Inverted
QT interval: 0.20 second
Other: None
Interpretation: Junctional tachycardia

113.

Rhythm: Regular
Rate: 47 beats/minute
P wave: Inverted and retrograde
PR interval: Unmeasurable
QRS complex: 0.12 second
T wave: Normal
QT interval: 0.52 second
Other: None
Interpretation: Junctional escape rhythm

114.

Rhythm: Regular
Rate: 250 beats/minute
P wave: Absent
PR interval: Unmeasurable
QRS complex: 0.04 second
T wave: Inverted
QT interval: 0.12 second
Other: Possible SVT
Interpretation: Junctional tachycardia

115.

Rhythm: Regular
Rate: 43 beats/minute
P wave: Absent
PR interval: Unmeasurable
QRS complex: 0.12 second
T wave: Normal
QT interval: 0.40 second
Other: ST-segment elevation
Interpretation: Junctional escape rhythm

116.

Rhythm: Regular
Rate: 50 beats/minute
P wave: Indiscernible
PR interval: Unmeasurable
QRS complex: 0.12 second
T wave: Distorted
QT interval: Unmeasurable
Other: None
Interpretation: AIVR

117.

Rhythm: chaotic
Rate: greater than 300 beats/minute
P wave: Indiscernible
PR interval: Unmeasurable
QRS complex: Abnormal
T wave: Indiscernible
QT interval: Unmeasurable
Other: None
Interpretation: Torsades de pointes

118.

Rhythm: Irregular
Rate: 40 beats/minute
P wave: Indiscernible
PR interval: Unmeasurable
QRS complex: 0.06 second
T wave: Normal
QT interval: 0.24 second
Other: None
Interpretation: Atrial fibrillation with periods of asystole

119.

Rhythm: Irregular
Rate: 60 beats/minute
P wave: Normal
PR interval: 0.16 second
QRS complex: Normal
QT interval: 0.60 second
Other: None
Interpretation: Sinus bradycardia with unifocal PVCs

120.

Rhythm: Regular
Rate: 75 beats/minute
P wave: Normal
PR interval: 0.36 second
QRS complex: 0.08 second
T wave: Normal
QT interval: 0.52 second
Other: None
Interpretation: Sinus bradycardia

Quick guide to arrhythmias

Guide to cardiovascular drugs

ACLS algorithms

Selected references

Index

Quick guide to arrhythmias

Sinus arrhythmia

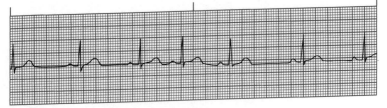

Features
◆ Rhythm irregular; varies with respiratory cycle
◆ Normal P wave preceding each QRS complex
◆ P-P and R-R intervals shorter during inspiration and longer during expiration

Causes
◆ Normal variation in athletes, children, and older adults
◆ Digoxin or morphine use, increased intracranial pressure (ICP), and inferior wall myocardial infarction (MI)

Treatment
◆ Typically no treatment necessary
◆ Possible correction of underlying cause

Sinus tachycardia

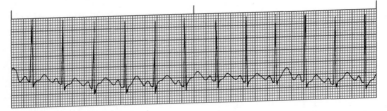

Features
◆ Rhythm regular
◆ Atrial and ventricular rates equal; rate > 100 beats/minute
◆ Normal P wave preceding each normal QRS complex

Causes
◆ Normal physiologic response to fever, exercise, stress, fear, anxiety, pain, dehydration; may accompany shock, left-sided heart failure, pericarditis, hyperthyroidism, anemia, pulmonary embolism (PE), or sepsis
◆ Atropine, isoproterenol, aminophylline, dopamine, dobutamine, epinephrine, quinidine, caffeine, alcohol, amphetamine, or nicotine use

Treatment
◆ No treatment necessary if patient is asymptomatic
◆ Correction of underlying cause
◆ Beta-adrenergic blocker or calcium channel blocker administration, if cardiac ischemia occurs

Sinus bradycardia

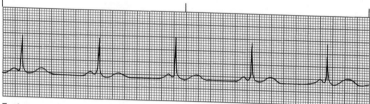

Features
◆ Rhythm regular
◆ Rate < 60 beats/minute
◆ Normal P wave preceding each normal QRS complex

Causes
◆ Normal during sleep and in well-conditioned heart (such as in athletes)
◆ Increased ICP, Valsalva's maneuver, carotid sinus massage, vomiting, hypothyroidism, hyperkalemia, hypothermia, cardiomyopathy, or inferior wall MI
◆ Beta-adrenergic blocker, calcium channel blocker, lithium, sotalol, amiodarone, digoxin, or quinidine use

Treatment
◆ No treatment needed (patient is usually asymptomatic); if drugs are cause, possible discontinuation of use
◆ Temporary pacemaker and atropine administration for low cardiac output, dizziness, weakness, altered level of consciousness, or low blood pressure
◆ Dopamine or epinephrine infusion, if indicated
◆ Temporary or permanent pacemaker may be needed if condition becomes chronic

Sinus arrest

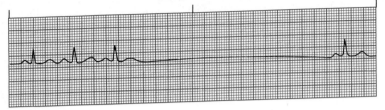

Features
◆ Rhythm regular, except for missing PQRST complexes (irregular as result of missing complexes)
◆ Normal P wave preceding each normal QRS complex

Causes
◆ Coronary artery disease (CAD), acute myocarditis, or acute inferior wall MI
◆ Increased vagal tone (Valsalva's maneuver, carotid sinus massage, or vomiting)
◆ Digoxin, quinidine, procainamide, or salicylate use (especially if given at toxic levels)
◆ Excessive doses of beta-adrenergic blockers
◆ Sinus node disease

Treatment
◆ No treatment needed if patient is asymptomatic
◆ For mild symptoms, possible discontinuation of drugs that contribute to arrhythmia
◆ Atropine administration, if patient is symptomatic
◆ Temporary or permanent pacemaker for repeated episodes

Premature atrial contractions (PACs)

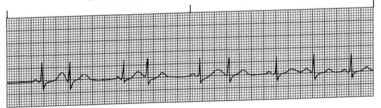

Features
◆ Premature, abnormal P waves (differ in configuration from normal P waves)
◆ QRS complexes after P waves, except in blocked PACs
◆ P wave often buried or identified in preceding T wave

Causes
◆ Triggered by alcohol or cigarette use, anxiety, fever, or infectious disease in normal heart
◆ Heart failure, coronary or valvular heart disease, acute respiratory failure, chronic obstructive pulmonary disease (COPD), electrolyte imbalance, or hypoxia
◆ Digoxin toxicity

Treatment
◆ No treatment needed if patient is asymptomatic
◆ Beta-adrenergic blockers, calcium channel blockers, or digoxin, if occurs frequently
◆ Treatment of underlying cause; avoidance of triggers (caffeine or smoking) and use of stress-reduction measures

Atrial tachycardia

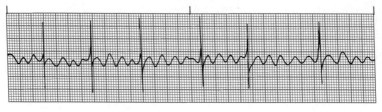

Features
◆ Rhythm regular if block is constant; irregular if not
◆ Rate 150 to 250 beats/minute
◆ P waves regular but hidden in preceding T wave; precede QRS complexes
◆ Sudden onset and termination of arrhythmia

Causes
◆ Physical or psychological stress, hypoxia, electrolyte imbalances, cardiomyopathy, congenital anomalies, MI, valvular disease, Wolff-Parkinson-White syndrome, cor pulmonale, hyperthyroidism, or systemic hypertension
◆ Digoxin toxicity; caffeine, marijuana, or stimulant use

Treatment
◆ Vagal stimulation, Valsalva's maneuver, and carotid sinus massage
◆ Priority is decreasing ventricular response with calcium channel blocker, beta-adrenergic blocker, digoxin, or cardioversion
◆ If other treatments are ineffective, amiodarone or procainamide

Atrial flutter

Features
◆ Atrial rhythm regular; ventricular rhythm variable, depending on degree of atrioventricular (AV) block
◆ Atrial rate 250 to 400 beats/minute; ventricular rate depends on degree of AV block
◆ Sawtooth P-wave configuration (known as flutter or F waves)
◆ QRS complexes uniform in shape

Causes
◆ Heart failure, severe mitral valve disease, hyperthyroidism, pericardial disease, COPD, systemic arterial hypoxia, and acute MI

Treatment
◆ Treatment of underlying cause
◆ Calcium channel blocker or beta-adrenergic blocker administration, if stable and heart functions normally
◆ Amiodarone, ibutilide, flecainide, propafenone, or procainamide administration, if arrhythmia is present for less than 48 hours
◆ Synchronized cardioversion (treatment of choice)
◆ Anticoagulation prior to cardioversion
◆ Ablation therapy for recurrent rhythm

Atrial fibrillation

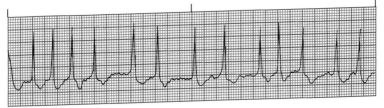

Features
◆ Atrial and ventricular rhythm grossly irregular
◆ Atrial rate > 400 beats/minute; ventricular rate varies
◆ No P waves; replaced by fine fibrillatory waves
◆ No PR interval
◆ QRS complexes uniform in configuration and duration

Causes
◆ Ischemic heart disease, hypertension, heart failure, valvular heart disease, and rheumatic heart disease
◆ Diabetes
◆ Alcohol abuse
◆ Thyroid disorders
◆ Lung and pleural disorders

Treatment
◆ Follow treatment guidelines for atrial flutter

Junctional escape rhythm

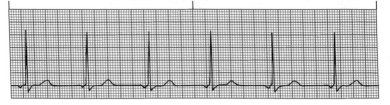

Features
- ◆ Rhythm regular
- ◆ Rate 40 to 60 beats/minute
- ◆ P waves before, hidden in, or after QRS complex; inverted if visible
- ◆ PR interval < 0.12 second (measurable only if P wave appears before QRS complex)
- ◆ QRS configuration and duration normal

Causes
- ◆ Inferior wall MI and rheumatic heart disease
- ◆ Digoxin toxicity
- ◆ Sick sinus syndrome
- ◆ Vagal stimulation

Treatment
- ◆ Treatment of underlying cause
- ◆ Atropine administration, for symptomatic slow rate
- ◆ Pacemaker insertion, if refractory to drugs

Premature junctional contractions

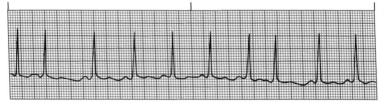

Features
- ◆ Rhythm irregular
- ◆ P waves before, hidden in, or after QRS complexes; inverted if visible
- ◆ PR interval < 0.12 second, if P wave preceding QRS complex
- ◆ QRS configuration and duration normal

Causes
- ◆ Inferior wall MI or ischemia, swelling of AV junction after surgery, rheumatic heart disease, and valvular disease
- ◆ Digoxin toxicity (most common) and excessive caffeine intake

Treatment
◆ No treatment if patient is asymptomatic
◆ Correction of underlying cause
◆ Discontinuation of digoxin, if appropriate
◆ Possible elimination of caffeine

Junctional tachycardia

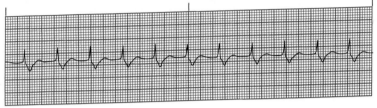

Features
◆ Rhythm regular
◆ Rate 100 to 200 beats/minute
◆ P wave before, hidden in, or after QRS complex; inverted if visible
◆ QRS configuration and duration normal

Causes
◆ Congenital heart disease (in children)
◆ Digoxin toxicity
◆ Swelling of AV junction after heart surgery
◆ Inferior- or posterior-wall MI or ischemia

Treatment
◆ Correction of underlying cause
◆ Discontinuation of digoxin, if applicable and appropriate
◆ Vagal maneuvers, adenosine, amiodarone, beta-adrenergic blocker, or calcium channel blocker, to slow rate
◆ Ablation therapy, if recurrent, followed by permanent pacemaker insertion

Wandering pacemaker

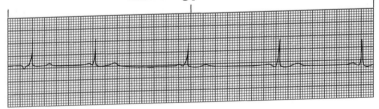

Features
◆ Rhythm irregular
◆ P waves change in configuration, indicating origin in sinoatrial node, atria, or AV junction
◆ *Hallmark:* At least three different P wave configurations
◆ PR interval varies
◆ QRS configuration and duration normal

Causes
◆ Possibly normal in young patients, common in athletes with slow heart rates
◆ Increased vagal tone
◆ Digoxin toxicity
◆ Inflammation of atrial tissue, valvular heart disease

Treatment
◆ No treatment if patient is asymptomatic
◆ Treatment of underlying cause if patient is symptomatic

First-degree AV block

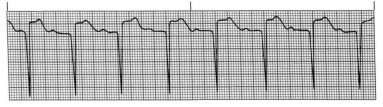

Features
◆ Rhythm regular
◆ P wave preceding each QRS complex; QRS complex normal
◆ PR interval > 0.20 second and constant

Causes
◆ Possibly normal in healthy person
◆ Myocardial ischemia, MI, myocarditis, or degenerative heart changes
◆ Digoxin, calcium channel blocker, and beta-adrenergic blocker use

Treatment
◆ Cautious use of digoxin, calcium channel blockers, and beta-adrenergic blockers
◆ Correction of underlying cause

Second-degree AV block Type I (Mobitz I, Wenckebach)

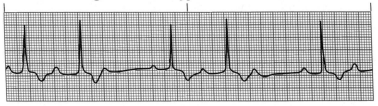

Features
◆ Atrial rhythm regular
◆ Ventricular rhythm irregular
◆ Atrial rate exceeds ventricular rate
◆ PR interval progressively, but only slightly, longer with each cycle until a P wave appears without a QRS complex

Causes
◆ Inferior wall MI, CAD, rheumatic fever, or vagal stimulation
◆ Digoxin toxicity
◆ Beta-adrenergic blockers or calcium channel blockers

Treatment
◆ Treatment of underlying cause
◆ Atropine administration or temporary pacemaker, for symptomatic bradycardia
◆ Discontinuation of digoxin, if appropriate

Second-degree AV block Type II (Mobitz Type II)

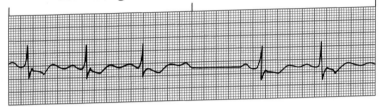

Features
◆ Atrial rhythm regular
◆ Ventricular rhythm possibly irregular, varying with degree of block
◆ P waves normal size, some not followed by a QRS complex
◆ PR interval is constant for conducted beats
◆ QRS complexes periodically absent

Causes
◆ Severe CAD, anterior MI, or degenerative conduction system changes
◆ Digoxin toxicity

Treatment
◆ Treatment of underlying cause
◆ Atropine, dopamine, or epinephrine administration, for symptomatic bradycardia (use atropine cautiously, it may worsen ischemia with MI)
◆ Temporary or permanent pacemaker
◆ Discontinuation of digoxin, if appropriate

Third-degree AV block (complete heart block)

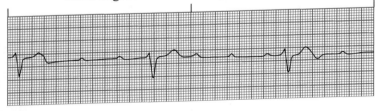

Features
◆ Atrial rhythm regular
◆ Ventricular rhythm regular and rate slow; if escape rhythm originates in AV node, rate is 40 to 60 beats/minute; if it originates in Purkinje system, rate is < 40 beats/minute

- No relationship between P waves and QRS complexes
- PR interval can't be measured
- QRS complex normal (originating in AV node) or wide and bizarre (originating in Purkinje system)

Causes

- Inferior or anterior wall MI, CAD, degenerative changes in heart, congenital abnormality, or hypoxia
- Digoxin toxicity

Treatment

- Treatment of underlying cause
- Atropine, dopamine, or epinephrine administration, for symptomatic bradycardia (*Note:* Don't use atropine with wide QRS complexes.)
- Temporary (transcutaneous or transvenous) or permanent pacemaker

Premature ventricular contractions (PVCs)

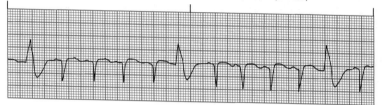

Features

- Atrial and ventricular rhythms may be regular in underlying rhythm; irregular during PVCs
- QRS premature
- QRS complex wide and bizarre, usually > than 0.12 second in premature beat
- T wave opposite direction to QRS complex
- PVCs may occur singly, in pairs, or in threes; alternating with normal beats; possibly unifocal or multifocal
- Most ominous when clustered, multifocal, and with R wave on T pattern
- PVC may be followed by full or incomplete compensatory pause

Causes

- Heart failure; myocardial ischemia, infarction, or contusion; myocarditis, myocardial irritation by ventricular catheter (such as pacemaker); hypokalemia; hypomagnesemia; metabolic acidosis; or hypocalcemia
- Drug intoxication, particularly with cocaine, tricyclic antidepressants, and amphetamines
- Caffeine, tobacco, or alcohol use
- Psychological stress, anxiety, pain, or exercise

Treatment

- If warranted, amiodarone, procainamide, or lidocaine administration
- Treatment of underlying cause
- Discontinuation of drug causing toxicity
- Potassium chloride I.V., if induced by hypokalemia
- Magnesium replacement, if due to hypomagnesemia

Ventricular tachycardia

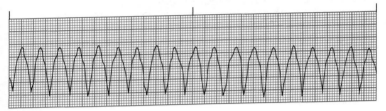

Features
◆ Atrial rhythm can't be determined; ventricular rhythm usually regular, may be slightly irregular
◆ Ventricular rate 100 to 250 beats/minute
◆ P waves indiscernible
◆ QRS complexes wide and bizarre; duration > 0.12 second
◆ May start and stop suddenly

Causes
◆ Myocardial ischemia, or infarction, CAD; valvular heart disease; heart failure; cardiomyopathy; ventricular catheterization; hypokalemia; hypercalcemia; or PE
◆ Digoxin, procainamide, quinidine, or cocaine toxicity

Treatment
◆ If patient is pulseless, immediate defibrillation and resuscitation
◆ If monomorphic VT, give amiodarone; if unsuccessful, or if the patient is symptomatic, synchronized cardioversion
◆ If polymorphic VT with a long QT interval, stop drugs that may prolong QT interval and treat electrolyte imbalances; if normal QT interval, give amiodarone
◆ If episodes of VT unresponsive to drugs recur, may need a cardioverter-defibrillator

Ventricular fibrillation

Features
◆ Ventricular rhythm rapid and chaotic
◆ No discernible P waves, QRS complexes, or T waves
◆ Fine or coarse fibrillatory waves

Causes
◆ Myocardial ischemia, MI, untreated ventricular tachycardia, hypokalemia, acid-base imbalances, hyperkalemia, hypercalcemia, electric shock, or severe hypothermia
◆ Digoxin, epinephrine, or quinidine toxicity

Treatment

◆ Rapid resuscitation defibrillation and cardiopulmonary resuscitation (CPR)
◆ Epinephrine or vasopressin administration followed by defibrillation and CPR
◆ Implantable cardioverter-defibrillator, if at risk for recurrent ventricular fibrillation
◆ Treatment of underlying cause

Asystole

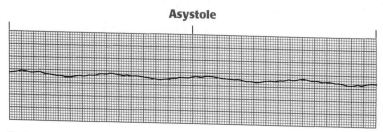

Features

◆ No atrial or ventricular rate or rhythm
◆ No discernible P waves, QRS complexes, or T waves

Causes

◆ Myocardial ischemia or infarction, heart failure, prolonged hypoxemia, severe electrolyte disturbances (such as hyperkalemia), severe acid-base disturbances, electric shock, ventricular arrhythmias, AV block, PE, or cardiac tamponade
◆ Cocaine overdose

Treatment

◆ After verification of rhythm (by checking more than one lead), CPR (following ACLS protocol)
◆ Endotracheal intubation
◆ Transcutaneous pacemaker
◆ Treatment of underlying cause
◆ Repeated doses of epinephrine and atropine, as ordered

Guide to cardiovascular drugs

This table details the drugs most commonly used to improve cardiovascular function and includes indications and special considerations for each.

DRUGS	INDICATIONS
Adrenergic blockers	
Alpha-adrenergic blockers Phentolamine, prazosin	◆ Hypertension ◆ Peripheral vascular disorders ◆ Pheochromocytoma
Beta-adrenergic blockers *Nonselective* Carvedilol, labetalol, nadolol, pindolol, propranolol, sotalol *Selective* Acebutolol, atenolol, bisoprolol, esmolol, metoprolol	◆ Prevention of complications after myocardial infarction (MI), angina, hypertension, supraventricular arrhythmias (such as paroxysmal supraventricular tachycardia [PSVT]), anxiety, essential tremor, cardiovascular symptoms associated with thyrotoxicosis, migraine headaches, pheochromocytoma
Adrenergics	
Catecholamines Dobutamine	◆ Increase cardiac output in short-term treatment of cardiac decompensation from depressed contractility ◆ Adjunct in shock to increase cardiac output, blood pressure, and urine flow
Epinephrine	◆ Bronchospasm ◆ Hypersensitivity reactions ◆ Anaphylaxis ◆ Restoration of cardiac rhythm in cardiac arrest

SPECIAL CONSIDERATIONS

◆ Monitor vital signs and heart rhythm before, during, and after administration.
◆ Instruct the patient to rise slowly to a standing position to avoid orthostatic hypotension.
◆ Assess pulse rate before administering dose.

◆ Monitor apical pulse rate before administration. Monitor blood pressure, electrocardiogram (ECG), and heart rate and rhythm frequently.
◆ Beta-adrenergic blockers can alter the requirements for insulin and oral antidiabetic agents.
◆ Signs of hypoglycemic shock may be masked; watch patients with diabetes for sweating, fatigue, and hunger.

◆ Monitor cardiac rate and rhythm and blood pressure carefully when initiating therapy or increasing the dose.
◆ Correct hypovolemia before administering drug.
◆ Incompatible with alkaline solution (sodium bicarbonate); don't mix or give through same line, and don't mix with other drugs.
◆ Administer continuous drip on infusion pump.
◆ Give drug into a large vein to prevent irritation or extravasation at site.

◆ Monitor cardiac rate and rhythm and blood pressure carefully when initiating therapy or increasing the dose.
◆ Correct hypovolemia before administering drug.
◆ Incompatible with alkaline solution (sodium bicarbonate); don't mix or give through same line, and don't mix with other drugs.
◆ Administer continuous drip on infusion pump.
◆ Give drug into a large vein to prevent extravasation; if extravasation occurs, stop infusion and treat site with phentolamine infiltrate to prevent tissue necrosis.

DRUGS	INDICATIONS

Adrenergics *(continued)*

Catecholamines *(continued)*
Norepinephrine

◆ Maintain blood pressure in acute hypotensive states
◆ GI bleeding

Noncatecholamines
Ephedrine

◆ Maintain blood pressure in acute hypotensive states, especially with spinal anesthesia
◆ Treatment of orthostatic hypotension and bronchospasm

Phenylephrine

◆ Maintain blood pressure in hypotensive states, especially hypotensive emergencies with spinal anesthesia

Antianginal drugs

Nitrates
Isosorbide dinitrate, isosorbide, mononitrate, nitroglycerin

◆ Relief and prevention of angina

Calcium channel blockers
Amlodipine, diltiazem, nicardipine, nifedipine, verapamil

◆ Long-term prevention of angina (especially Prinzmetal's angina)

Antiarrhythmics

Class IA antiarrhythmics
Disopyramide phosphate, procainamide hydrochloride, quinidine sulfate, quinidine gluconate

◆ Ventricular tachycardia
◆ Atrial fibrillation
◆ Atrial flutter
◆ Paroxysmal atrial tachycardia (PAT)

SPECIAL CONSIDERATIONS

- ◆ Monitor cardiac rate and rhythm and blood pressure carefully when initiating therapy or increasing the dose.
- ◆ Correct hypovolemia before administering drug.
- ◆ Incompatible with alkaline solution (sodium bicarbonate); don't mix or give through same line, and don't mix with other drugs.
- ◆ Administer continuous drip on infusion pump.
- ◆ Give drug into a large vein to prevent irritation or extravasation at site.

- ◆ Monitor cardiac rate and rhythm and blood pressure carefully when initiating therapy or increasing the dose.
- ◆ Correct hypovolemia before administering drug.
- ◆ Incompatible with alkaline solution (sodium bicarbonate); don't mix or give through same line, and don't mix with other drugs.
- ◆ Administer continuous drip on infusion pump; can be given by I.V. push in cardiac arrest situations.
- ◆ Give drug into a large vein to prevent extravasation; if extravasation occurs, stop infusion and treat site with phentolamine infiltrate to prevent tissue necrosis.

- ◆ Monitor cardiac rate and rhythm and blood pressure carefully when initiating therapy or increasing the dose.
- ◆ Correct hypovolemia before administering drug.
- ◆ Don't mix with other drugs.
- ◆ Administer continuous drip on infusion pump.
- ◆ Give drug into a large vein to prevent extravasation; if extravasation occurs, stop infusion and treat site with phentolamine infiltrate to prevent tissue necrosis.

- ◆ Monitor the patient's blood pressure before and after administration.
- ◆ Only sublingual and translingual forms should be used.

- ◆ Monitor cardiac rate and rhythm and blood pressure carefully when initiating therapy or increasing the dose.
- ◆ Calcium supplementation may decrease the effects of calcium channel blockers.

- ◆ Check apical pulse rate before therapy. If you note extremes in pulse rate, withhold the dose and notify the practitioner.
- ◆ Use cautiously in patients with asthma.
- ◆ Monitor for ECG changes (widening QRS complexes, prolonged QT interval).

DRUGS	INDICATIONS

Antiarrhythmics *(continued)*

Class IB antiarrhythmics
Lidocaine, mexiletine, tocainide
◆ Ventricular tachycardia
◆ Ventricular fibrillation

Class IC antiarrhythmics
Flecainide, moricizine, propafenone
◆ Ventricular tachycardia
◆ Ventricular fibrillation
◆ Supraventricular arrhythmias

Class II antiarrhythmics
Acebutolol, esmolol, propranolol
◆ Atrial flutter
◆ Atrial fibrillation
◆ PAT

Class III antiarrhythmics
Amiodarone, dofetilide, ibutilide, sotalol
◆ Life-threatening arrhythmias resistant to other antiarrhythmics

Class IV antiarrhythmics
Diltiazem, verapamil
◆ Supraventricular arrhythmias

Miscellaneous
Adenosine
◆ PSVT

Anticoagulants

Heparins
Heparin and low-molecular-weight heparins, such as dalteparin and enoxaparin
◆ Deep vein thrombosis (DVT)
◆ Embolism prophylaxis
◆ Disseminated intravascular coagulation
◆ Prevention of complications after MI

Oral anticoagulants
Warfarin
◆ DVT prophylaxis
◆ Prevention of complications of prosthetic heart valves or diseased mitral valves
◆ Atrial arrhythmias, such as atrial fibrillation and atrial flutter

SPECIAL CONSIDERATIONS

◆ IB antiarrhythmics may potentiate the effects of others.
◆ Administer I.V. infusions using an infusion pump.
◆ Monitor for ECG changes (widening QRS complexes, prolonged PR interval).

◆ Correct electrolyte imbalances before administration.
◆ Monitor the patient's ECG before and after dosage adjustments.
◆ Monitor for ECG changes (widening QRS complexes, prolonged PR and QT interval).

◆ Monitor apical heart rate and blood pressure.
◆ Abruptly stopping these drugs can exacerbate angina and precipitate MI.
◆ Monitor for ECG changes (prolonged PR interval).

◆ Amiodarone increases the risk of digoxin toxicity in patients also taking digoxin.
◆ Monitor for signs of pulmonary toxicity (dyspnea, nonproductive cough, and pleuritic chest pain) in patients taking amiodarone.
◆ Monitor blood pressure, heart rate, and rhythm for changes.
◆ Monitor ECG before and after dosage adjustments.
◆ Monitor for ECG changes (prolonged QT interval) in patients taking dofetilide, ibutilide, and sotalol.

◆ Monitor heart rate and rhythm and blood pressure carefully when initiating therapy or increasing dose.
◆ Calcium supplements may reduce effectiveness.

◆ Adenosine must be administered over 1 to 2 seconds, followed by a 20-ml flush of normal saline solution.
◆ Record rhythm strip during administration.
◆ A brief period of asystole (up to 15 seconds) may occur after rapid administration.

◆ Monitor partial thromboplastin time (PTT); the therapeutic range is 1½ to 2½ times the control.
◆ Monitor the patient for signs of bleeding.
◆ Concomitant administration with nonsteroidal anti-inflammatory drugs, iron dextran, or an anti-platelet drug increases the risk of bleeding.
◆ Protamine sulfate reverses the effects of heparin.

◆ Monitor prothrombin time (PT) and International Normalized Ratio (INR) in patients receiving warfarin; the effects of oral anticoagulants can be reversed with phytonadione (vitamin K_1).
◆ Monitor the patient for signs of bleeding.

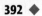

DRUGS	INDICATIONS

Anticoagulants *(continued)*

Antiplatelet drugs
Aspirin, dipyridamole, ticlopidine, clopidrogel
- ◆ Decreased risk of death after MI
- ◆ Prevention of complications of prosthetic heart valves

Antihypertensives

Vasodilators
Diazoxide, hydralazine, minoxidil, nitroprusside
- ◆ Moderate to severe hypertension (in combination with other drugs)

Angiotensin-converting enzyme inhibitors
Benazepril, captopril, enalapril, enalaprilat, fosinopril, lisinopril, perindopril, quinapril, ramipril, trandolapril
- ◆ Hypertension
- ◆ Heart failure

Angiotensin II receptor blockers
Candesartan, eprosartan, irbesartan, losartan, olmesartan, telmisartan, valsartan
- ◆ Hypertension
- ◆ Valvular disease

Antilipemics

Bile-sequestering drugs
Cholestyramine, colesevelam, colestipol
- ◆ Hyperlipidemia
- ◆ Hypercholesterolemia

Fibric acid derivatives
Fenofibrate, gemfibrozil
- ◆ Hyperlipidemia
- ◆ Hypercholesterolemia
- ◆ Hypertryglyceridemia

HMG CoA inhibitors
Atorvastatin, fluvastatin, lovastatin, pravastatin, simvastatin
- ◆ Hyperlipidemia (types IV and V)

SPECIAL CONSIDERATIONS

◆ Monitor the patient for signs of bleeding.
◆ Aspirin, and ticlopidine should be taken with meals to prevent GI irritation.
◆ Dipyridamole should be taken with a full glass of fluid at least 1 hour before meals.

◆ Monitor blood pressure before and after administration.

◆ Monitor blood pressure before and after administration.
◆ In patients whose renal function may depend on the renin-angiotensin-aldosterone system, such as those with severe heart failure, treatment with angiotensin-converting enzyme (ACE) inhibitors and angiotensin-receptor blockers has been related to oliguria or progressive azotemia and (rarely) to acute renal failure or death.

◆ Monitor blood pressure before and after administration.
◆ In patients whose renal function may depend on the renin-angiotensin-aldosterone system, such as those with severe heart failure, treatment with ACE inhibitors and angiotensin-receptor blockers has been related to oliguria or progressive azotemia and (rarely) to acute renal failure or death.

◆ Monitor blood cholesterol and lipid levels before and periodically during therapy.
◆ Monitor liver function studies and creatine kinase (CK) throughout therapy.
◆ Advise the patient to drink 2 to 3 qt (2 to 3 L) of fluid daily and to report persistent or severe constipation.

◆ Monitor blood cholesterol and lipid levels before and periodically during therapy.
◆ Monitor liver function studies and CK throughout therapy.
◆ Advise the patient to drink 2 to 3 qt of fluid daily and to report persistent or severe constipation.

◆ If being administered with bile sequestrants, give at least 4 to 6 hours apart.
◆ Administer with meals (or at bedtime when using extended release forms).
◆ Monitor blood cholesterol and lipid levels before and periodically during therapy.
◆ Monitor liver function and CK levels throughout therapy.

DRUGS	INDICATIONS

Cardiac glycoside and phosphiodiesterase (PDE) inhibitors

Cardiac glycoside
Digoxin
- ◆ Heart failure
- ◆ Supraventricular arrhythmias

PDE inhibitors
Inamrinone, milrinone
- ◆ Heart failure refractory to digoxin, diuretics, and vasodilators

Diuretics

Thiazide and thiazide-like diuretics
Bendroflumethiazide, chlorthalidone, hydrochloro-thiazide, hydroflumethiazide, indapamide
- ◆ Hypertension
- ◆ Edema

Loop diuretics
Bumetanide, ethacrynic acid, furosemide
- ◆ Hypertension
- ◆ Heart failure
- ◆ Edema

Potassium-sparing diuretics
Amiloride, spironolactone, triamterene
- ◆ Edema
- ◆ Diuretic-induced hypokalemia in patients with heart failure
- ◆ Hypertension

Thrombolytics

Alteplase, reteplase, streptokinase
- ◆ Acute MI
- ◆ Acute ischemic stroke
- ◆ Pulmonary embolus
- ◆ Catheter occlusion
- ◆ Arterial thrombosis

SPECIAL CONSIDERATIONS

◆ If immediate effects are required, a loading dose of digoxin is required.
◆ Check apical pulse for 1 minute before administration; report pulse less than 60 beats/minute.
◆ Therapeutic serum levels are 0.5 to 2 ng/ml.

◆ These drugs are contraindicated in the acute phase of MI and after MI.
◆ Serum potassium levels should be within normal limits before and during therapy.

◆ Monitor serum potassium levels.
◆ Monitor intake and output.
◆ Monitor blood glucose values in patients with diabetes. Thiazide diuretics can cause hyperglycemia.

◆ Monitor for signs of excess diuresis (hypotension, tachycardia, poor skin turgor, and excessive thirst).
◆ Monitor blood pressure, heart rate, and intake and output.
◆ Monitor serum electrolyte levels.

◆ Monitor ECG for arrhythmias.
◆ Monitor serum potassium levels.
◆ Monitor intake and output.

◆ Monitor PTT, PT, INR, hemoglobin, and hematocrit before, during, and after administration.
◆ Monitor vital signs frequently during and immediately after administration. Don't use an automatic blood pressure cuff to monitor blood pressure.
◆ Monitor puncture sites for bleeding.
◆ Monitor for signs of bleeding.
◆ Monitor for reperfusion arrhythmias when used to treat acute MI.

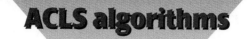

ACLS algorithms

Bradycardia

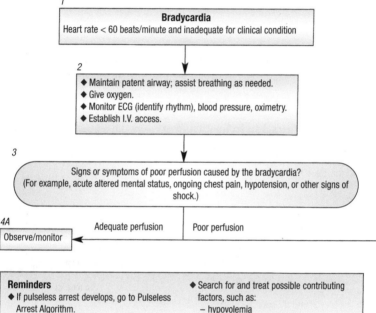

1

Bradycardia
Heart rate < 60 beats/minute and inadequate for clinical condition

2

◆ Maintain patent airway; assist breathing as needed.
◆ Give oxygen.
◆ Monitor ECG (identify rhythm), blood pressure, oximetry.
◆ Establish I.V. access.

3

Signs or symptoms of poor perfusion caused by the bradycardia?
(For example, acute altered mental status, ongoing chest pain, hypotension, or other signs of shock.)

Adequate perfusion   Poor perfusion

4A
Observe/monitor

Reminders
◆ If pulseless arrest develops, go to Pulseless Arrest Algorithm.

◆ Search for and treat possible contributing factors, such as:
  – hypovolemia
  – hypoxia
  – hydrogen ion (acidosis)
  – hypokalemia/hyperkalemia
  – hypoglycemia
  – hypothermia
  – toxins
  – tamponade, cardiac
  – tension pneumothorax
  – thrombosis (coronary or pulmonary)
  – trauma (hypovolemia, increased ICP).

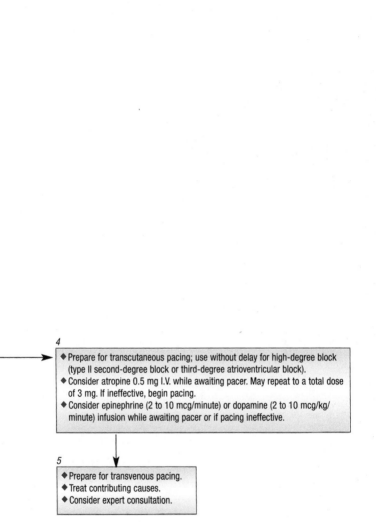

4

- ◆ Prepare for transcutaneous pacing; use without delay for high-degree block (type II second-degree block or third-degree atrioventricular block).
- ◆ Consider atropine 0.5 mg I.V. while awaiting pacer. May repeat to a total dose of 3 mg. If ineffective, begin pacing.
- ◆ Consider epinephrine (2 to 10 mcg/minute) or dopamine (2 to 10 mcg/kg/minute) infusion while awaiting pacer or if pacing ineffective.

5

- ◆ Prepare for transvenous pacing.
- ◆ Treat contributing causes.
- ◆ Consider expert consultation.

Pulseless arrest

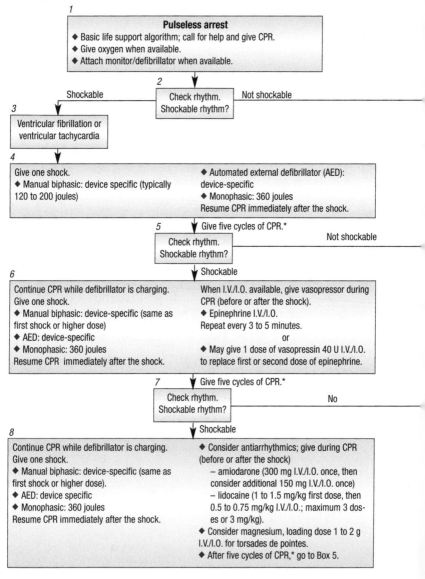

1

Pulseless arrest
◆ Basic life support algorithm; call for help and give CPR.
◆ Give oxygen when available.
◆ Attach monitor/defibrillator when available.

2

Shockable   Check rhythm.   Not shockable
Shockable rhythm?

3

Ventricular fibrillation or
ventricular tachycardia

4

Give one shock.
◆ Manual biphasic: device specific (typically 120 to 200 joules)

◆ Automated external defibrillator (AED): device-specific
◆ Monophasic: 360 joules
Resume CPR immediately after the shock.

5   Give five cycles of CPR.*

Check rhythm.   Not shockable
Shockable rhythm?

6   Shockable

Continue CPR while defibrillator is charging.
Give one shock.
◆ Manual biphasic: device-specific (same as first shock or higher dose)
◆ AED: device-specific
◆ Monophasic: 360 joules
Resume CPR immediately after the shock.

When I.V./I.O. available, give vasopressor during CPR (before or after the shock).
◆ Epinephrine I.V./I.O.
Repeat every 3 to 5 minutes.
or
◆ May give 1 dose of vasopressin 40 U I.V./I.O. to replace first or second dose of epinephrine.

7   Give five cycles of CPR.*

Check rhythm.   No
Shockable rhythm?

8   Shockable

Continue CPR while defibrillator is charging.
Give one shock.
◆ Manual biphasic: device-specific (same as first shock or higher dose).
◆ AED: device specific
◆ Monophasic: 360 joules
Resume CPR immediately after the shock.

◆ Consider antiarrhythmics; give during CPR (before or after the shock)
   – amiodarone (300 mg I.V./I.O. once, then consider additional 150 mg I.V./I.O. once)
   – lidocaine (1 to 1.5 mg/kg first dose, then 0.5 to 0.75 mg/kg I.V./I.O.; maximum 3 doses or 3 mg/kg).
◆ Consider magnesium, loading dose 1 to 2 g I.V./I.O. for torsades de pointes.
◆ After five cycles of CPR,* go to Box 5.

*After an advanced airway is placed, rescuers no longer deliver "cycles" of CPR. Give continuous chest compressions without pauses for breaths. Give 8 to 10 breath/minute. Check rhythm every 2 minutes.

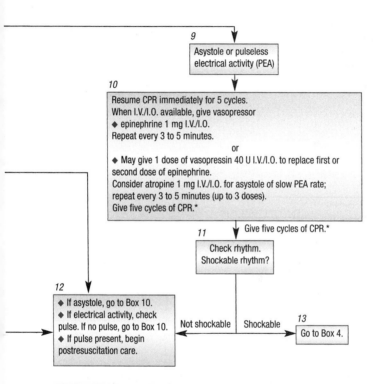

9
Asystole or pulseless
electrical activity (PEA)

10
Resume CPR immediately for 5 cycles.
When I.V./I.O. available, give vasopressor
◆ epinephrine 1 mg I.V./I.O.
Repeat every 3 to 5 minutes.

or

◆ May give 1 dose of vasopressin 40 U I.V./I.O. to replace first or
second dose of epinephrine.
Consider atropine 1 mg I.V./I.O. for asystole of slow PEA rate;
repeat every 3 to 5 minutes (up to 3 doses).
Give five cycles of CPR.*

Give five cycles of CPR.*

11
Check rhythm.
Shockable rhythm?

12
◆ If asystole, go to Box 10.
◆ If electrical activity, check
pulse. If no pulse, go to Box 10.
◆ If pulse present, begin
postresuscitation care.

Not shockable   Shockable

13
Go to Box 4.

During CPR
◆ Push hard and fast (100/minute).
◆ Ensure full chest recoil.
◆ Minimize interruptions in chest compressions.
◆ One cycle of CPR: 30 compressions then 2
breaths; five cycles = 2 minutes.
◆ Avoid hyperventilation.
◆ Secure airway and confirm placement.
◆ Rotate compressors every two minutes with
rhythm checks.

◆ Search for and treat possible contributing
factors, such as:
 – hypovolemia
 – hypoxia
 – hydrogen ion (acidosis)
 – hypokalemia/hyperkalemia
 – hypoglycemia
 – hypothermia
 – toxins
 – tamponade, cardiac
 – tension pneumothorax
 – thrombosis (coronary or pulmonary)
 – trauma.

Tachycardia

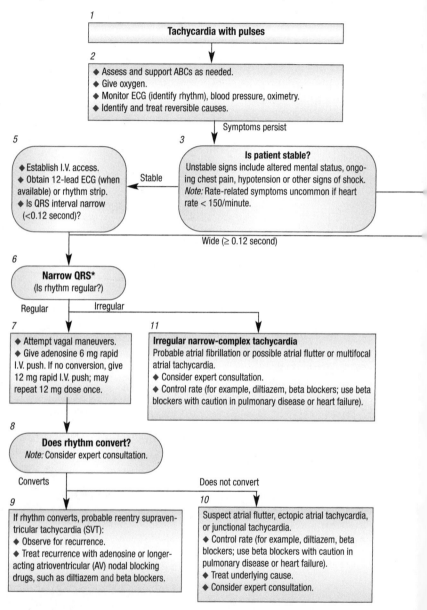

1

Tachycardia with pulses

2
- ◆ Assess and support ABCs as needed.
- ◆ Give oxygen.
- ◆ Monitor ECG (identify rhythm), blood pressure, oximetry.
- ◆ Identify and treat reversible causes.

Symptoms persist

5
- ◆ Establish I.V. access.
- ◆ Obtain 12-lead ECG (when available) or rhythm strip.
- ◆ Is QRS interval narrow (<0.12 second)?

Stable

3
Is patient stable?
Unstable signs include altered mental status, ongoing chest pain, hypotension or other signs of shock.
Note: Rate-related symptoms uncommon if heart rate < 150/minute.

Wide (≥ 0.12 second)

6
Narrow QRS*
(Is rhythm regular?)

Regular   Irregular

7
- ◆ Attempt vagal maneuvers.
- ◆ Give adenosine 6 mg rapid I.V. push. If no conversion, give 12 mg rapid I.V. push; may repeat 12 mg dose once.

11
Irregular narrow-complex tachycardia
Probable atrial fibrillation or possible atrial flutter or multifocal atrial tachycardia.
- ◆ Consider expert consultation.
- ◆ Control rate (for example, diltiazem, beta blockers; use beta blockers with caution in pulmonary disease or heart failure).

8
Does rhythm convert?
Note: Consider expert consultation.

Converts   Does not convert

9
If rhythm converts, probable reentry supraventricular tachycardia (SVT):
- ◆ Observe for recurrence.
- ◆ Treat recurrence with adenosine or longer-acting atrioventricular (AV) nodal blocking drugs, such as diltiazem and beta blockers.

10
Suspect atrial flutter, ectopic atrial tachycardia, or junctional tachycardia.
- ◆ Control rate (for example, diltiazem, beta blockers; use beta blockers with caution in pulmonary disease or heart failure).
- ◆ Treat underlying cause.
- ◆ Consider expert consultation.

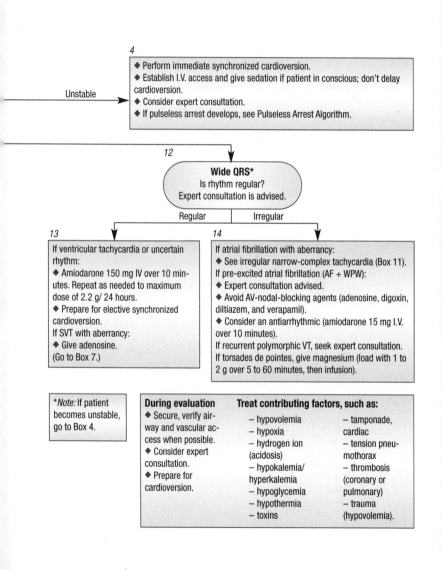

4
◆ Perform immediate synchronized cardioversion.
◆ Establish I.V. access and give sedation if patient in conscious; don't delay cardioversion.
◆ Consider expert consultation.
◆ If pulseless arrest develops, see Pulseless Arrest Algorithm.

Unstable →

12
Wide QRS*
Is rhythm regular?
Expert consultation is advised.

Regular | Irregular

13
If ventricular tachycardia or uncertain rhythm:
◆ Amiodarone 150 mg IV over 10 minutes. Repeat as needed to maximum dose of 2.2 g/ 24 hours.
◆ Prepare for elective synchronized cardioversion.
If SVT with aberrancy:
◆ Give adenosine.
(Go to Box 7.)

14
If atrial fibrillation with aberrancy:
◆ See irregular narrow-complex tachycardia (Box 11).
If pre-excited atrial fibrillation (AF + WPW):
◆ Expert consultation advised.
◆ Avoid AV-nodal-blocking agents (adenosine, digoxin, diltiazem, and verapamil).
◆ Consider an antiarrhythmic (amiodarone 15 mg I.V. over 10 minutes).
If recurrent polymorphic VT, seek expert consultation.
If torsades de pointes, give magnesium (load with 1 to 2 g over 5 to 60 minutes, then infusion).

***Note:** If patient becomes unstable, go to Box 4.

During evaluation
◆ Secure, verify airway and vascular access when possible.
◆ Consider expert consultation.
◆ Prepare for cardioversion.

Treat contributing factors, such as:
– hypovolemia
– hypoxia
– hydrogen ion (acidosis)
– hypokalemia/ hyperkalemia
– hypoglycemia
– hypothermia
– toxins

– tamponade, cardiac
– tension pneumothorax
– thrombosis (coronary or pulmonary)
– trauma (hypovolemia).

Selected references

"2005 American Heart Association Guidelines for Cardiopulmonary Resuscitation and Emergency Cardiovascular Care, Part 7.2: Management of Cardiac Arrest," *Circulation* 112(suppl IV):IV-58-IV-66, 2005.

"2005 American Heart Association Guidelines for Cardiopulmonary Resuscitation and Emergency Cardiovascular Care, Part 7.3: Management of Symptomatic Bradycardia and Tachycardia," *Circulation* 112(suppl IV):IV-67-IV-77, 2005.

"2005 American Heart Association Guidelines for Cardiopulmonary Resuscitation and Emergency Cardiovascular Care, Part 8: Stabilization of the Patient with Acute Coronary Syndromes," *Circulation* 112(suppl IV):IV-111-IV-120, 2005.

"AHA Scientific Statement: Practice Standards for Electrocardiographic Monitoring in Hospital Settings," *Circulation* 110(17):2721-46, October 2004.

Albert, N.M. "Cardiac Resynchronization Therapy through Biventricular Pacing in Patient with Heart Failure and Ventricular Dyssynchrony," *Critical Care Nurse* 23(3 Suppl.):2-13, June 2003.

Brantman, L., and Howie, J. "Use of Amiodarone to Prevent Atrial Fibrillation After Cardiac Surgery," *Critical Care Nurse* 26(1):48-56, 58; quiz 59, February 2006.

Coady, E. "Managing Patients with Non-ST-Segment Elevation Acute Coronary Syndrome," *Nursing Standard* 20(37):49-56, May 2006.

Cuisset, T., et al. "Benefit of a 600-mg Loading Dose of Clopidogrel on Platelet Reactivity and Clinical Outcomes in Patients with Non-ST-Segment Elevation Acute Coronary Syndrome Undergoing Coronary Stenting," *Journal of the American College of Cardiology* 48(7):1339-45, October 2006.

DeBoor, S., et al. "Nonrespiratory Sinus Arrhythmia," *American Journal of Critical Care* 14(2):161-62, March 2005.

ECG Interpretation: A 2-in-1 Reference for Nurses. Philadelphia: Lippincott Williams & Wilkins, 2005.

ECG Interpretation Made Incredibly Easy, 3rd ed. Philadelphia: Lippincott Williams & Wilkins, 2005.

Jones, S. *Always At Your Side ECG Notes: Interpretation And Management Guide.* Philadelphia: F.A. Davis Co., 2005.

Lim, W., et al. "Reliability of Electrocardiogram Interpretation in Critically Ill Patients," *Critical Care Medicine* 34(5):1338-43, May 2006.

Pyne, C. "Classification of Acute Coronary Syndromes Using the 12-Lead Electrocardiogram as a Guide," *AACN Clinical Issues* 15(4):558-67, October-December 2004.

Index

i refers to an illustration; t refers to a table.

◆